FLORENCE NIGHTINGALE
and the MEDICAL MEN

FLORENCE NIGHTINGALE
and the
MEDICAL MEN

Working Together for Health Care Reform

Lynn McDonald

McGill-Queen's University Press

Montreal & Kingston • London • Chicago

ISBN 978-0-2280-1092-0 (cloth)
ISBN 978-0-2280-1203-0 (paper)
ISBN 978-0-2280-1319-8 (ePDF)
ISBN 978-0-2280-1320-4 (ePUB)

Legal deposit third quarter 2022
Bibliothèque nationale du Québec

Printed in Canada on acid-free paper that is 100% ancient forest free (100% post-consumer recycled), processed chlorine free

This book has been published with the help of a grant from the Canadian Federation for the Humanities and Social Sciences, through the Awards to Scholarly Publications Program, using funds provided by the Social Sciences and Humanities Research Council of Canada.

Funded by the Government of Canada   Financé par le gouvernement du Canada   Canada   Canada Council for the Arts   Conseil des arts du Canada

We acknowledge the support of the Canada Council for the Arts.

Nous remercions le Conseil des arts du Canada de son soutien.

Library and Archives Canada Cataloguing in Publication

Title: Florence Nightingale and the medical men : working together for health care reform / Lynn McDonald

Names: McDonald, Lynn, 1940- author.

Description: Includes bibliographical references and index.

Identifiers: Canadiana (print) 20220171963 | Canadiana (ebook) 20220172013 | ISBN 9780228010920 (cloth) | ISBN 9780228012030 (paper) | ISBN 9780228013198 (ePDF) | ISBN 9780228013204 (ePUB)

Subjects: LCSH: Nightingale, Florence, 1820-1910. | LCSH: Nursing – Great Britain – History – 19th century. | LCSH: Mentoring in medicine – Great Britain – History – 19th century. | LCSH: Hospital care – Great Britain – Safety measures – History – 19th century. | LCSH: Medical statistics – History – 19th century.

Classification: LCC RT37.N5 M32 2022 | DDC 610.73092 – dc23

This book was designed and typeset by Peggy & Co. Design in 11/14 Adobe Garamond Pro.

In 1897, to hospital reformer Sydney Holland Nightingale said: "Keep what you know is right before you, and never cease trying to get it. Aim high and people will follow you in the end ... No, no, no one can be neutral in this life; you are either doing good or bad, and the very fact of not trying to do good is bad in itself."

– Sydney Holland, Viscount Knutsford, *In Black and White*, 154

CONTENTS

FIGURE AND TABLES

Figure

Tables

PREFACE

This book closes my work on Florence Nightingale, or at least book-length publication. My work on her began in the 1970s when – as a social scientist, not a nurse or doctor – I began to search for the women who made serious contributions to sociological and political theory, but were ignored in the standard textbooks and books of reading on those subjects. Nightingale was one of many "missing persons" I found. She was a particularly fine example, an early social scientist and adept at statistics. Sociology students were pleased to hear about her work. She, accordingly, appears, a mere four pages, in my *Early Origins of the Social Sciences* (McGill-Queen's University Press, 1993). She was given substantial sections in my next two books, on the women founders themselves, in 1994 and 1998. A 16-volume *Collected Works of Florence Nightingale* made available the full range of her writing, published and unpublished, from all over the world (Wilfrid Laurier University Press, 2001–12). That might have done it, but four more non-peer-reviewed, invited books, with different publishers, appeared in 2010, 2017, 2018, and 2020.

This book closes the gap that remained: Nightingale's work with doctors, evident throughout but not dealt with explicitly.

A word of explanation may be required on the use of "Medical Men" in the title with, if not, for a feminist author, an apology. Nightingale supported women's entry into medicine, although she never made it a cause, as she did reducing high hospital death rates in war, founding the nursing profession, making regular, civilian hospitals safer, and promoting sanitation and social conditions in India. Women come into this book, then, but in small numbers, in chapter 6. Yet it is clear that the great breakthroughs Nightingale made – the causes just mentioned – occurred in collaboration with leading men, doctors. This book, with a return to McGill-Queen's University Press as the publisher, tells that story.

Thanks are due to the director of McGill-Queen's, Philip Cercone, for seeing this through, over many years. Thanks go to Janice Hicks, at the University of Guelph, and to Lesley Mann, for technical assistance, and to Ken Simons, for assistance on the index. Finally, I express my appreciation to friends and colleagues in the Nightingale Society, formed in 2012 to promote knowledge of her work and legacy.

Lynn McDonald
Toronto, March 2022

DRAMATIS PERSONAE

Dr Henry Dyke Acland (1815–1900), Regius professor of
medicine, Oxford

Dr Elizabeth Garrett Anderson (1836–1917), first woman to qualify in
medicine in England

Dr Thomas Graham Balfour (1813–1891), director, Army
Statistical Department

Dr John Shaw Billings (1838–1913), Civil War doctor, designer of
Johns Hopkins University Hospital

Dr Elizabeth Blackwell (1821–1910), first woman doctor, friend

Henry Bonham Carter (1827–1921), cousin, secretary, Nightingale
Fund Council

Dr Sir James Clark (1788–1870), physician to Queen Victoria

Dr John Croft (1833–1905), medical instructor to the nurses,
St Thomas' Hospital, London

Dr William Farr (1807–1883), superintendent of statistics, General
Register Office

Dr C.H. Fasson (c. 1821–1892), medical superintendent, Edinburgh
Royal Infirmary

(Sir) Douglas Galton (1822–99), RE, hospital architect, major colleague

Sidney Herbert (Lord Herbert) (1810–1861), MP, secretary of state for
war, head of royal commission

Dr Thomas Gilham Hewlett (1831–1889), medical officer of
health, Bombay

Sir John McNeill (1795–1883), head of Supply Commission,
Crimean War

Dr Sir William Mure Muir (1819–1905), director-general, Army
Medical Department

Dr (Sir) James Paget (1814–1899), surgeon, St Bartholomew's Hospital, London, surgeon to Queen Victoria

Dr Edmund A. Parkes (1819–1876), first professor of military hygiene, Army Medical School

(Sir) William Rathbone (1819–1902), MP, workhouse-infirmary philanthropist, Liverpool

Dr (Dame) Mary Ann Scharlieb (1845–1930), pioneer woman doctor in India

Dr James Y. Simpson (1811–1870), pioneer of chloroform use, hospital reformer

Dr Andrew Smith (1797–1872), director-general, Army Medical Department

Dr John Sutherland (1808–1891), head of Sanitary Commission, major colleague

Sir Harry Verney (1801–1894), brother-in-law, chair of Nightingale Fund Council

Dr C.J.B. Williams (1805–1889), physician at University College Hospital, London

FLORENCE NIGHTINGALE
and the MEDICAL MEN

THE LIFE *and* TIMES
of FLORENCE NIGHTINGALE

Florence Nightingale was born on 12 May 1820 in Florence, Italy, the younger daughter of William Edward Nightingale (1794–1874), who had inherited a vast lead fortune from his great-uncle Peter Nightingale, on condition of his taking the Nightingale name, and of Frances Smith (1788–1880), daughter of a radical MP and abolitionist, William Smith. The elder daughter, Frances Parthenope (1819–1890), later Lady Verney, was born the previous year in Naples ("Parthenope" in Greek). The Nightingales returned to England in 1821.

The family divided its time between two large, beautiful country homes: Lea Hurst, in Derbyshire, and, beginning in 1826, Embley Park, in Hampshire, with occasional stays at rented accommodation in London. The girls were taught at home by governesses and their classically educated father.

Florence Nightingale was baptized in the Church of England. Three grandparents were Unitarians, but the only one she knew, her paternal grandmother, was vehemently evangelical Church of England (Anglican). The parents had been married in the Church of England – the established, state church – by an evangelical priest. They attended Methodist chapels in Derbyshire and the local parish church (Church of England) in Hampshire, where Mr Nightingale was patron of the living. When travelling, they liked to visit other churches, including Roman Catholic. Florence remained in the Church of England all her life, read widely, and had liberal views theologically. She disliked her church's social conservatism and the paltry expectations it had of its members, especially women. Roman Catholicism had serious expectations and at least a role for women, as nuns, but she disagreed with much of its theology.

At age sixteen, Florence experienced a "call to service," from God, as she understood it. The call she took to mean nursing, especially of the poor, but nursing patients of any class was then a lower-class occupation, unthinkable for anyone in her family. She did not have a chance to nurse until age thirty-three, in London, just before the Crimean War.

A family trip back to Europe, 1836–38, while Embley was being massively expanded, renewed acquaintance with Florence's namesake city and included lengthy stays in Rome, Genoa, Geneva, and Paris.

While not permitted to work, the young Nightingale was allowed to take other extensive trips, with suitable family friends as chaperones. Charles H. and Selina Bracebridge were a childless couple, sympathetic to her calling – they later accompanied her to the Crimean War (1854–56). These trips did much to expand Nightingale's horizons, when university was not an option for women. The three visited Rome in 1847–48, when a friendship was forged with the newly married Sidney Herbert (1810–1861) and Elizabeth Herbert (1822–1911), both of whom would be instrumental in sending Nightingale to the Crimean War.

In 1849–50 Nightingale, again with the Bracebridges, visited Egypt, including a trip up and down the Nile, recorded in detail in her (privately printed) *Letters from Egypt*. They next went on to Greece for an extended period, then across Europe to Germany, where Nightingale had her first (of two) stays at the Deaconess Institution at Kaiserswerth-am-Rhein, near Düsseldorf. All these expeditions were far more than ordinary tourism, including visits to hospitals and orphanages as well as to art museums, plus many opera performances. In Egypt, the party attended a service at a mosque and saw a slave market, where Nubians, captured as girls, were sold.

These various travels also exposed the young Nightingale to the political upheavals of the day: the uprisings of 1838 in both Paris and Rome while with her family, then the greater one in 1848 in Rome with the Bracebridges. The 1836–38 trip deepened her fondness for the country of her birth, Italy. In Geneva the party met exiled Italian independence leaders. Nightingale's progressive and liberal values, and sympathy for the oppressed, were fostered through all these experiences. In due course, she became fluent in French, German, and Italian. Her Bible is annotated with quotations in those languages, plus Latin and Greek, even a few words in Hebrew.

Nursing Experience

There was no nurse training at Kaiserswerth when she visited it, briefly, in 1850, nor during her three-month stay in 1851, when she did obtain experience in the wards and apothecary.

In Britain, before nurse-training schools, the only way to learn the subject was by working alongside a doctor at a hospital. Nightingale hoped to receive exactly that at the Salisbury Infirmary with a respectable, elderly family friend, Dr Richard Fowler (1765–1863). Her family, however, said no. Dr Fowler none the less continued to foster her interest. The two discussed science and metaphysics.

Nightingale was allowed to travel to Ireland in 1852 in the company of the Fowlers. She hoped for hospital experience at St Vincent's Hospital, Dublin, which she visited with them. Dr Fowler then accompanied her to Harold's Cross to meet the mistress of novices of the Sisters of Charity, the order that nursed St Vincent's. The hospital, however, was set to close for renovations, and nothing came of the plan. She and the Fowlers had a wonderful time touring Dublin, then went up to Belfast for meetings of the British Association for the Advancement of Science.

In 1853, she acquired experience in several Paris hospitals nursed by Roman Catholic religious orders – again, no formal training. The intermediary for Paris was Henry Edward Manning, then a prominent convert to Catholicism, whom she had met in Rome.

That was her hospital background when she became lady superintendent of the Establishment for Gentlewomen during Illness, in Upper Harley Street in London in 1853. Three doctors provided their services to it, two of whom became her lasting colleagues: William Bowman, later a baronet (1816–1892), an ophthalmic surgeon who served on the board of the Nightingale Fund Council from its inception, and Henry Bence Jones (1913–1873), who later encouraged her to reform the notorious workhouse infirmaries.

The Crimean War

In October 1854, Nightingale was asked by her friend Sidney Herbert, MP, then secretary at war, to lead the first team of British women to nurse in war. Elizabeth Herbert, who served on the Ladies' Committee at the Harley Street hospital, urged her to accept, to fulfil her old calling. Nightingale, thirty-four and with limited experience, was none the less the most qualified person to head the team.

Nightingale and her nurses, as we see in chapter 2, had also to contend initially with the overt hostility of army doctors. The nurses, however, soon earned their respect and were given greater responsibilities. Nightingale was asked to take on hospitals in the Crimea as well as those in Turkey, where she and her team started. They arrived on 5 November 1854, at the Barrack Hospital in Scutari (now Uskadar), across the Bosphorous from Constantinople (now Istanbul), capital of the Ottoman Empire. Much of her work was improving infrastructure at that unsanitary, defective hospital, then the largest in the world. She established laundries and kitchens, purchased beds and bedding – for which she paid through a fund raised by the *Times* newspaper. In May 1855, on the first of her several visits to the Crimea, she fell ill and nearly died of "Crimean fever," probably brucellosis. She recovered and returned to work, but would suffer a major relapse back home.[1]

Late in 1855, a fund was established in recognition of her work. Army officers, soldiers, and the public at large contributed, not only at the war, but in England, Scotland, Ireland, France, India, Australia, and New Zealand. The £50,000 (a vast fortune) the Nightingale Fund raised was duly employed to start the first nurse-training school in the world,

Her priority on return to Britain, in August 1856, however, was not nursing but ascertaining the causes of the high death rates at the war, to ensure that they did not happen again. Soon after her return, she was invited to meet Queen Victoria, Prince Albert, and Lord Panmure, the secretary of state for war (having replaced the Duke of Newcastle in February 1855), at Balmoral Castle in Scotland, where the royal family spent much of the summer. She agreed to prepare a short "précis" on the war, which turned into an 853-page confidential report, which was never published but which she had printed and sent to numerous people, always stressing its confidentiality. She also produced a public statement, "Answers to Written Questions," as a brief to the Royal Commission on the Crimean War, for which she also did much work behind the scenes, as well as influencing the appointment of members.

In 1858, Nightingale became the first woman elected a fellow of the Royal Statistical Society. She was nominated by medical statistician Dr William Farr for her work on the various reports. To persuade her to accept, he recalled that "learned ladies" in Florence had "worthily filled academical seats," and quoted Socrates.[2]

Nightingale's original "Notes on Hospitals" was presented as two papers at the second annual meeting of the National Association for the Promotion of Social Science (also known as the Social Science Association), held in Liverpool in 1858. They articulate the lessons she learned from the war hospitals, with comparative material from civil hospitals. Substantially revised and expanded, they became *Notes on Hospitals* (1863). Her most famous book, *Notes on Nursing*, appeared in January 1860, an expanded edition later that year, and a cheap *Notes on Nursing for the Labouring Classes* in 1861.

In June 1860, the first nurse-training school in the world opened, at St Thomas' Hospital, then located near Tower Bridge, London. In 1861, her second school opened, for midwifery nursing, at King's College Hospital, London. Lesser sums (all from the Nightingale Fund) helped set up nurse training in several other hospitals. Nightingale did not run any training school but met with matrons and nurses at her home. She continued to mentor leading nurses, British and others, until late in life.

Faith as Foundation

Nightingale's deep religious faith can be seen in so much of her work, from methodology to her professional associations. Her approach to research and policy formulation builds on her belief that "God governs by His laws, but so do we, when we have discovered them. If it were otherwise, we could not learn from the past for the future." This statement comes from her tribute to the Belgian statistician L.A.J. Quetelet, who influenced her work, and whom she met when he visited London to chair the International Statistical Congress in July 1860.[3]

Nightingale's faith similarly grounded her decades of activism. God made the world, and it was good. However, things went wrong. While the Great Litany in the *Book of Common Prayer* petitioned God: " ... from plague, pestilence, and famine, Good Lord, deliver us," she disagreed. Instead of praying "that anything should be otherwise," people should act to repair the damage themselves. As she explained in her *Suggestions for Thought*, she wanted children to be inspired with the idea that one can "second God!"[4] "Submitting" to God's will, the standard goal for church people then, assumed a harsher God than Nightingale's. If people believed, as she did, that God's laws were perfect, then we would not so much need to "obey" them as to "second" them, the "perfect will" and "perfect love" of God.[5]

Medical Condition and Working Style

Nightingale had only one relatively healthy year after the Crimean War, when, probably, the brucellosis she suffered in 1855 reappeared in its chronic form. The disease would be treated by antibiotics now, but there was then no cure or effective treatment. Opiates reduced the pain, but caused drowsiness. Nightingale learned to do without, to work around her illness as much as possible. She described herself as variously a "prisoner to my room" or a "prisoner to my bed." She also enjoyed respites, when she could go out. Simplistic statements that she "took to her bed" for the rest of her life are wrong.

There is virtually no information on Nightingale's health status in childhood and early adulthood. There is mention of her being treated with leeches and blistering, for unspecified illnesses. Her family was keen on water cures, and she took several, notably seven weeks at the spa town of Malvern in Worcestershire in 1851. Incidentally, it was at a water cure in Umberslade Hall, Warwickshire, in 1852 that she learned from the doctor, Walter Johnson, himself the son of a doctor, Edward Johnson, that all the nurses were "drunkards, without exception, sisters and all, and that there were only two nurses whom the surgeon can trust to give the patients their medicines."[6]

After Crimea, Nightingale took further water cures, to no avail. When she had to have "peccant" teeth extracted in 1870, the surgeon (Edwin Saunders, later Sir Edwin) and a surgeon / anaesthetist came with nitrous oxide, as advised by her physician, C.J.B. Williams.[7]

For many years, Dr William Miller Ord (1834–1902), who worked at St Thomas' for half a century and with whom Nightingale had dealings, was also her personal physician. In 1892, his son, William Wallis Ord (1869–1940), "young Dr Ord," came "every day to galvanize me."[8] He also had a distinguished medical career, receiving an OBE. "Young Dr Ord" appears also below in connection with Dr John Shaw Billings of Johns Hopkins University Hospital, as he married a daughter of Billings's and discussed the Baltimore hospital situation with Nightingale. This book does not take up speculation about Nightingale's medical condition, or her "clinicopathology," as conferences like to put it.[9]

Nightingale would always prefer conservative, low-intervention doctors, possibly a lesson learned from her own experiences. She lived during the period of "heroic" medicine, when doctors, desperate to counter raging fevers, turned to ever-more-powerful substances, discussed in chapter 1. Anaesthetics were new and controversial during the Crimean War (Nightingale took a supply with her). Antiseptic surgery dates from the mid-1860s, aseptic practices later, after the appearance of her main books.

Nightingale developed an effective way of conducting research, writing, and meeting with people in her home. She saw visitors one on one: experts and officials from India, matrons and nurses, and a great variety of people asking her for help in finding nurses, planning a new hospital, or some other worthy project. Time with family and friends took second place for her, fitted around this "business," "my Father's business," as she called it, acknowledging that old calling. People who were declined personal interviews normally received a letter in response, sometimes with detailed advice and even a (modest) donation.

Nightingale's own network of colleagues and advisers was impressive, and it continued to grow as new cabinet members and MPs came into office and new medical talent emerged. She always worked collectively, seeking advice and having her own questionnaires, draft articles, and reports vetted by suitable experts.

The only member of her family to become a doctor was Samuel Shore Smith (1861–1925), later Shore Nightingale, elder son of her favourite cousin, William Shore Smith. In 1895, Nightingale asked for him to be appointed to the Nightingale Fund Council, and he duly attended meetings except when in India. He volunteered for plague service in Bombay 1898–1904 and rejoined the council on his return.

Philanthropy and Celebrity

Nightingale supported many charities, hospital building funds, and schools, paid people's doctors' and grocers' bills, and gave money privately to all sorts of needy people. As a celebrity, she was often asked to give her name to charitable projects. She usually declined, reluctant to let her name appear without her work, as she put it. She was also wary of her name assisting dubious causes, and could not spare the time to check organizations' credentials, supporters, and actual work.

Nightingale was partial to unfashionable causes. She let her name be used frequently in *Times* advertisements by the "London Dispensary for Diseases and Ulceration of the Legs." Its advertisement in 1860 stated that she "was well aware of the sufferings of our brave soldiers in the Crimea from this disease" and came forward "most generously" as a patron. The Earl of Shaftesbury and the Lord Bishop of Ripon were listed after her.[10] In 1872, the wording of the ad was changed to: "Established in 1857 under the distinguished patronage of Miss Florence Nightingale and many members of the aristocracy."[11]

Causes she supported publicly included British or local charities for the poor, famine, and war relief. Newspaper accounts during the years from 1857 to 1898 show her donations, sometimes with a letter or comment in support, to: a hospital for women and children in Chatham (fifty guineas),[12] Neapolitan exiles in England (£20),[13] Indian famine relief (£20),[14] relief for destitute sick or wounded Polish patriots,[15] £20 for a wreck register for the Lifeboat Institution,[16] four guineas for a ragged school,[17] the British and Colonial Emigration Society,[18] distress in Paris (siege in the Franco–Prussian War),[19] a "mite" for the Livingstone Expedition, with a letter, "If it cost £10,000 to send him a pair of boots, England ought to give it,"[20] £50 for relief in Bosnia and Herzegovina, her name at the top,[21] £25 for the Russian Sick and Wounded Fund,[22] a training ship for pauper boys,[23] a cheque and a letter for atrocities in Bulgaria,[24] more famine relief in India, with a public letter,[25] a volunteer ambulance (£25 and a letter),[26] distress in Sheffield,[27] toys for school children,[28] a coffee house (as an alternative to the pub),[29] shipwreck survivors,[30] a convalescent hospital for East End poor (her name as a referee),[31] ten guineas for the New Hospital for Women, London, her second donation, noting that £9,000 was still needed,[32] and the last, in 1898, ten guineas for the relief of hurricane victims in the West Indies.[33] She made donations and gave her name for memorials to valued colleagues, notably for Sidney Herbert,[34] and one later for Sir Bartle Frere, a progressive governor of Bombay.[35]

Evidently Nightingale's name helped to raise money. It presumably helped also to sell books, for advertisements of books for which she wrote an introduction feature her name as much as the author's.

For hospital building funds, Nightingale sometimes held out her good name as a bribe: the hospital could use it only if it made crucial improvements in design or site. For the Winchester Infirmary in Hampshire, for example, she made her donation contingent on a new site,[36] and even persuaded a wealthy donor, Lord Ashburton,[37] to make his contingent as well. For others, such as the New Hospital for Women, Euston Road, there were no strings attached.[38]

Nightingale could not stop her name from appearing in ads for commercial products, such as lithographs, a waltz named after her, and a perfume, Florence Nightingale's Bouquet. In the United States, there was "soothing syrup" for teething babies, called "the Florence Nightingale of the Nursery," in numerous ads in the *New York Times* 1860–61. Valid causes used her name, such as a Florence Nightingale Society in Brooklyn, which raised money for a nursing school at what became the Methodist Episcopal Hospital, and duly graduated trained nurses.[39] Two examples also from the American Civil War are noted in chapter 4.

Last Days and Death

Nightingale continued to produce papers and reports well into her seventies, in the 1890s. By her eighties, failing eyesight and mental faculties limited her to sending out brief messages of support. She died at age ninety on 13 August 1910 at her London home, attended by a nurse. The death certificate was signed by her last doctor, Louisa Garrett Anderson, daughter of the first woman to qualify as a doctor in England. Nightingale was buried with her parents at St Margaret of Antioch Church, East Wellow, near the family home, Embley Park, in Hampshire. The small monument, as per her instructions, gives only her initials and dates of birth and death. An offer of burial at Westminster Abbey was declined, in accordance with her wishes. Services for her, however, were held at St Paul's Cathedral and many churches, in Britain and around the world. Her birthday, 12 May, became International Nurses' Day and is still celebrated, now often as part of "Nursing Week."

INTRODUCTION

Working with Doctors

Nightingale's Bicentenary (2020) and the Coronavirus Pandemic

When this book was in the planning stages, 2020 was in view, the bicentenary of Florence Nightingale's birth, designated the Year of the Nurse and Midwife by the World Health Organization (WHO) in her honour. Only the first few celebrations actually happened as planned, for in 2020 coronavirus soon became a pandemic. When the European Association for the History of Nursing convened in Florence, Italy, 13–15 February 2020, delegates did not know that COVID-19 had hit northern Italy. The Florence Nightingale Museum, at St Thomas' Hospital, opened its new exhibition on its honourée on 28 February, but the secretary of state for health cancelled his appearance, suddenly taken up with the pandemic. Lockdown followed in March, and bicentennial events were cancelled, delayed, or turned into virtual meetings.

The new plague duly sparked interest in Nightingale's groundbreaking example as she dealt with high rates of disease and death in the Crimean War, 1854–56. She, with medical colleagues, learned the lessons of the war hospitals. They tracked the decline of the death rates in them and identified why, determined that such extensive disease and death should not recur in war or peace. Nightingale was celebrated as a leader in what we call "data visualization" for her use of persuasive visuals, which helped her to press for sweeping, effective changes in practice and became a model for future reformers.

One 2020 article in the *Guardian* asked: "How would Florence Nightingale have tackled COVID-19?,"[1] while another answered with "fresh air."[2] In the *Financial Times*, an expert in data visualization called her "the pandemic hero we need."³ The author of this book proposes that we look to her on "disease prevention parallels and principles."⁴

The WHO continues to advocate frequent handwashing as a crucial measure for prevention of disease; Nightingale's advocacy of that (and washing the face, too) dates back to her *Notes on Nursing* (1860), with additional points she added in later papers. As understanding increased of how air-borne droplets transmit COVID-19, it became only more obvious how much proper ventilation was needed – a theme for Nightingale from her Crimean days on through her later publications.

It seems that Nightingale had in mind some sort of "early warning system." The WHO of course did not exist in her lifetime, but the British Empire covered a great deal of the earth's territory, with at least one colony on every continent and explorers frequently in Antarctica. Pandemic was not the issue then, but there were sizable epidemics of diseases whose causes (bacilli) were not yet identified. The British Army collected statistics on hospital admissions and deaths for its own personnel. Nightingale recommended upgrading of that to weekly reports, which would become daily during an epidemic. In a memo to the Army Sanitary Commission, she proposed a "Sanitary Intelligence Commission" in the field to gather data on local conditions and dangers and recommend necessary measures.⁵ Nightingale's simple proposal reflects high ambition: not merely to collect annual data and report them, but to present an early warning when a disease was spreading, in order to put measures into place to stop it.

Nightingale's Productive Collaborations with Doctors

While Florence Nightingale is well recognized as the principal founder of the nursing profession, a pioneer theorist of environmental health, and an effective hospital reformer, few analysts have mentioned her extensive collaboration with physicians in all these concerns. Zachary Cope's *Florence Nightingale and the Doctors* (1958) reports mainly on her early relations with doctors but does not show how her views evolved along with changes in medical science and practice. Indeed, one would think that she published northing after 1863, while she was still producing major essays in 1893. Cope's chapter 14 challenges the view that she had any chronic organic disease herself and suggests a "breakdown," an inference countered in 1995 by Young and noted in the preceding "Life and Times of Florence Nightingale."⁶

The present book relates Nightingale's working relationships with a sizable number of doctors, in many countries, and over the whole course of her very long life. Chapter 1 sets the stage with the earliest physicians, including those who encouraged her to reform nursing and public health. Chapters 2–6 report on specific areas of work from the Crimean War (1854–56) in chapter 2, with civilian doctors after Crimea in chapter 3, with military doctors in chapter 4, and in hospital design in chapter 5. Chapter 6 covers midwifery and the entry of women into medicine.

Chapter 7 deals with Nightingale's late writing for doctors (in the 1880s and 1890s), a health-visitor project run with the medical officer of health of Buckinghamshire, the state registration of nurses (on which doctors were prominent both for and against), and bacteriology and germ theory (where Nightingale's work is frequently misrepresented).

Chapter 8 reflects on Nightingale's enduring legacy worldwide. It begins with comparative material on William Osler, often considered the founder of modern medicine. It examines her insights on sunlight and healing in relation to recent work on neuroplasticity. It relates the old "hospitalism" of her day with current studies of hospital-acquired infections. Finally, it explores how her principles might apply to dealing with current challenges in health care worldwide.

Substantial correspondence between Nightingale and doctors survives and covers her entire working life. She kept letters, and many of her correspondents kept hers, some with envelopes, and some with the signature cut off for friends who collected. Her letters were typically well written, often witty, and sometimes touching. This sizable correspondence shows mutual respect and professionalism, and the significant role doctors played in the origins of professional nursing. It reveals further how closely she worked with them on hospital safety and health promotion.

The exchange of observations and insights went both ways. Nightingale required medical information and data, and doctors often needed nurses, or advice on hospital design or renovation. Each person sent the other their latest books. Some doctors became friends, along with their wives, children, and grandchildren. There is warmth and humour in many exchanges.

Nightingale's relations with nurses were quite different. She was head of the Nightingale Fund, which paid for her nurse-training school at St Thomas' Hospital and, to a lesser extent, for those at several other hospitals. She mentored matrons (nursing directors) and senior nurses after their training, some for decades. They approached her for advice and help. She gave it, strategized with anxious matrons and nurses, and sent them home with gifts. Several leading matrons ran into problems with their hospital administration, and Nightingale had to enlist support from senior doctors and hospital governors and board members. These mentoring relationships are overwhelmingly of dependence on her, with much expression of affection on both sides.

By late in her life, there were nursing leaders who could provide Nightingale with useful information, without evident anxiety. With doctors, in contrast, the exchanges were always matter of fact, often with personal messages, but never the desperate pleas for help so characteristic of letters from nurses. Doctors tended to reply promptly to her requests for information, or apologized profusely. She was happy to help when called on, and similarly apologetic with any delay.

While in politics Nightingale was a staunch liberal, in medicine she was consistently conservative, opting for the least intervention possible. She had seen "heroic medicine" in the cholera outbreak of 1854, when arsenic, bleeding, mercury, and opiates were used, and killed many patients.[7] As we saw in the biographical sketch above (p. 12), she had herself been bled and blistered. Her letters throughout her life on finding a doctor for a relative, employee, or friend show favourable references to cautious, conservative doctors. When she recommended surgeon James Paget to her brother-in-law, Sir Harry Verney, for example, she said, "No one is so safe as he."[8]

Medical Science in the Nineteenth Century

When Nightingale did her first nursing, in 1851, anaesthetics were new, antiseptics unknown, and germ theory yet a quarter-century and more in the future. There were few effective drugs and much recourse to harmful substances, like arsenic, lead, and mercury, as doctors tried aggressive measures against diseases they did not understand.

Vast specialization developed in the twentieth century, but in Nightingale's time, there was little beyond medicine and surgery as fields of practice, anatomy and physiology as subjects. The Army Medical School, which opened in 1860, had three chairs (professorships): in military medicine, military surgery, and military hygiene. At about mid-century, such specialties as obstetrics / gynaecology, ophthalmology, and pathology were emerging. The Pathological Society was founded in 1846; the London Obstetric Society held its first meeting in 1859. Bacteriology became a specialty even later, with discoveries beginning only in the late 1870s, discussed further in chapter 7. Great advances in medical science were made after Nightingale had produced her major books. Her insistence on medicine and nursing assisting in the "restorative" process makes sense in the light of how severely limited medicine and pharmaceuticals were at the time.

Even late in the century, when so many major breakthroughs were made, there was an obvious lag between identifying a disease's cause and developing effective treatment or vaccine. Sturdy measures for prevention remained essential.

Deleterious Treatments

It is well known in our time that harmful drugs and treatments were frequently used throughout the nineteenth century (and earlier), and continued well into the twentieth.[9] Bloodletting, or venesection, is a major example, one that Nightingale never challenged. Nurses had to learn how to apply leeches, but there is nothing to suggest that she or they facilitated bleeding with the more draconian lancet.

Bloodletting and blistering, as we see below, both date back to ancient times, and make sense in Galen's theory of humans' (and animals') "four humours": yellow bile, blood, phlegm, and black bile. An imbalance in these caused disease, so reducing the excess treats the condition. The imbalance in blood was the most common form, hence bloodletting. The amount taken varied greatly by practitioner and disease, and could be enormous, totalling litres in successive bleedings.

Bloodletting to treat such diseases as pneumonia was "convincingly challenged in the mid-nineteenth century," but, thanks to "medical conservatism," continued well into the twentieth. Using the technique for pneumonia appears in such a "modern" medical textbook as Osler's *Principles and Practice of Medicine* (1892), and even in the 1942 (posthumous) edition.[10]

Blistering, or vesiculation, entailed the application of caustic agents, such as mustard plaster, to the skin. In theory, the blister it created drained the toxins and thus the infection's source. Mustard plasters also warm muscle tissue and can thus reduce pain. A more extreme form used a heated iron rod.

Both emetics, to cause vomiting, and purging through the bowels were believed to extract the toxins by removing bodily fluids. Calomel, or mercury chloride, was a common purgative. Chapter 2 notes its frequent use during the Crimean War for bowel diseases, especially cholera, along with Nightingale's negative views.

Advances in medical science later in the century reshaped nurse training, which is noticeable in Nightingale's later works. A major theme of this book is the interplay between advances in medical science and in nursing practice. Nightingale had no medical training and did not attempt to make up for it. Doctors themselves were experimenting, for patients became sick and required care, which necessitated scrupulous collection of data and monitoring of results.

As we see in chapter 7, bacteriology emerged in late century, and gradually the great killer fevers were identified. The major cause of maternal mortality, puerperal fever (discussed in chapter 6), was not known until after Nightingale's working life. The term is no longer used, as several pathogens are involved. The "Crimean fever" that nearly killed Nightingale in 1855 was probably brucellosis, identified in 1883, but not ever known by name to her.

Ineffective Treatments

Given the paucity of effective treatments available for the common infectious diseases and fevers, it is not surprising that the sick, and their doctors, turned to such measures as water cures. That is, qualified medical doctors themselves ran spas with concerted programs of (often cold-) water cures, typically allied with healthful diet and exercise. Nightingale and her family themselves used water cures, as we saw above.

A medical appliance that presumably caused no harm, but neither prevented nor cured, was the "cholera belt." Sir James McGrigor, a surgeon in the Napoleonic Wars and later director-general of the Army Medical Department, recommended its use, while not purporting that it was a cure. Also called a "flannel belt," the device was a flannel bandage wound round the abdomen, supposed to protect the wearer against cholera. Europeans sweated a lot in hot climates, and these belts may at least have reduced the discomfort from profuse sweat, then cooling. They were routinely advised for use in hot climates, and in the Crimea, which was not hot. During the Crimean War, both Drs William Aitken and Edmund A. Parkes advised their use. Nightingale, as per her custom, provided what the doctors wanted. "Miss Nightingale's Store" (inventory) included forty-three dozen flannel belts.[11]

Cholera belts were again said to be "wanted" in 1879, for the Anglo–Zulu War.[12] They appear in 1882, as articles omitted, for the Egyptian campaign. As Nightingale explained to a volunteer for the National Aid Society: "Every man has one or two properly made flannel cholera belts to tie on with tapes, and usually the company officers see that the men wear them."[13] These devices were still considered "necessary" in 1888 for a Verney (a member of Nightingale's sister's family) going to India.[14]

From Hygiene and Sanitary Science to State Medicine and Public Health

Between about 1800 and the 1850s, state measures to prevent disease and promote health were markedly improved.[15] After years of inquiries and agitation, the Health of Towns Act (1848) was the first proactive, preventive legislation for England (excluding London) and Wales. Governments had acted to curtail epidemics, to protect their borders with quarantines, and to fumigate and burn diseased materials, but not to prevent epidemics. In that and later measures, "the state became guarantor of standards of health and environmental quality." Government financed necessary local structural changes, especially in water and sewerage.[16] The Health of Towns Act as adopted (after Parliament rejected an earlier bill) was a compromise, merely permissive, not mandatory, but many towns appointed medical officers of health and launched reforms.

Nightingale knew many of the experts and advocates and pushed behind the scenes on the next advances. She worked for years with Edwin Chadwick, Britain's leading "sanitarian," who had been prominent since the 1830s. She greatly respected, but did not know, Dr Southwood Smith, the founder of the Health of Towns Association and a force behind the 1848 legislation. She wanted him to give evidence on mortality and sickness in model lodging houses to the Royal Commission on the Crimean War,[17] but he had retired in 1854. She had a copy of her confidential report sent to him,[18] and hoped he would do a review of it,[19] which he did not. She owned a copy of his influential two-volume *Philosophy of Health, or, an Exposition of the Physical and Mental Constitution of Man* (1836–37).

Liverpool was the first city to institute strong public-health measures, prompted by the influx of ill and starving Irish immigrants from the

Irish Potato Famine (1845–52). It is no coincidence that the Sanitary Commission set up by Lord Palmerston's government in 1855, which did so much to save lives during the Crimean War, was staffed mainly by Liverpudlians, and that Nightingale knew and appreciated them.

Terminology was evolving. "Hygiene" was the name then for the discipline of disease prevention. Nightingale and Dr John Sutherland, head of the Sanitary Commission during the Crimean War, often used the French spelling, *hygiène*, recognizing the early work of French doctors, although *hygiea* was the Greek word for health and the goddess of health. "Sanitary science" was a common nineteenth-century usage, its practitioners "sanitarians." "Sanitary" derives from the French *santé* (health).

"State medicine" came into use after 1850. W.H. Rumsey used it in his *Essays on State Medicine in Great Britain and Ireland* (1856) to indicate laws and regulations enforced by government. De Chaumont gave his *Lectures on State Medicine* in 1875 to the Society of Apothecaries. The British Institute of Public Health, later the Royal Institute of Public Health, launched its *Journal of State Medicine* in 1892. "Public health" in time became the usual term.

Rumsey's 1867 paper on state medicine for the British Medical Association meetings in Dublin led to a proposal to cooperate on its promotion with the Social Science Association's Section on Public Health, and a Joint Committee on State Medicine and the Organization of Sanitary Laws met first in 1868. It helped launch the Royal Sanitary Commission in 1869 to investigate enforcement of Britain's myriad sanitary laws and to ensure an efficient sanitary authority for every region, excepting the metropolis, which was regulated separately.[20] It reported first in late 1870, and the first bill was introduced in 1871. A second report came out in 1871.

With new legislation pending, Edwin Chadwick suggested to Nightingale that she become personally acquainted with James Stansfeld – an "honest man" – president of the Local Government Board and in effect England's minister of social welfare. His post combined sanitary purposes with administering the Poor Laws, and he would put sanitary administration onto a "better footing."[21] Nightingale indeed would work with him assiduously for some years on this, and then further on the repeal of the Contagious Diseases Acts, which discriminated against women in the attempt to reduce venereal disease in the armed forces.

W.H. Wyatt, chair of the Board of Guardians at St Pancras Workhouse, also admired Stansfeld, who, he told Nightingale, had made "beneficial" changes.[22] The next year, he wrote her that Stansfeld could appoint six managers to the Poor Law hospitals, and that judicious choices could be very helpful.[23] Stansfeld would soon be highly criticized by doctors and medical organizations for defects in the legislation.

Publicity given to poor sanitation by the near-death in November 1871 of the Prince of Wales (later Edward VII) from typhoid fever gave Nightingale some hope of action. He had fallen ill of typhoid fever, the disease that killed his father, Prince Albert, in 1861. She noted sardonically to her brother-in-law, Sir Harry Verney:

> Now that they have all but killed an heir apparent to the Throne, perhaps they may listen (as to one 'risen from the dead').
>
> The question now is: Can we, in the act of next session, obtain a clause or clauses to empower local boards to require not only plans of houses to be submitted to them, but all the details of house drainage and of water supply. At present, there is no security or safety. And yet no sewer gas ought ever to enter a house (and no water pipe ought ever to burst by frost). The whole can be done. But it has been no one's business hitherto to do it. Will Mr Stansfeld begin? Scarcely a family is safe.

Nightingale thought that the local boards should have the power "to enter and inspect and direct improvements in all existing houses, as well as in new houses. It is terrible to think that the lives of the people are entrusted to bricklayers and common plumbers, and even footmen. Yet it is vain to deny that such is the case." Verney, to whom she was writing, was a long-time MP and a widower who married her sister, Parthenope, in 1858.

On drainage, the local boards then had the power "to drain streets, courts, houses, and other buildings," "to require that water be laid on to all houses not having a sufficient supply," and "to sanction plans of new houses and to see that the plans provide for drainage." But that was "mere outside work," taking "the means of health, cleanliness and convenience up to the outer walls of the house." Yet it might happen, as the notorious example in Scarborough had shown, "that the whole work was simply a *perfectly contrived* apparatus for *killing the inmates*."[24] At Lord Chesterfield's Londesborough Lodge, in Scarborough, Yorkshire, both the owner and the visiting Prince of Wales had fallen ill of typhoid, and only the prince survived. The press attacked the home's sanitary defects.

In the same letter, Nightingale outlined her questions for Stansfeld:

Are the entire inside drainage and water supply arrangements
within houses to be left as at present in the hands of plumbers'
apprentices or journey men? ... Would it not be worthwhile to
give powers to local boards to examine not only the plans of new
houses before sanction, but also all the internal water supply and
drainage arrangements, water closets, baths, sinks, etc., proposed to
be adopted in these houses, with the view of ensuring (1) that water
pipes shall be thoroughly protected from frost and so arranged as
not to injure the house in case of accidents, and so that all water
escapes may be directed outside the house; (2) that the connections
of all water closets, sinks, baths, etc., shall be so made with the
outside drainage works that no foul air shall enter the house from
the drains and that all W.C. pipes and other drain connections are
ventilated into the open air?

Would it not also be desirable to give the boards power of entry
on all existing houses, and a right to all necessary information as to
the drainage and water supply arrangements within existing houses
such as shall enable them to judge whether such arrangements fulfil
the requirements 1. and 2. above?[25]

The first sanitary law to ensue from the Royal Sanitary Commission
compelled every county, urban and rural, to appoint a medical officer of
health. Yet gaps in enforcement remained substantial, as was pointed out
in the medical press.[26]

Stansfeld told Sir Harry Verney in 1872 that he concurred with Nightingale's views "entirely" and would do "as near what she proposes" as he
could.[27] In a letter to Sir Harry, she expressed her pleasure that Stansfeld
had "inserted 'our' clause in his Sanitary Bill, and some say it is one of
the best clauses in it."[28] However, much was still lacking.

Dr Francis Anstie's death in 1874 from poor sanitation, related in
chapter 3, resulted from his work in a charitable institution, another
cogent reminder of the dangers of "sewer gas." It was obvious that
strong, comprehensive legislation was needed, for preventable deaths
occurred in all classes, from the very poorest homes to charitable institutions, elite public schools, and the country estates of the very rich
(e.g., Lord Chesterfield's).

The near-death of the Prince of Wales came up in another of Nightingale's letters, to Dr John Sutherland, when she was revising text for a new edition of her *Notes on Nursing*. She asked for "base data" on how sewer air entered houses, and how to prevent that, both for "our own houses" and such as the "grand country house by the sea where the *heir to the throne* was all but murdered [word struck through] killed." Other examples were schools and universities, such as Caius College, Cambridge, the Royal Hibernian School, and homes, "*even among noblemen's children*, from the cause, finding out how the sewer air comes in *and how it can be prevented.*"[29] The hoped-for new material in the chapter on housing was never published.[30] Sutherland did not write it up in a way she could use, and she evidently did not think she could do it herself.

It took many years for medical faculties to start teaching public health. Dublin was the first university to hold examinations in "state medicine," in 1871, while Cambridge and Edinburgh followed in 1875. Not until late century were programs in various medical schools made comparable, and students were few. The topics echo Nightingale's in *Notes on Nursing*, on ventilation, water purity, housing, food, and so on, with one on "the history of sanitation," covering the advances made by British commissions, which led to laws to prevent and limit disease.

Nightingale's Earliest Medical Contacts

The eminent American doctor Samuel Gridley Howe (1801–1876), pioneer of education for the blind, was one of the first people to encourage Florence Nightingale in her mission to become a nurse. He and his new wife, Julia Ward Howe – both were abolitionist leaders – visited the Nightingale family on their honeymoon in England in 1844. Nightingale had already studied his reports. A record of their early conversation survives:

> FN: Dr Howe, you have had much experience in the world of philanthropy; you are a medical man and a gentleman; now may I ask you to tell me, upon your word, whether it would be anything unsuitable or unbecoming to a young Englishwoman, if she should devote herself to works of charity, in hospitals and elsewhere, as the Catholics sisters do?"

SGH: "My dear Miss Florence, it would be unusual, and in England whatever is unusual is apt to be thought unsuitable, but I say to you, go forward if you have a vocation for that way of life; act up to your aspiration and you will find that there is never anything unbecoming or unladylike in doing your duty for the good of others. Choose your path, go on with it, wherever it may lead you, and God be with you!"[31]

Howe evidently knew Dr Fowler, the physician in whom Nightingale confided about learning nursing, for he told him that it was "rare" to find a woman with the grace and charm of youth seeking to know "the *laws* as well as the operations of nature." He felt "a redoubled interest in our pursuit from the consciousness that fair and pure young spirits are also centering upon them."[32]

Back in Boston, Howe "ardently desired a son," but told his wife that he would forgive her if she had a girl, "if you will name her for Florence Nightingale." Born in August 1845, the daughter was duly named Florence. Nightingale sent, with her letter to the Howes, "a golden cup," reported to be "now a precious heirloom."[33]

A follow-up letter to Mrs Howe thanks Dr Howe for his interesting letter, with illustrations of mesmerism.[34] Another 1845 letter, to both of them, has amusing remarks about Queen Victoria (having a baby), politics (anti-Tory), and religious trends (people going Catholic). Nightingale joked about forming a society "for ameliorating the condition of young ladies of fortune and education," for which she would be secretary, at £500 a year, then a good income. She recounted her attendance at the death of her own old "nurse." The only observation about nursing as such is a reference to a woman who died from "ignorant nursing."[35]

The correspondence ends with a condolence letter to Mrs Howe on Dr Howe's death in 1877. Julia Ward Howe by then was famous as a suffrage leader and writer of the towering "Battle Hymn of the Republic," which inspired Union soldiers during the American Civil War.[36]

One other doctor from Nightingale's pre-Crimea days was William Bowman, FRS, later a baronet (1816–1892), a distinguished ophthalmic surgeon, whom she assisted in a difficult operation at her small hospital in Harley Street. He wanted her to become superintendent of nursing at King's College Hospital, which she agreed to do, but had to withdraw when asked to go to the Crimean War. Bowman, in other words, had confidence in her ability before she was famous.

Bowman was a member of the original Nightingale Fund Council. He attended its first meeting in 1859 and most until his death in 1892, often chairing. He also served on the committee delegated to do much of the work. Many of the meetings were held at his home. Nightingale, however, was disappointed with his handling of the crisis when the matron, Anglican nun Mary Jones, left King's College Hospital and her order over a dispute with the council. Bowman had been one of the founders of the order, St John's House, and Nightingale thought that the matter could have been resolved.

Bowman continued to be a good adviser. On the death of Agnes Jones, the first trained matron of a workhouse infirmary, he sent Nightingale his condolences for her "heavy loss," noting that Jones had been "one of the very few who enjoyed your full confidence and in whom you looked to carry on your system in the future." He admitted to being "perhaps too hopeful," believing that others would be forthcoming, and that "all that is sound and good in our work will survive individuals, however worthy."[37] When her tribute to Jones, "Una and the Lion," appeared, he wanted her to publish it separately, as a "touching notice," "golden words" to show at St John's House.[38]

Nightingale was (early) impressed with the ideas of two Edinburgh doctor brothers who were advocates of phrenology, George Combe (1788–1858) and Andrew Combe (1797–1847), both of whom it seems she met on pre-Crimea trips. Phrenology, the science of determining mental characteristics from the size and shape of the skull, had an enormous following then and into the early twentieth century. Meetings of the Phrenology Society lasted for days and were well attended, including aristocrats and fellows of the Royal Society. Nightingale was intrigued with the subject and took extracts from Andrew Combe's book. It seems that she met George Combe again in 1847, when he lent her his *Phrenological Journal*, which she read "with the greatest of interest," commenting on "cerebration" as discussed by Dr Engledue, a leading phrenologist.[39]

However, both Andrew and George Combe devoted most of their time to regular medical subjects. Andrew produced the solid, oft-reprinted *Principles of Physiology Applied to the Preservation of Health and to the Improvement of Physical and Mental Education* (1834) and *A Treatise on the Physiological and Moral Management of Infancy* (1840). Both were used at the Nightingale School of Nursing, and Nightingale gave copies as gifts to nurses. Sir James Clark put out a further edition of Combe's book on infancy as *The Management of Infancy* (1860), adding an introduction with quotations from Nightingale's *Notes on Nursing* and appreciation of her for originating the nursing school.[40] He went further than Combe in holding that "no family" should be without her *Notes on Nursing*. It was comprehensive and judicious, and its advice applied even more to children than to patients in general.[41]

Late in 1856, Nightingale sought advice from George Combe on medical education. She asked him to write down "the subjects which now compose medical education … excluding as they do *sanitary* instruction."[42] Introducing health promotion or disease prevention into medical education would be a lifelong preoccupation of hers. He sent her details, enclosing a copy of his biography of his brother, Andrew, which contained material "on the *defects* of medical education." Sir James Clark could tell her "how far they still exist."[43]

Sir James Clark (1788–1870) was a pre-Crimea doctor friend and a member of the royal commission that studied it later. Nightingale stayed with him and his wife at Birk Hall, near Balmoral, Scotland, when he was treating her sister, Parthenope, in 1852. Clark, as physician to Queen Victoria, had the use of Birk Hall, then owned by the Prince Consort, and later a Scottish residence of Queen Elizabeth, the Queen Mother, and then of the current Prince of Wales. The Clarks hosted Nightingale again in 1856 when she went, after Crimea, to meet Queen Victoria, Prince Albert, and War Secretary Lord Panmure about post-war strategy.

Clark was an original supporter of the Nightingale Fund and a member of its first council. He was invited to meet L.A.J. Quetelet at one of Nightingale's breakfasts for the delegates to the International Statistical Congress in London in July 1860. On her own poor health, Clark advised spreading out her work over time.[44] He shared her great appreciation of Sidney Herbert, who chaired the Royal Commission on the Crimean War (1857–58), on which he sat. Yet she was also critical of him, finding him weak in dealing with Andrew Smith, director of the Army Medical Department.[45]

Nightingale's 1856 trip to Balmoral was arranged as a visit to Birk Hall. Only two weeks after her return to England, Sir James Clark wrote Samuel Smith, Nightingale's uncle, who acted for her far more than her father. He had heard from Sidney Herbert of her "fatigue" and need to "mend" for a short time. When she "has recovered her full health," he hoped that she would travel to Scotland "to rest and be braced by our mountain air." As a physician, he was concerned about the effects of "anxious brain work." The queen wanted to see her (he wrote this from the royal residence at Osborne, Isle of Wight), "and this she can do very conveniently and quietly when both are in Scotland. The queen knows that we have asked her to come."[46] The visit took place in September 1856.

Clark continued to be Nightingale's intermediary with the royal family. She sent him an early copy of her *Notes on Matters Affecting the Health, Efficiency and Hospital Administration of the British Army* (1858), asking him to present a copy, currently being bound, to the queen. She asked his advice on transmitting copies to other members of the royal family.[47] She later sent Clark her (improved) edition of *Notes on Nursing* for the queen and the princess royal (also Victoria).[48]

In due course, Nightingale sent Clark copies of her India report for transmission to Leopold I, king of the Belgians (uncle of both Queen Victoria and Prince Albert), and to Victoria, with a letter for the latter, to send or burn as he likes, and two for himself. She wondered also about sending the queen her short paper on India: "She might look at that, because it has pictures. And she certainly will not look at the report." She expressed also her disappointment that not one review had "seized our main point, viz., reform your stations first – it is not your climate – it is not even mainly your sites – it is your living like beasts, not civilized men, without water supply, without drainage, etc., heightened by climate and by sites, which kills you."[49]

Clark was sympathetic and helpful in her numerous struggles with the War Office, especially on starting the Army Medical School (opened 1860) at Fort Pitt, Chatham, in Kent, with the right appointments and conditions. She shared with him her concerns about pathology at the school: "Pathologists are apt to get into the way of considering the main end of such a school to be that of making good pathological preparations. But, if the Chatham school produces many good pathological preparations, you must report it to the Statistical Congress *as bad*. Pathology is doubtless essential. But the aim of our Army School is the prevention of disease, not the record of the harm disease has done."[50]

Sir James was Nightingale's great facilitator, thanks to his position and his general agreement with her views. He could intervene and propose – Nightingale fed him lines. The support he gave her was valuable, but not at the level of that of Drs John Sutherland and William Farr, who provided her with ideas and gave critical feedback on her proposals. On Clark's death, his son, Sir John Clark, became a diligent member of the Nightingale Fund Council.

Dr John Sutherland, Colleague from the Sanitary Commission to Old Age

For much of her working life, Nightingale had the benefit of the advice of Dr John Sutherland (1808–1891), an Edinburgh-trained doctor and public-health expert, whom she had met in 1855 when he headed the Sanitary Commission. He served as a sort of research assistant, answering her questions succinctly and drafting material for her. Mrs Sutherland gave practical assistance as well, to become a friend herself, and Nightingale's "favourite wife."

After the war, Dr Sutherland became a civilian employee, on contract, at the War Office. He never held another post and published little in his own name, although he wrote many useful reports, apparently content to play second fiddle to Nightingale. The two agreed on the basics and could work out their differences. Both were careful about details – he, of course, grounded with a sound medical education. He frequently spent full days at Nightingale's home, going over papers for her and drafting notes and replies to correspondence. Since he was profoundly deaf, they communicated often by note, thereby recording many of these exchanges. Other colleagues visited to confer when he was there.

While Nightingale was largely an invalid, Sutherland could travel. He was sent to inspect army hospitals and barracks in the Mediterranean – Gibraltar, Malta, the Ionian Islands – and to see French hospitals in Algeria. Yet he deferred to her on general goals and vision. She was the better writer, so that her finished version sparkles in comparison with his draft.

Members of Parliament occasionally complained about Sutherland's remuneration, saying that other doctors in the department could do his work at no extra cost. Ministers always defended him. Lord Hartington, for example, as undersecretary for war, said: "These duties were better performed by Dr Sutherland than they could be by any other person."[51] Nightingale sometimes had to remind ministers to be ready to speak up when questioned in the House about the expenditure.

She and Sutherland also shared a deep religious faith. She disagreed with his sabbatarianism – she routinely worked on Sundays. On one occasion, to prepare for advising a new Indian viceroy, Lord Dufferin, she urged Sutherland to make an exception: "If you did a little on Sunday, the Recording Angel would drop not a tear but a smile."[52] He declined.

Early in their work together, Nightingale sent him a draft of a section of her religious-philosophical speculations, *Suggestions for Thought*. He was scandalized at her departure from accepted doctrine, especially on free will, which was always free, in his view, while Nightingale, at this point, was entertaining the idea of its being caused by other conditions. Sutherland wrote detailed objections on the manuscript, but tactfully sent it back via Nightingale's aunt, Mai Smith (her father's sister Mary, who had wed her mother's brother, Samuel Smith). He confessed that he had perhaps "expressed my opinions sometimes too strongly, but my excuse must be that I have felt strongly. The points at issue would never separate us in any practical work. They are therefore harmless so far as that is concerned." He added that they might not be so harmless "in other hands ... and it is for such a reason that I have felt strongly about them ... In our work we have enough of difference of opinion to make it desirable not to have more. I regret that, on this most important of all subjects, we should differ at all."[53]

It appears that the two never discussed the matter. Nightingale never published *Suggestions for Thought*, but had it printed and circulated privately – presumably she did not send Sutherland a copy. She kept his objections in, adding her own comments: "It is said that," or "It is objected that," followed by her refutation.[54]

A deeply felt common faith, however, remained a bond between the two, shared as well with Mrs Sutherland. In a letter after Dr Sutherland's death in 1891, his widow recalled his "talking of death, resting in Jesus, peace." He liked to look at "the engraving of the crucifixion you gave me, and which has always hung opposite our bed." He "always tried to lead an 'inner life' apart and, while in the world, doing its work, not to be of the world,"[55] His last words to his wife were for Nightingale: "Give her my love and blessing."[56] This part of their relationship has been entirely missed in coverage of their work by other authors, who like to stress their differences.

Dr Sutherland was strong on priorities and tactics, what to take on and when. He gave Nightingale sage advice as early as August 1856, just after her return to England, about not proceeding quickly on nursing. Her letter to him is not extant, so we know only that it related to nursing in military hospitals and acting on the Nightingale Fund. He wrote her that there was no hope of improving nursing without improving the hospitals, which would take time. She, in fact, proceeded promptly on statistical analysis of the war hospitals and hospital reform, before making any decisions on using the Fund to start a nursing school.

On dealing with the war secretary, Lord Panmure, Sutherland advised her to stick to defects that she could document: "Facts are always facts, while advice may be returned without thanks, which in your case it is better to avoid. Unfortunately, there are great differences of opinion as to what is required to reform the Army Medical Department."[57] Certainly her reports were heavy on facts, introducing proposals for change with care. Sutherland's assistance to her will be clear throughout the rest of this book.

On his death, Nightingale wanted suitable obituaries published. When she wrote to the editor of the *Times* with a notice on his death, she called herself "his pupil both in sanitary administration and practice ... anxious for my master's fame."[58] She thought him "one of the leading sanitarians of this century," not given the credit he deserved for either of the royal commissions on which he served. While Sidney Herbert wrote "almost all" of the 1858 report of the Royal Commission on the Crimean War, "Dr Sutherland got up the evidence," while for India, he wrote "nearly the whole of the report" – *Report of the Royal Commission on the Sanitary State of the Army in India* (1863). Further, on all of the sub-committees to implement the recommendations of the Crimean War report, again Herbert chaired them, but Sutherland "was the active member." This work improved the health not only of soldiers, but of "the *whole native population*" in India.[59]

Statistical Analysis with Dr Farr

Dr William Farr (1807–1883) was Britain's leading medical statistician when Nightingale met him, soon after the Crimean War. He rose from a humble background, aided by a local squire and mentoring by the utility theorist Jeremy Bentham, to become superintendent of statistics, the second position in Britain's General Register Office. Nightingale met him through Sidney Herbert, who told her that Farr would be "a most valuable witness" for the royal commission.[60] A lively correspondence between the two began in January 1857, which she carried on after his death with his wife and daughters. A Farr daughter was named after her, and Nightingale left a legacy to the unmarried daughter at home.

As becomes clear in the chapters to follow, Farr left his mark on her work, as did Sutherland. Farr and his office did the statistical work on the Crimean War data. He had published charts much earlier, but those he prepared on the Crimean data – the iconic "polar area charts" – were far better. Clearly the two colleagues had a synergy that worked.

Farr was sick and at home one day when Nightingale wanted his advice on her own (written) evidence for the royal commission. He asked her to call on him: "I should like very much to go through your evidence with you and to find as much fault as I can."[61] Clearly his office was working up the data for her: "The calculation for the period from October 15 to January 31st will reach you by 4 o'clock. I will do February for you afterwards." (Secondary sources often, incorrectly, have Nightingale collecting and analyzing the data on her own.)

One batch he sent her contained "a new note for your diagrams submitted for approbation! The *radial lines* show the *rates of mortality*; the *dark* area represents the *culpability* of the authority, which in an army increases (at least as fast) as *the square of the rate of mortality*."[62] As the work progressed, he said how much he and his colleagues prized her approval, and sought "*future* work in the great cause, which we are bound by sacred vows to promote to our lives' end."[63]

Farr and his assistants did the background work not only for the Crimean War and the Indian commissions, but also for her "Sanitary Statistics of Native Colonial Schools and Hospitals" (1863).[64] For years he gave her considerable help on civilian hospitals. He reported to her what he had picked up in meetings he attended that she could not. A letter of his apologizes for not being able "to do anything for you" that day, but he hoped "to be able to work for you" on the Monday.[65]

They shared the belief that diagrams should be able to tell the story. He described "the effect of the display of the appalling subject," mortality rates, in a diagram. "It is, however, the perspective of writing with diagrams and tables before you, to render any reference to them by the reader unnecessary. This you have done."[66]

When Nightingale asked for a critical read of material in preparation, he gave "much care and much interest," but found little to fault: "The just indignation is expressed with natural eloquence. I have ventured to point out every fault I could find, but my criticisms are only made so freely because I know you will treat them merely as suggestions with the due number of ??? after them in your own careful revision of the whole work."[67] Soon he was on to "important sources of evidence" to be elicited that could halve the mortality of the army.[68]

Farr also sent Nightingale his own material and asked for advice, for example, on improvements in police data.[69] She found a mistake – 28 per cent should have been 28 per 1,000 – duly corrected, as an assistant informed her.[70] Farr also asked her for favours, such as supporting worthy causes he favoured, but later apologized for troubling her. On Sidney Herbert's death, Farr gave a paper in tribute, and asked Nightingale to give a copy to Elizabeth Herbert.[71] She duly returned Lady Herbert's appreciation.

Farr's letters are whimsical in places, with quotations from Greek mythology, the Bible, Chaucer, Shakespeare, Milton, Turgenev. He quoted Goethe, in German, on the world being "governed by numbers, whether well or badly."[72] On Christmas day 1857, he thanked her for the "six copies of your precious oration illustrated, to be placed next in merit and utility to Milton's on unlicensed printing."[73] The six copies included several for distribution to the clerks who worked on the data; they wanted their copies autographed.[74]

Farr once asked her where Sutherland was, so that he could look in on him: "We shall consult and fly to you, be assured, if we stump into any inextricable difficulty."[75] When she sent him the new, cheap edition of her *Notes on Nursing for the Labouring Classes*, he replied that the inexpensive version would be "dearer than ever."[76] He wrote her "a short epistle" on the "longest day of the year."[77] He asked her opinion on books, "a single line."[78] The Farrs appreciated the "fine birds" (game) Nightingale sent them. Her family often sent her partridge, grouse, and pheasant from their grounds, and she liked to pass them on.

Nightingale returned Farr's compliments. When he was working on the 1871 British census, she called this "putting forth your beneficent feelers all over this land, spinning your web, to tell us how many we are – not how many we have killed and lost in horrid war."[79] When he returned to England after a trip for his health, she said: "To you is due a great part of the saving of lives effected by the immense strides sanitary progress has made in the last forty years, as far as this depended on statistical work, all over England and Europe. London – the healthiest large city in the world, I suppose – owes this to you mainly, inasfar as you have pointed out and tested our way and our progress."[80] When she thanked him for a New Year's message, she said that his encouragement was "always the most welcome" she received.[81] In 1878, she subscribed to the fund to commission a portrait of him.[82]

Nightingale had tried assiduously, but unsuccessfully, in 1864–65, to have Farr appointed to the prestigious Institut de France. When, in 1879, it appeared that Britain's top statistical position, registrar general, would soon become vacant, she tried to get him the post. "I lost no time," she told him, in asking Lord Beaconsfield (Benjamin Disraeli) to appoint him: "You cannot wish more than I that you should be registrar general." However, the position had not yet been vacated.[83] As it happened, ill health forced Farr to retire later that year.[84]

She then approached Sir Stafford Northcote, chancellor of the Exchequer, to ask that Farr receive full pay on his retirement, after forty-one years' service, she noted. Farr had "created" the General Register Office, she told Northcote, as he preceded its head, Major Graham. "Dr Farr's name and work are synonymous with rise and progress in sanitary and statistical science, whether in England, India or Europe." He was responsible for producing "a great part" of the statistics for both the Crimean and Indian royal commissions. She had worked with him for twenty-five years.[85]

What pension he received is not clear in the correspondence. (Farr in his later years was in financial difficulties from bad investments.) On a last attempt to have him honoured, she inquired from a colleague what he thought Farr would like – a CB or a knighthood? He received neither. On his death, she sought a pension for his wife and daughters.[86] She gave £100 to a testimonial fund, in effect for his widow and daughters, and offered to make her support public, if that would help bring in more subscribers. She considered that the world was in Farr's debt as much as in Quetelet's, that they together, "we may say, originated the practical application (or at least organized it) of a science without which all other sciences – moral, social, political or administrative – could not exist as sciences at all."[87]

Daughter Florence Farr (1860–1917) became a famous actress. George Bernard Shaw wrote the lead role for her in his *Arms and the Man* (1894), his much-performed spoof on war. In a key scene, the captain declaims: "I've no ammunition. What use are cartridges in battle? I always carry chocolate instead." Florence Farr was the first actress to call him "the chocolate cream soldier!" Nightingale's only correspondence with her, however, concerns a pension for her mother and the daughter at home.

The one biography of Farr skimps on his work with Nightingale.[88] There is also a memorial volume of his work and a biographical sketch.[89]

Doctors' Demand for Trained Nurses

Some doctors had articulated the need for skilled nurses long before Nightingale. They were aware that the untrained "nurse" or family member often failed to carry out their orders and missed important changes in the patient's condition. Yet others thought that the quality of "nursing" was adequate – an example from St Thomas' appears in chapter 3. Enough, however, wanted a capable person at the bedside.

A System of Clinical Medicine (1843), by a leading Irish physician, Robert James Graves, gives numerous instances of good and bad nursing. He advised doctors not to undertake a fever case without "a regular fever nurse," training unspecified. He had regretted having done so in the past. Family members and friends could give "sympathy," but without the "strict sense of duty" or "laudable desire of increasing her own reputation." He now made it "a general rule to refuse attending any dangerous and protracted case of fever without a properly qualified nurse," but without saying how to find such a person.[90] His examples show the value of the nurse's observations reported to the physician.

A decade later, similar views appeared in a review of a book on nursing in the *British Medical Journal*: "We doctors well know that the life of the patient is often far more in the hands of the nurse than it is in the hands of the doctor. For example, in cases of fever, what avail all the minute directions of the physician, if there be not an intelligent and *honest* nurse at hand to carry them out?"[91]

In 1867, the Norwich Board of Guardians, in charge of care for the city's destitute, appointed a committee to inquire "into systems of nursing for the sick poor at home." Nightingale's correspondent, Dr Joseph Allen, who had previously practised at the Liverpool Workhouse Infirmary, wrote her about the inadequate nursing care available, that those who fall ill "are nursed according to no system, but anyhow, leaving all to Providence." He was "desirous that such a state of things should no longer exist" and asked her to point out "some systematic way of nursing the outdoor sick poor"[92] (those not in a workhouse). District (home-visiting) nursing was not established until about 1873, and her paper on providing such care dates to 1876.

For Nightingale, nursing, medicine, surgery, and hygiene, or health sciences, were separate professions. Nursing was necessarily subordinate, for nurses, as women, were excluded from a university education, and few had anything close to secondary schooling. Women were permitted in British universities only in the 1880s, and then in small numbers. Nurses were not junior doctors – perish the thought! – but a new profession with distinct, and worthy, functions. To Dr John Croft, who instructed the Nightingale nurses at St Thomas', she called the field a "branch of hospital work."[93]

Many nurses of today dislike Nightingale's insistence on a subordinate role for nurses. Some even deny any difference in level of knowledge or status – lumping doctors in with "other health professionals." In Nightingale's time, however, it could not have been otherwise. Physicians had a university education and a medical degree, and some had further specialist training. Many wrote books and gave papers. Some nurses needed coaching in basic reading, writing, and arithmetic. Few even owned a professional book; Nightingale often gave them their first, as numerous letters of thanks attest. By late in her life, there were exceptions – nurses who published – but they often needed help with the manuscript. A number gave papers at conferences, for example at the Congress on Hospitals, Dispensaries, and Nursing at the world congress in Chicago in 1893 – thirty-three years after her nursing book appeared and her school opened. Nightingale couldn't attend but sent a paper.

She was content to start her school with apprenticeship training, requiring only that applicants be literate. Even then, the tutor had to sit in on classes and take her own notes in order to help pupils learn the material. The doctor / instructor did the examining. The nursing profession made enormous strides in Nightingale's lifetime, but the start was difficult. Nurses, when her school at St Thomas' opened in 1860, were not allowed to take a patient's temperature – the task of a medical student or dresser. Over the next decades, they increasingly took on the tasks of junior doctors in tests and dressings, as related in chapter 7. Medicine, of course, was also moving ahead, so that the gulf in knowledge and skills between nurses and physicians remained substantial. Doctors found Nightingale's approach acceptable: they themselves diagnosed and prescribed, while nurses carried out their orders, administered food, drink, and medicines as required, observed, took notes, and reported back to them.

Nightingale, however, was insistent that nurses run their own profession. Only a nurse (matron, superintendent, or nursing director), but not a doctor, could hire, dismiss, discipline, or promote a nurse. A doctor with a complaint about a nurse's conduct took it to the matron, who answered to the head of the hospital administration, as did the medical superintendent. One suspects that this separation was also intended to prevent sexual harassment by doctors, although nothing so unsavoury appears on paper.

Nightingale preferred lay hospital administration to medical. At one level, this was a compliment to doctors – that they would want to spend their time practising their profession, not in bureaucracy. It also reflects her firm belief that they were inept at administration. The great improvements in the running of English hospitals came from lay input, she thought. She joked to Sidney Herbert: "There must be something in the smell of the medicines which induces absolute administrative incapacity."[94] When a new initiative on district nursing was being considered in 1874, Nightingale was asked her views on a list of doctors. She knew several of them personally and had had a "voluminous correspondence" with them: Drs Burgess, Lechmere, Rumsey, and Sieveking. But they were "nearly the most unbusiness-like men I have ever known." Not a one on the list could she recommend.[95]

In 1879, Nightingale claimed that "leading" physicians and surgeons were the first to admit that the regular, *lay* administration of the hospital should "not be in the hands of the medical staff."[96] A year later, she told Henry Bonham Carter (1827–1921), her first cousin (through her mother) and secretary of the Nightingale Fund Council, "Doctors have no idea of administration."[97]

Apart from the great gap in education between doctors and nurses, their personal conduct and ethics differed notably. Physicians were professionals, most of them "gentlemen." Many "nurses" of the time – no trademark on the job title – were allegedly often slatternly, sexually available, drunk on the job, and notorious for stealing their patients' food and drink. Even worse, some demanded bribes for services. Nightingale observed in an appendix to her *Notes on Hospitals*: "The cardinal sin of paid nurses, of all classes, of all nations, is taking petty bribes and making petty advantages (of many different sorts and sizes) out of the patients."

Members of religious orders were exempt, but not their servants.[98] It is difficult for medical and nursing personnel today to realize the scope of the moral challenge Nightingale faced in establishing professional nursing. Medicine was an ancient profession, typically dated back to the Hippocratic school in fifth-century-BCE Greece. Trained nursing dates only to the second half of the nineteenth century.

Nightingale knew from experience that nuns and deaconesses were the exception to the slovenly drinkers in British hospitals. They gave devoted, sober care in hospitals, but without training. Nightingale found their standards of hygiene badly lacking. Many orders fitted patient care into their schedule of prayer and meditation. Some orders did not permit nuns to touch men or pregnant women. Most forbade night work. A leading American doctor who had experience of Sisters of Charity as nurses before the Civil War described them as "kind and gentle, but not trained."[99] Nuns and deaconesses could not be models for Nightingale in the creation of the new profession.

The stress on the necessary *moral* qualities often rankles contemporary nurses. "A good nurse must be a good woman," Nightingale told a community leader in Vienna seeking to start training there. Too many were not, and physicians often failed to notice their errant conduct, knowing little "how nurses hoodwink them: the bad woman, the clever nurse, must be an idiot if she cannot hoodwink the doctor."[100] When Nightingale had reason to complain about bad standards at a hospital, as she did for the Vienna General, she did not blame the doctors, nor did she for the "lawless" Edinburgh Royal Infirmary, related in chapter 3.

Finally, Nightingale wanted nurses to be like physicians in taking up advocacy when needed. She greatly admired the Crimean War doctors who stuck their necks out to report problems. She wanted nurses, too, to be patients' advocates and defenders when things went wrong. They "ought to be the patients' defender and keeper," she told her Vienna correspondent, but in some cases "you have to defend the patient against the nurse." Hence the need for a high moral standard. In that same (long) letter, she noted that cruelty occurred in "the best medical-staffed hospitals."[101]

Nightingale's Definitions of Health and Healing

In the Conclusion of every edition of her *Notes on Nursing*, Nightingale set out her position on healing:

It is often thought that medicine is the curative process. It is no such thing; medicine is the surgery of functions, as surgery proper is that of limbs and organs. Neither can do anything but remove obstructions; neither can cure; nature alone cures. Surgery removes the bullet out of the limb, which is an obstruction to cure, but nature heals the wound. So it is with medicine; the function of an organ becomes obstructed; medicine, so far as we know, assists nature to remove the obstruction, but does nothing more. And what nursing has to do in either case is to put the patient in the best condition for nature to act upon him.

She repeated her plea for fresh air, quiet, and cleanliness, against the view that medicine was the *sine qua non*, the panacea.

In an encyclopaedia article in 1890, Nightingale again put her position clearly:

Nursing is putting us in the best possible conditions for nature to restore or to preserve health, to prevent or to cure disease or injury. The physician or surgeon prescribes these conditions; the nurse carries them out. Health is not only to be well, but to be able to use well every power we have to use. Sickness or disease is nature's way of getting rid of the effects of conditions which have interfered with health. It is nature's attempt to cure – we have to help her. Partly, perhaps mainly, upon nursing must depend whether nature succeeds or fails in her attempt to cure by sickness. Nursing is therefore to help the patient to live. Nursing is an art, and an art requiring an organized practical and scientific training. For nursing is the skilled servant of medicine, surgery and hygiene.[102]

Nightingale used similar wording in her 1893 paper for the congress in Chicago: "The physician prescribes for supplying the vital force, but the nurse supplies it." Training in the laws of health and disease, God's laws, as she thought them, was essential.[103]

Nightingale had one early medical contact, Sir John Forbes (1787–1861), on the key point that nature, not chemicals, cured. He was a neighbour of hers in London for several years at the end of his distinguished career. The two exchanged books and corresponded, but never met. His last book, the polemical *Of Nature and Art in the Cure of Disease* (1857), antedated her *Notes on Nursing* by three years. His was aimed at junior doctors, to improve their practice "by strengthening their confidence in nature's powers and by mitigating ... the evils of Polypharmacy."[104] He condemned the "want of trust in nature and the over-trust in art prevalent among the members of the medical profession."[105] They should, instead, "assist Nature" in her operation, cooperating with her and excluding obstructive agencies, very much what Nightingale believed.[106] The number of cases that were "directly" curable was small, Forbes stated, while "restorative powers" were inherent in the system itself. Physicians took credit for cures that were simply the effect of time, that is, that nature finally "conquered" the disease.[107] The book ends with rejection of the doctor as the "heroic character of a controller of nature and a conqueror of disease."[108]

Forbes's book saw a second English edition, an American edition, and translation into Swedish, but it was promptly attacked. A physician wrote the *Lancet* that it was "preposterous" that a doctor of Forbes's reputation should "wilfully disparage the value of our art and, under the name of heroic and perturbative, attempt to depreciate some of the most valuable adjuncts we profess."[109]

When Nightingale's *Notes on Nursing* appeared early in 1860, Forbes promptly wrote her with his compliments. The letter is not extant, but she told Dr Sutherland that he had said that he "went along" with her book entirely – "a great deal for a *medical man* to say." Forbes's own tome, she said, was "the only medical book I know in *our* sense at all."[110] It contains, however, no mention of nursing. Nightingale wrote Forbes diffidently:

> Nothing has given me half so much pleasure as a note from you about my little nursing book. That you, to whom the world is so much indebted in the matter of its health, should endorse it with your imprimatur is a very great satisfaction to me. All I can say for the book is that there is not one word of theory in it. Every sentence of it is the fruit of bitter experience. That your experience as a physician should coincide with mine as a nurse gives it value.
>
> The great object I had in view was to recall the art of observation which has, I think, deteriorated, even in my day, under the load of supposed science. People have eyes "and they see not."
>
> My conclusions were arrived at by looking at disease simply from the practical side. If people who have science too (which I

wish I had) would do the same, how much might not be done for
the world's health!

I know your book "Nature and Art in the Cure of Disease"
well. But should it not be a trouble to you to send me a copy, as
you so kindly offer, I should consider it a great honour to have one
from you ...

P.S. You encourage me by your kindness to send you another
little book of my hospital experience.[111]

Nightingale, in contrast with Forbes, never presumed to reprimand
doctors. Far from accusing them of failure in observation, she stressed,
positively, how much they counted on nurses for observation, and directed
her admonitions to nurses to get it right.

Working Relationships with Doctors and Nurses Compared

There were nursing leaders Nightingale esteemed, like Mary Jones, mother
superior and matron at King's College Hospital. However, Jones soon
began to defer to her, called on her for help in administrative problems,
but then left both her order and nursing. Sarah E. Wardroper, the matron
at St Thomas', who had started improving nursing standards when she
took over in January 1854, was a "hospital genius," for her ability to
allocate staff and plan. However, she had never nursed herself and had
no gift for or interest in nurse training. When she was appointed, she
was a doctor's widow with young children to support. She had the status
of "gentlewoman," unusual then for a hospital matron.

It was only late in Nightingale's life that a few nurses emerged who
related to her somewhat as peers, reporting their experiences to her with
some assurance, albeit still with diffidence. She considered Florence
Lees (1840–1922) to be the founder of district, or home-visiting nursing,
although Lees herself for years needed enormous encouragement to
start in it. Nightingale learned much about asepsis in 1896 from Finnish
nurse Ellen Ekblom. Letters from Georgina Franklin, a nurse in India
during a plague epidemic, reported confidently and in detail on what she
had learned there. Elizabeth Vincent, the matron at the St Marylebone
Workhouse Infirmary, was exceptional in her matter-of-fact reports, which
highlighted progress made and problems solved.

The fact of Nightingale having good, working relationships with doctors (men), but not with nurses (women), has been grossly misinterpreted. Superficial accounts have her not liking women and preferring to work with men. For example, the entry in the *Oxford Dictionary of National Biography* has Nightingale considering women to be "selfish ... and though she adulated a chosen few, she preferred working with men."[112] The essay's senior author, Monica Baly, was, in earlier works, highly positive about Nightingale's work and person. Feminist authors have been particularly firm on the matter. Karen Armstrong, for example, said that Nightingale "hated women and wanted co-operation only of men,"[113] Martha Vicinus, a professor of English and women's studies, held that Nightingale had a "low" opinion of women, citing no sources.[114]

These assessments are based on a statement Nightingale made in 1861, that her doctrines had "taken no hold among women," that not one of the Crimean nurses would help "to carry out the lesson of that war or those hospitals," although many men did. She told a close friend that this was because "*Women have no sympathy.*"[115] Yet her statement of lack of help from women, while much from men, was correct for the time; it was not a principle to follow. In 1861, she had steady support from Drs Sutherland and Farr, civil engineer Rawlinson, royal engineer and cousin-in-law Douglas Galton, and of course Sidney Herbert until his death, precisely on applying the lessons of the war. Earlier, 1854–56, she had respected women colleagues, in Lady Cranworth and Lady Canning, capable women, her superiors at the Harley Street hospital, who assisted her with selecting nurses for the Crimean War. Her correspondence with them is on a par with that with men colleagues. She would have a respected woman colleague again in 1865, when Agnes Jones launched professional nursing at the Liverpool Workhouse Infirmary. Indeed, beginning about then, women emerged who did help on her mission, and from whom she learned many things, although typically she gave more to them than they to her.

Gaining Professional Status for Nurses

Nurses were first mentioned in the census in 1861, grouped in "Domestic" service – a new occupational classification designed by Dr Farr about the time Nightingale's school opened. Nurses remained in that category in 1871, but in 1881 were moved to "Subordinate medical service." In

1891, they were labelled "Sick nurses," "sandwiched between the medical suborder and their subordinate workers," as "Sick nurse, midwife or invalid attendant." Left in "Domestic" were nursemaids and children's nurses, classed as "Indoor servants."[116] The situation was similar in the United States, where nurses were first named as a category in 1860.

Today's nurses, however, are fond of imagining a golden past, of equal relations between doctors and nurses before Nightingale. They then blame her for making nurses subservient. For example, her stress on nursing being a profession for women, and the nurse being a "good woman," it is said, "deprofessionalized" relations between medicine and nursing.[117] Nightingale, in a British nursing journal, is accused of "unwittingly" creating "the subservient role of nurses to doctors."[118] Is there any profession, then or now, that admits persons with less than a secondary-school education as equals to those with a university education and specialist qualifications?

Doctors' Orders: Discretion versus Obedience

In "Nightingale nursing," the nurse carries out the doctor's medical orders, with discretion. Nightingale always contrasted the "intelligent obedience" required of nurses with the "blind obedience" of nuns and soldiers. In 1868, when discussing the introduction of professional nursing at the Sydney Infirmary in New South Wales, she remarked to the colonial secretary: "The days of blind obedience, whether it was ever desirable or not, are entirely over and can never come back. Amongst free and independent people (which is our tone and spirit, ever-increasing), there must be much forbearance ... Co-operation must take the place of obedience."[119]

She emphasized this also in a letter to Queen Victoria's daughter Princess Alice (Princess Louis of Hesse) in Darmstadt, who was very supportive of nursing: "Inspiring *intelligent* obedience to the orders of the medical authorities" had to be the "governing spirit" of the hospital: "We cannot, and do not wish to, make use of the Roman Catholic arts for enforcing obedience, *blind* obedience."[120] In an 1872 address to nurses, she criticized the "blind, unconditional obedience" required in religious orders, preferring the greater freedom, individual responsibility and self-command, "greater thought in each, more discretion and higher, not less, obedience. For the obedience of intelligence, not the obedience of slavery, is what we want."[121] Her address to nurses of 1876 similarly commended "the freedom of action you enjoy by that *intelligent* obedience to rules and orders," which alone was "worthy of the name of 'trained nurse.'"[122] In a paper read at the Chicago congress in 1893, she referred to "strict, intelligent, obedience to the physician's or surgeon's power and knowledge." Training was to make the nurse not "servile," but rather "loyal" to medical orders and authorities.[123]

A doctor's article on nurse training in the *Glasgow Medical Journal* in 1889 expanded on "intelligent obedience" as the accurate and intelligent carrying out of instructions, not as a mere automaton or machine: "Nurses are officers in the army drawn up to do battle with disease, and in the absence of the commander much will frequently be left to the trained intelligence and skill of the nurse."[124] Nowhere, however, did Nightingale or the article's author, Dr John Lindsay Steven (who became the journal's editor in 1890), give any criteria for or concrete examples of not following the doctor's orders. This was the time of "heroic medicine," which harnessed blistering, bloodletting, intestinal purging, sweating, and vomiting and used medicines such as mercury, lead, antimony, bismuth, camphor, and arsenic, substances "which scientists now know to be highly toxic."[125] Nightingale is not known to have administered any of these materials, nor to have been directed to. She was clearly aware of the harm of some, as we see in chapter 2, when both she and army doctors opposed the use of calomel (mercury chloride).

Sceptical as she was about conventional medical treatment, Nightingale was no advocate for anything else. She opposed homeopathy, which was then gaining support as alternative medicine. Practitioners who were not medically trained were, for her, "quacks," their remedies "quack medicine." For her, the nurse's ability to provide the doctor with detailed observations of the patient's condition was key to treatment, as she set out in the chapter "Observation of the Sick" in *Notes on Nursing*. The requirements for observation then became increasingly complex. Nurse training had to keep up with medical knowledge and doctors' demands. In an 1876 letter to nurses, Nightingale could report the usefulness of a good standard of observation. She noted a physician's statement that "he knew when an operation ought to be performed by reading the nurse's report on the case." Another recounted that, on "reading the nurse's history of the case, he found patients to be suffering from typhoid fever who had been reported as consumptive." Another doubted if many of their medical students could have sent a better report than the nurse's history.[126]

Doctors' Attack on Nightingale's Views of Contagion

Nightingale's views on contagion were promptly attacked by doctors. An Edinburgh doctor criticized her statements in *Notes on Nursing for the Labouring Classes* (1861), which were the same as in the earlier versions and indeed in *Notes on Hospitals*. Dr Gairdner cited her statement that diseases were not "separate things," but "conditions, just as much under our own control, or rather as the reactions to a kindly nature." He also expressed respect for her and approved of the rest of the book, but wished that she had considered "whether the facts stated and the opinions expressed are consistent with the modesty and reticence of true science as regards the unknown." The "doctrine of specific contagion" was not to be settled in her "offhand manner." Given that the doctrine in which she was brought up was "extreme and irrational and devoid of evidence," we must "equally withhold assent from her curiously vague statements." He disparaged her "simple assertion" about seeing and smelling smallpox: "We must surely admit of some doubt and difficulty in settling the question of the origin of morbid poison, without being thereby committed to the preposterous doctrine that they grow up indiscriminately out of mere dirt and overcrowding. Her experience of fevers is entirely opposed to mine ... The *degree* of overcrowding has nothing to do with the type of fever produced, nor do these diseases 'begin, grow up and pass into one another' in the manner stated." Because her labours were "so valuable, I feel it necessary thus to refer to them as the expression of a too confident and indeed wholly untenable medical theory."[127]

It is not evident that Nightingale ever saw that criticism. Certainly she had not changed her views on contagion for her revised, book-length *Notes on Hospitals* (1863). It was promptly attacked by several doctors, for similar, good reasons, beginning with an anonymous review in the *Medical Times and Gazette*. This was followed by editorial comment and letters to the editor. An editorial on comparative hospital mortality in the *Lancet* included critical comments on *Notes on Hospitals*. Both journals also gave the book much praise.

Most provocative was her intrepid statement on "contagion and infec-tion," in chapter 1 of *Notes on Hospitals*: "In certain hospitals it has been the custom to set apart wards for what are called 'infectious' diseases, but in reality there ought to be no diseases so considered. With proper sanitary precautions, diseases reputed to be the most 'infectious' may be treated in wards among other sick without danger." Much of Nightingale's objection to the word "contagion" was etymological: the word's root makes it "with the fingers." "Infection" had no such defect, she said, and represented "fact," not superstition or hypothesis. Her real objection was to the use of contagion as implying inevitability, and hence an excuse for inaction.

The anonymous, rather sexist reviewer for the *Medical Times and Gazette* noted Nightingale's "wholesale denunciation of 'contagion and infection.'" She would deserve "rough treatment" for her comments, he suggested, if she had not been a lady. He praised her sections on convalescent and children's hospitals and Indian army hospitals. Like other doctors who wrote in, he criticized also her treatment of mortality statistics and hospital comparisons. Nightingale was "incorrect, illogical, and impulsive."[128] Following Farr, Nightingale had given mortality rates of deaths per bed for a year. Using this indicator, rates as high as 90 could appear, which meant not that 90 per cent of patients died, but that 90 patients over the year died for each bed – not nearly so bad – and a meaningful number. The same *e* review commended the book, as "of great service to our profession." It also agreed with her campaign for a different site for the new St Thomas' Hospital.

Dr Farr wrote Nightingale promptly on the appearance of the first review to say that he would insert something of his own: he agreed neither with the reviewer nor with her on all points, but valued discussion.[129] In his rebuttal, he stated that he would not defend Nightingale, as she could take on any comers, but then did, at length. He cited a number of alternative ways of presenting mortality data, and noted how challenging it was to compare hospitals that experienced radically different patient stays. Farr concluded unambiguously: "She probes all the ways which make hospitals ways of death to their inmates. She collects plans; she consults engineers; and she brings the whole of the facts together in a clear, practical form, and holds out hopes that general hospitals may yet benefit mankind directly, and not merely as pathological observatories and medical schools." Her new edition, in his opinion, was "the most judicious, complete and masterly treatise that has recently appeared on any subject."[130] He sent in a shorter letter with further points two weeks later.[131]

The editor followed up Farr's comment with further, ruder objections. He repeated the points condemning Nightingale's view of "contagion" and "infection," especially "the notion of setting apart wards for diseases

INTRODUCTION 45

so reputed," that infectious patients "may be safely treated in wards with the other sick, 'with proper sanitary precautions.'" Her statements about contagion would lead to "hazardous practice and they are marred by rhetorical artifice," which the editor was sorry to see Farr approve. He turned the problem of Nightingale's hyperbole back to Farr, highly commending the book:

> Now we leave it to Dr. Farr to decide how far Miss Nightingale's views are consistent with his own of the existence of specific zymotic poisons, and whether he will take the responsibility of advising hospital committees to follow her dictum, and not to isolate "infectious" cases ... We object to Miss Nightingale's doctrines about contagion, as ignoring one truth to exalt another ... If our reviewer attacked Miss Nightingale, he would sign his name, but what he attacks are the fallacies which disfigure a valuable work – fallacies which may lead to the loss of many a life, if anyone shall be found rash enough to treat scarlet fever as not infectious, because Miss Nightingale has said that "no diseases ought to be considered infectious." ... All this fight has been about one or two incidental matters on which we conceive Miss Nightingale to be wrong, and to have been justly criticised. As regards the whole aim and scope of her labours, and the immense value of "Notes on Hospitals," there cannot be two opinions. She is too plain spoken herself to object to fair criticism of its few *maculae*.[132]

Fever expert Charles Murchison, who was then at the London Fever Hospital, later at St Thomas' Hospital, wrote a nuanced critique. He unambiguously accepted the separation of fever patients from others in general hospitals. He acknowledged the defects in many hospitals in ventilation, but defended the admission of fever patients to general hospitals as necessary to give medical students adequate experience. Isolation within the hospital then was essential. "Valuable lives ought not to hang upon the absolute perfection of hospital nurses." He agreed that much could be done to prevent fevers from spreading, but the "amount of ventilation" needed "would be absolutely fatal to many of the patients in the wards of a general hospital – to patients, for example, suffering from bronchitis or acute renal anasarca."[133] Nightingale frequently purchased copies of Murchison's *Treatise on the Continued Fevers of Great Britain* for nurses.

John Syer Bristowe (1827–1895), another physician with objections, was then on the staff at St Thomas' Hospital. He was critical of Farr's support of Nightingale's accusations against hospitals, words that "insinuate a very grave charge against existing hospitals." This was, he said, a particularly serious matter for someone in Dr Farr's position (he was superintendent of statistics at the General Register Office).[134] The anonymous reviewer weighed in again, now complaining of Farr's "confused and violent letter," his "arithmetical flights of fancy," which constituted "a gross misuse of figures."[135]

A *Lancet* editorial discussed *Notes on Hospitals* at length, with great general approval, but pointed objection on contagion. The book was "the most instructive and complete treatise on hospital construction which has yet appeared." Its author was "more than justified in laying the greatest stress on internal and external sanitary conditions, satisfactorily explained."[136] However, on contagion, "Her doctrines are not stated in a manner which admits easily of discussion; we cannot accept them; and no effort is made to place them in a form which can convince." Even so "illustrious" a person as she could not expect to find "converts amongst our ranks" without explaining at greater length and with better arguments.

Miss Nightingale would distribute fever patients over well-ventilated wards. Dr Murchison has shown that practically contagion is disregarded by the physicians of London, who distribute fever patients through the wards as a less evil than that resulting from their concentration. They are bolder than Miss Nightingale.

Pregnant with a great truth – that health in hospital, as out, depends upon the strictest sanitary regulations, instinct with an earnest purpose, rich in the results of manifold experience, and warmed with the vital usefulness of incomparable practical energy, these notes by Miss Nightingale must henceforth be studied by everyone who would build, modify or administer any hospital for the sick.[137]

Much of the considerable discussion in the *Lancet* was between Farr and Dr Timothy Holmes at St George's Hospital, Hyde Park Corner, most of it not involving Nightingale. In one letter to the editor, Holmes made it clear that he had not written the review of *Notes on Hospitals*, which, he said, Farr had insinuated he did.[138] Farr, again, said that Nightingale needed no defence on her use of mortality statistics, a method of his that she had adopted on "careful examination," and which her critic had not understood.[139]

On contagion, one can only suppose that Farr took the hint of the editor of the *Medical Times and Gazette* and pursued with Nightingale her opposition to it, for she never repeated that "dictum" again. For years thereafter, indeed, she approved of hospital designs that provided for small wards separate from regular wards for such cases. "Isolation" and "separation" wards would appear frequently in her correspondence and publications on hospitals.

Nightingale's hyperbolic rant on not isolating infectious patients did not prevent the book from wide use. It seems no hospital acted on her position, and virtually everything else in the book was sound, some of it still today. Royal engineer Douglas Galton, himself an eminent hospital architect, cited it.[140] Nursing historians said that it had "probably done more than any other treatise to promote sound views of hospital economy."[141] *Notes on Hospitals* was used for advice in the building of hospitals during the American Civil War, as we see in chapter 4.

Nightingale's material was much quoted in medical works, for example in a chapter on hospital construction and arrangement in Timothy Holmes's edited collection, *A System of Surgery*. Its author, J. Ranald Martin, a former member of the Royal Commission on the Crimean War, said that *Notes on Hospitals* afforded "at once the largest and most matured experience, with the best descriptions that I am acquainted with."[142] Also in that chapter, he used material from Nightingale's *Notes on Nursing* on her environmental approach and much on nutrition. Nightingale never had *Notes on Hospitals* reprinted, although it was soon out of print, and she continued to work on hospital design for the rest of her working life.

PART ONE

Close Working Relationships
(1850s–1880)

TRIAL BY FIRE

The Crimean War (1854–1856)

Background to the War

In March 1854, the British government joined France in declaring war on Russia in support of Turkey. Russia, then expanding "south of the Danube," constituted a threat to British interests. Troops began to go to "the East" in April 1854, first to Turkey, then to the Bulgarian coast, near Varna, where unsanitary conditions resulted in large numbers of deaths.

The Russians in fact retreated back north of the Danube, whereupon the taking of Sebastopol became the object of the war. In September 1854 the British Army, with the French and Turkish, landed unopposed in the Crimea. The first battle took place at the Alma on 20 September. The allies won, and began to move towards Sebastopol. The second, at Balaclava, 26 October 1854, would become famous for the misunderstood orders leading to the suicidal "Charge of the Light Brigade." Finally, Inkermann, on 5 November 1854, moved the Allies close to Sebastopol, short of taking it. They settled in for what became a ten-month siege "before Sebastopol," as dispatches would call it. Having expected to be in and out of "the East" fast, they were entirely unequipped for a Crimean winter.

The British Army initially rejected the idea of taking women nurses to the war, but had to reconsider when frequent, detailed newspaper reports flagged the inadequate care and appalling conditions in the hospitals. The Crimean War was the first with war correspondents; news reached London in roughly ten days (there was no direct telegraph). That the French Army had Sisters of Charity as nurses was well known. The French, the main instigators of the war, were also better prepared and equipped for it.

The British Army was poorly prepared – it had not fought a powerful enemy since the defeat of Napoleon in 1815. The commander-in-chief,

Lord Raglan, famously lost his arm in that war – the raglan sleeve is named after him. The available medical equipment was inadequate. The supply system was grossly defective, with different departments responsible for procurement, delivery, reception, and use of medicines, bedding, clothing, food, everything. The British Army had no field hospitals, but was given Turkish barracks, 300 miles (480 kilometres) across the Black Sea from the Crimea, to serve as makeshift hospitals. They lacked running water, laundries, and kitchens. The sewers and drains were plugged. Beds were non-existent at the start.

The director-general of the Army Medical Department, Dr (later Sir) Andrew Smith (1797–1872), was closely involved in the decision to send women nurses to the war in autumn 1854. He did not see any need for them, but did not oppose the project, explaining that, while it would be impossible to take women into the field with the army, with a fixed hospital at Scutari, "no military reason exists against their introduction." When Lady Maria Forester called on him to propose sending women nurses, and offered funds for the purpose, he sent her to see Nightingale.[1]

Smith saw Nightingale's role as limited to ensuring that the nurses "did their duty" and did not interfere with medical arrangements. She, of course, did much more, notably to make up for deficiencies in organization, to make sure needed supplies reached the right hospital fast. Asked if women nurses would be an advantage to the public service, Smith answered that they would be, "if good nurses could be obtained," adding: "I was perfectly aware that females can see many things in which there might be a deficiency of cleanliness and comfort that men do not see."[2] Clearly he was out of touch with actual conditions in the hospitals, where bedding and clothing were lacking, the men lay on floors with vermin-infested clothing, and there was no laundry. He did not order soap for soldiers' use until the second year of the war.

Prior to leaving for the war in October 1854, Nightingale had "two or three" interviews with him at his office, taken there by Sidney Herbert, the secretary at war, or junior war minister, who spoke on war matters in the House of Commons (and left office before year's end), or by the Duke of Newcastle, the secretary of state for war, or senior war minister, who dealt with the House of Lords, or possibly by both officials. After the war, she recalled that Smith "never looked upon me with favour … but … as a caprice of these two men which he was obliged to submit to." He was "a very honest man, without vanity, conscientious and abhorring popularity, without benevolence, sincerely believing old ways the best, and that there is no great improvement to be made in this world ... the most impracticable of human instruments."[3]

The Duke of Newcastle was much more amenable to sending out women nurses. He was asked at the 1855 hearings of the Select Committee on the Army before Sebastopol (Roebuck Commission) about how the decision was reached:

> The question of the employment of nurses in the hospital had been mooted at a very early stage (before in fact, the army left this country) and the general opinion of military men was adverse to their employment. It had been tried upon former occasions and I believe the class of women that had been tried had been ordinary hospital nurses, and they had been found to be very much addicted to drink, and often much more callous to the sufferings of the soldiers than those male attendants who had been employed more recently. Under these circumstances, they were very averse to it ...
>
> The difficulty was to find any lady who was competent to undertake so great a task as the organisation of such a body, and I confess I despaired, having seen one or two, of making the attempt, until Mr Sidney Herbert, then secretary at war, being personally acquainted with Miss Nightingale, with whom I had also the honour of being acquainted, suggested that it might be possible to induce her to undertake so great a task, though we felt great delicacy in proposing it. We found, however, at once, that she was willing, and we felt that anything which she undertook would be successful.[4]

Dr Smith's two-volume report after the war refers only briefly to the work of the "lady nurses" and states that the men were grateful for their "kind treatment," neglecting to acknowledge the much greater scope of their work and Nightingale's obtaining supplies and establishing laundries and kitchens.[5]

Dr Smith would be fully exonerated in the investigations after the war of responsibility for the gross defects in the hospitals. His defence was that he had ordered adequate supplies, and could not be held responsible for the failure of other departments to deliver them without undue delay to the right hospital. He was correct. Nightingale herself always pointed to organizational defects, rather than personal failure, as responsible. She, Herbert, and other reformers worked assiduously after the war to change the system.

Smith retired in 1858, when Nightingale and the royal commission were finishing their reports and she and Herbert were keen to move on to implementation. It was crucial to find a good replacement, a doctor who had been efficient and was ready to challenge the system, which Dr Thomas Alexander did, as we see in chapter 4.

Conditions at Scutari

Nightingale and her nurses arrived at the Barrack Hospital, Scutari (now Uskudar), in the Asiatic side of Constantinople (now Istanbul), on 5 November 1854 – it would be her base of operations through the war. No provision had been made for them, and the hospital, a converted Turkish barracks, was already crowded from the first two battles of the war – Alma (20 September) and Balaclava (26 October). More wounded were due to arrive from Inkermann (5 November). As well, many soldiers were there for diseases caught in the staging ground near Varna, Bulgaria, before invading the Crimea.

Nightingale and her team were the first British women to nurse in war. That the British Army had previously employed women as "nurses" did not help, for they did not give patient care, but were, in effect, hospital cleaners, recruited from the wives or widows of private soldiers and non-commissioned officers, paid less than laundresses and cooks, and given the status of a private soldier. They reported to a sergeant, not a doctor.[6] For Nightingale, the nurse had to know how to clean in order to ensure that it was properly done. However, as she put it succinctly in *Notes on Hospitals*: "A nurse must not be a scrubber. And a scrubber cannot be a nurse."[7] She would direct much of her time and energy to ensuring high standards of cleanliness.

The principal medical officer, Dr Duncan Menzies (1803–1875), was not only hostile to Nightingale and women nurses, but not up to the task of organization and was soon found to be corrupt. He was censured and sent home. Nightingale found out about the corruption from the American missionary in Constantinople, whose bakery, which he had set up to employ his poor Christian parishioners, supplied bread to the hospitals. He told her that Menzies, with the second purveyor, had demanded a portion of the contract's proceeds. He refused. Their bread was spoiled (e.g., made sour and bedbugs inserted), and in due course they lost the large contract at the Scutari Barrack Hospital.[8] Nightingale found this out later at the hospital at Koulali, which had good bread, because its contract was still in force. She then had the Scutari contract reinstated at a decent price for the bakery.

Menzies was complacent, a major failing in Nightingale's eyes. She quoted a report of his, "General Remarks on the Prevailing Diseases":

> I have to report favourably of the buildings now denominated the general and supplementary hospitals, the former having been built for the purpose ... but the latter as a barrack for troops ... These buildings may be pronounced convenient for the reception of the sick and wounded, being roomy, well ventilated and supplied with excellent water, out offices and other necessary conveniences. There are, however, no doubt various improvements required, such as the construction of an additional kitchen for the General Hospital and a wash house and dead house at the barracks.

Menzies noted the need for rooms for nurses "who have recently been sent out by the government."[9]

A memoir "from the ranks" captures conditions at the hospital and transport to it just before the nurses arrived. Memoirs and correspondence by officers are plentiful, so the perspective of Sergeant-Major Timothy Gowing (1834–1908), Royal Fusiliers, wounded at Inkermann, is a welcome addition from a non-officer:

> As soon as it came to my turn I was attended to and my wounds dressed and bandaged. I remained for two days and then a number of us were sent to Scutari. We were taken down to Balaclava on mules, some of them lent by our chivalrous allies the French.
>
>   We got a good shaking, but eventually found ourselves on board an old steamer. It was a horrible scene – poor fellows having every description of wound, and many died before we left the harbour. We were packed on board anyhow – to live or die – and away we went. The sea was rather boisterous and I was not very comfortable with poor fellows dying fast all around me. There were not sufficient medical officers to look after fifty men, much less three or four hundred.[10]

The sergeant-major continued with the "heart-rending" sight of men who "had not the slightest thing done for them since they were wounded on that bloody field ... left to die in agony, their poor mangled bodies infested with vermin." He could give more details, but "enough has been said to afford a sufficient condemnation of British management."

When he recovered and returned to duty, the army was put on half rations of "half a pound of mouldy biscuit and half a pound of salt junk (beef or pork)," with coffee, in its raw, green state, with no means of roasting it: "No wood or firing was to be had ... Men would come staggering into the camp from the trenches soaked to the skin and ravenously hungry, when a half-pound of mouldy biscuit would be issued ... The whole camp was one vast sea of mud, the trenches in many places knee deep; men died at their posts from sheer exhaustion or starvation rather than complain, for it they reported themselves sick, the medical chests were empty."[11]

Dr Menzies's hostility to the nurses was the exception for his profession. Doctors would find out that Nightingale could provide supplies that the commissariat had failed to deliver, or which were stored unopened miles away. The nurses' services would be in increasing demand as doctors in other hospitals heard what they had achieved at Scutari. Nightingale, for her part, greatly respected the doctors for their dedication and hard work. She would defend them and look out for their interests, and, for some, later press for pensions for their widows.

Dr Menzies's replacement was Alexander McGrigor (1810–1855), who was pleased to have the nurses and worked effectively with Nightingale. She evidently secured a promotion for him through Sidney Herbert, whereupon she sent him a note of congratulations, warning him not to mention any connection with her, as it would cause "jealousy and dissatisfaction."[12] She commended him in a letter to Lord Raglan, the commander-in-chief, reporting on the visit the general, Sir George Brown, had made. Dr McGrigor took him around. She noted her "sense of the obligation which this hospital is under to him, as being virtually its founder, and still supporting it with unabated zeal, vigour, and assiduity." McGrigor died of cholera in 1855.

Nightingale remarked on the stoicism of the men on the trip to the hospital from the Crimea, who complained only of the lack of orderlies and utensils (bedpans), "by which a great amount of stench result." These last arrivals, 750, came down "in a wretched state of sickness." Then on to what was wrong:

Having been informed that there is a quantity of warm clothing in Balaclava Harbour, I nevertheless grieve to find that these men (all landed since the 19th) *are more ragged and even destitute of clothing than* any of the preceding. The number of frostbitten cases might, it appears to me, have been diminished by an examination of the state of the men on their return from the trenches. The majority of cases are those arrived from dysentery and exhaustion, sometimes both. These have suffered by the length of the time on board, ten days. The usual arrangements for landing the sick have certainly not been so prompt as they might have been. The authorities do not seem to perceive the importance of this for the saving of life.[13]

Times articles often noted Nightingale's personal care of soldiers. Two doctors who died at Scutari, for example, had been "tended in their last moments and had their dying eyes closed by Miss Nightingale herself." That story may have been the first to describe her as a "ministering angel": "Wherever there is disease in its most dangerous form and the hand of the spoiler distressingly nigh, there is that incomparable woman sure to be seen; her benignant presence is an influence for good comfort even amid the struggles of expiring nature. She is a 'ministering angel' without any exaggeration." This report also uses the "lady with the lamp" imagery. As she glided through the corridors, "every poor fellow's face softens with gratitude at the sight of her. When all the medical officers have retired for the night, and silence and darkness have settled down upon these miles of prostrate sick, she may be observed alone, with a little lamp in her hand, making her solitary rounds."[14]

Chef Alexis Soyer also saw the "lady with the lamp" in action one night, at about 2 a.m., now with a private soldier, a recovered patient, holding the lamp for her. The doctors had given up on the "poor fellow," Soyer noted, so she was writing a last letter for him, to send on to his relatives.[15]

While the coverage of Nightingale and her nurses was overwhelmingly positive, even hagiographic, there were exceptions. A captain of the King's Own Regiment of Foot wrote to his sister:

We have here now arrived from England a quantity of nurses and nuns to wait on the wounded and ill. They are useful, especially the latter, but they are such an enormous expense to the country, and they are hardly worth the money, for most soldiers prefer their comrades who make attentive nurses. The nurses and nuns are under the superintendence of a Miss Nightingale, a *young* lady (about thirty three) with a large fortune, she appears a very manly personage and talks quite in the strong-minded style. There is also a Mrs Bracebridge, a lady of very good family and rich; her husband is here and they do a great deal of good among the patients.[16]

All the while, nurses, Nightingale herself included, could do nothing in the hospitals without medical orders. She was attending a dying patient on a cold night in January 1856, one account states, to find that his feet were "stone cold." She asked an orderly to fetch a hot water bottle, but he declined, as there were no directions from a doctor: "Miss Nightingale stood corrected, and trudged off to find a doctor and make requisition for the bottle in due form."[17]

Nightingale was oddly protective of doctors during the worst times at the hospital. Before the cleanup of toilets and drains, tubs were kept in the wards, as many men could not walk to the toilets. Nightingale went in early in the morning to supervise their removal – two orderlies to a tub, with a pole between them: "Is it fair to ask medical officers to see to these details of drudgery?" she asked rhetorically.[18] The Sanitary Commission duly got the toilets working, and the tubs were permanently removed.

How bad the toilets were she could only describe indirectly – the stench went far, but she of course did not enter the men's toilets. Her source was the testimony of Augustus Stafford to a commission. He, a Conservative MP, happened to be in Turkey when the Crimean War began, and undertook to visit patients at the Barrack Hospital and write letters for them. He explained how it was that there was no running water in the toilets:

When the army was at the barracks in the summer, these taps were by the soldiers broken off, and in consequence the supply of water was stopped. When the barrack was reopened as a hospital, no sufficient pains were taken to repair those pipes, or secure a flow of water, and the pipes soon choked up and the liquid feces, the evacuations from those afflicted with diarrhea, filled up the pipes, floated up over the floor and came into the room in which the necessaries were, extended and flowed into the anteroom, and were more than an inch deep when I got there in the morning; men suffering from diarrhea, who had no slippers at the time and no shoes on as this flood of filth advanced, came less and less near to the necessary, and nearer and nearer to the door till at last I found them within a yard of the anteroom performing the necessary functions of nature, and in consequence the smell from this place was such that I can use no epithet to describe its horror.[19]

Conflict with Dr John Hall, Principal Medical Officer

Inspector General of Hospitals Dr John Hall (1795–1866) was sent from India to the Crimea to head up the medical services for the British Army as principal medical officer (PMO). As an experienced medical officer, his early duties included inspection of the Barrack Hospital at Scutari and the Military Hospital at Koulali, which he approved for hospital use, with some modifications. He seems to have missed the gross defects of the Barrack Hospital, and failed to act on officers' reports on defects when they revealed them, points Nightingale would cite in detail in her later analysis of what went wrong.

Hall's differences with Nightingale have been commented on ever since the war. He possibly resented her personal friendship with the junior war minister at the war's start, Sidney Herbert, and the high esteem held for her by his senior counterpart, the Duke of Newcastle. Hall called her a "petticoat impérieuse" when complaining of her to his superior, Dr Smith.[20] When Hall was made a KCB (knight commander of the Order of the Bath), she renamed the title "Knight of the Crimean Burial-grounds"; he also won the French Legion of Honour and the Turkish Medjidie medal. The two differed as well on the use of chloroform: he opposed it[21]; she, with many junior medical officers, approved it, and brought supplies with her.

Nursing academics have reproved Nightingale for not being deferential to Dr Hall in her writing. However, this is to miss entirely how much out of step he was with medical opinion. His opposition to chloroform was not unfounded, for anaesthetics were new, doses were uncertain, and an overdose could kill the patient. He cautioned his medical officers against using it, stating that few would survive if they did, for "the knife is a powerful stimulant, and it is much better to hear a man bawl lustily than to see him sink silently into the grave."[22] Eminent Edinburgh surgeon

James Syme wrote to the *Times* contesting this opinion, from "long and ample experience ... that pain, instead of being 'a powerful stimulant,' most injuriously exhausts the nervous energy on a weak patient, and that, therefore, chloroform should be used, the more necessary the degree of weakness."[23] Another Edinburgh surgeon, James Y. Simpson, sent many surgeons to the war who were experienced with chloroform. He provided the supply Nightingale took with her.[24]

The soldiers had long stays on the wharf awaiting transport, and the Black Sea crossing could take a week, described above by a sergeant-major. Official reports documented the lack of medical attendance, orderlies, food, and toilet facilities. Lord Raglan, the commander-in-chief, censured one doctor in a general order, while also noting that Dr Hall could not be exonerated; either he or his subordinates should have ensured that everything necessary was on board for the sick and wounded.[25]

Hall dealt directly with other nurses, notably Mary Francis Bridgeman, the superior of the Irish Sisters of Mercy. She had signed a contract that she and her nuns would serve under Nightingale, then reneged on it. A more serious complaint about Hall was his complacency about the bad conditions in the hospitals and the high death rates. Hall, as PMO, reported favourably to Lord Raglan on a rate of hospital admissions to army strength of 3.93 per cent, with a death rate of 0.38 per cent. Nightingale protested that the rate was only for a week, when normally rates were given per year. When annualized, the rates that so pleased Hall turn out to be more than double the size of the army.[26]

Nightingale argued that it was impossible for the most experienced person to judge matters because of the way Hall put them: "0.52, 3.93 percent look nothing. But multiply 3.9 by 52 = 2028, in order to get the annual admissions per 1000, and it will be found that the whole force will go twice through hospital in a year at that rate." William Farr told Nightingale that Hall's calculation was "singularly calculated to mislead."[27] Sidney Herbert, in his evidence to the royal commission, explained how Hall had misled Raglan and ministers back in London with his reports:

> Lord Raglan sent Dr Hall to inspect the hospitals, and Dr Hall
> went back giving a very flourishing account of the state of them,
> and that report was sent home to us, that "Lord Raglan had reason
> to believe that all was going on well," that "all the information
> which he (Lord Raglan) had was perfectly satisfactory to him, which

was the information given by the inspector general of hospitals, in whose statement he of course placed confidence," that Dr Hall's statement was founded upon what he had himself seen. "But I apprehend," adds Mr Herbert, "that people have looked upon the state of things at Scutari with very different eyes. I have received throughout extremely contradictory evidence from Scutari. Officers who were there, even quite at the beginning, wrote and said that they had never seen an army hospital more effective."[28]

When the Sanitary Commission reported in 1855,[29] with its devastating critique of the conditions Hall had considered adequate, Hall replied that everything had either been done, or was in progress, so that the "benefit of their labours was more assumed than real." As well, the effort was not worth the expense.[30]

John Hall still has his defenders, authors who consider that it was his measures, and those of the regular working of the Army Medical Department, that improved the hospitals – in effect, that the sanitary and supply commissions were not needed. Hall was the victim of "stigmatizing," while Nightingale failed to understand statistics, and was arrogant in her (ironic) explanation that the army would go through the hospitals at least twice in the year.[31] It seems more likely that her "twice" point, quoted above, was simply to stress how much Hall had misled his superiors by citing rates based on a week, contrary to the normal use of a year.

To Sir John McNeill, Nightingale described Hall as clever, almost as clever as General Airey, but guilty of "incredible apathy, beginning with the fatal letter approving of Scutari, October, 1854, continuing with all the negative errors of non-obtaining of lime juice, fresh bread, quinine, etc., up to his *not* denouncing the effects of salt meat." Except for the assistant quartermaster-general, he was "(morally) the worst of the liars."[32]

The First Investigation: The Cumming–Maxwell Commission

There would be many investigations of the Crimean War hospitals and medical services, conducted both during and after the war, in the east and back in London. The members of the first, the Cumming–Maxwell commission, went out on the same ship as Nightingale and her nurses in October 1854: Drs Alexander Cumming (c. 1790–1858) and

Thomas Spence, with a barrister third member, Peter Benson Maxwell. Dr Cumming was also appointed to the Barrack Hospital at Scutari, and Nightingale had to comply with his orders. This commission was sent by the War Office, to make inquiries on hospital conditions, but it had no power to make changes.

A letter of complaint in the *Times* by an Anglican nun / nurse, Elizabeth Wheeler, led to both her and Nightingale being called before the commission at Scutari to be questioned. Wheeler, appointed to the hospital there, had written to a friend in London with not only revelations of poor hospital conditions, but claims of poor care by doctors, whom she, a nurse, a mere week after arrival, presumed to judge. The friend forwarded the letter to the *Times*, which published it with a London address to which parcels of food and wine could be sent.

Wheeler's letter stated that men died from exhaustion, perhaps preventable with "such nourishment as I know they ought to have had." Readers were asked to send wine, chicken broth, preserved meat for soup, chocolate, gelatine, brandy, flannel, and warm clothing. Wine, she added, "would be of immense service to some of the nurses just before going into the wards." Since nurses were given free wine or a strong beer at lunch and dinner, this presumably was a plea for wine at breakfast. The nurses' food, Wheeler went on, lacked even a drop of milk, while the bread was "extremely sour," the bad bread, we know, from the corrupt baker who obtained the contract by bribery. The butter was "most filthy," decomposed, and the meat "more like moist leather than food."[33]

Wheeler was summoned to give evidence to the Cumming–Maxwell commission on 22 December 1854. Nightingale was called the following day, when she largely contradicted her nurse's statement. She did not share Wheeler's view that men had died from lack of "restoratives," but blamed poor distribution of them, so that some men took their ration all at once, even four gills (a pint) at a draught.[34] She reported that she inspected the wards under Wheeler every day. A double allowance of wine had been issued, but the orderlies drank the extra. Further, she had seen orderlies drink the port wine ordered for the patients, a point Wheeler had emphasized. The supply, however, Nightingale thought was adequate.

She also countered Wheeler's testimony as to the number of deaths: the nurses reported to her every day the number in their wards. Wheeler had had bad cases, but not "hopeless," and only one surgical case, when Nightingale herself dressed the wound.

Sarah Ann Terrot, another Anglican nun, kept a journal that records a more sympathetic account of Wheeler than Nightingale's. Terrot blamed the commission as unjust in its questioning (Nightingale said nothing either way on this). The editor of the journal, however, noted that Wheeler's letter in the *Times* was wrong and that she had exaggerated the number of deaths.[35]

While there is no surviving correspondence on Wheeler's dismissal, it seems most likely that Cumming insisted on it. No letters remain between Nightingale and Wheeler's superior in England, Lydia Priscilla Sellon, abbess of the Society of the Most Holy Trinity, Osnaburgh Street, Regent's Park, London, whom Nightingale knew, but it seems that it was arranged that Wheeler would leave voluntarily, to avoid dismissal. (The order's archives, at Pusey House, Oxford, include other correspondence and journal notes by and to the sisters and superior.) Nightingale spared Wheeler the disgrace of dismissal. In her report, she listed the departure under "Cause of Retirement … private reason."[36]

Cumming was also the doctor who told Nightingale that she could not accept the full second contingent of nurses, sent out without her or their knowledge or agreement, which arrived in December 1854. She must select from among them so as to keep the total number of nurses at the Barrack Hospital no higher than fifty.[37]

Doctors in the Crimean Hospitals: Drs Alexander and Longmore

In May 1855, when Nightingale finally travelled to Balaclava in the Crimea itself – Scutari was 300 miles (480 kilometres) distant, in Turkey – she was well known and well received. An army doctor who saw her reported that she went over the various hospital establishments, "where, of course, all the attention and respect she so well merits were paid to her."[38] A surgeon of the Light Infantry reported seeing her soon after her arrival, escorted by Lord Raglan, General Pélissier (the French commander-in-chief), and British and French staff officers. She visited the hospital, to see the poor conditions there. "But her visit was productive of much good. Through her report and her influence, the arrangements were improved and went on improving until the time came when, long before the war was over, we had almost a superabundance of medical comforts and even luxuries sent to the hospital."[39]

Two regimental surgeons posted in the Crimea stand out for their ability and bravery in speaking out on the poor conditions: Thomas Alexander, CB (1812–1860), and Thomas (later Sir Thomas) Longmore (1816–1895). Nightingale knew neither of them at the time, but sought both of them out after the war when seeking allies to bring in reforms.

Alexander, as surgeon to the Light Division in Bulgaria, saw enormous loss of life from disease. When the Cumming–Maxwell commission began its investigation, he promptly sent it a detailed, critical report, with numerous recommendations for improvement.[40] Inspector General of Hospitals Dr John Hall asked to borrow Nightingale's copy of that report and kept it for a year. When he returned it, as she told Sidney Herbert, she discovered that he had cut out almost all of Alexander's evidence.[41]

When Nightingale began to address the problems after the war, Alexander stood out as "one of the two deputy inspectors of whom I have formed the best opinion."[42] Dr Sutherland advised Nightingale, "Get Alexander. Nobody else if you cannot. He is our man."[43] She called him "pretty nearly the honestest man I know, and the only honest man in the department."[44] Sir John McNeill, co-head of the extremely effective Supply Commission, considered him independent, meaning not subservient, and "the most efficient man in the service." Sidney Herbert made his own chairing of the royal commission contingent on Alexander's being appointed to it. He was.

Nightingale had three other reform-minded physicians placed on the royal commission – Drs Sutherland, Sir James Clark, and J. Ranald Martin – and, as secretary, T. Graham Balfour, a doctor and statistician. They helped to offset the presence of Dr Andrew Smith, director-general of the Army Medical Department. Other sympathetic members were General Storks, a friend of Nightingale's from Crimea days, Augustus Stafford, MP, whom she knew from his visiting at the Scutari Barrack Hospital, and the legal member, Sir Thomas Phillips.

Soon after Alexander returned to London, early in 1857, he called on Nightingale, and the two met at length several times. She was pleased with him, as she told Sidney Herbert: "He is full of moral energy and directness of purpose. He knows what he wants and will go straight at it, without any disguise."[45] Meeting him again after he had conferred with Herbert, she "set him to work to 'index' his subjects" for the royal commission.[46] About the same time, she told the commission's secretary, Dr Balfour, that Alexander was "burning for the fight. And I hope we shall do well."[47]

Preparing for the questioning of Sir John Hall, Nightingale wanted Alexander to raise the choice of ground for the camp of the Light Division in Bulgaria, where it spent some months in the worst part of an area known to be pestilential. She suggested that he ask: "By whom was the ground chosen for the camp of the Light Division at Devna?"[48]

Nightingale facilitated meetings between key doctors and Sidney Herbert. She, for example, arranged for Sir John McNeill to "indoctrinate" him, as she told him, either at the Herberts' home or at hers.[49] This was the last year that she was able to travel and attend meetings, and her health broke down again before the Crimean work was finished.

Thomas Longmore was surgeon to the 19th Regiment. He too gave trenchant evidence to the Cumming–Maxwell commission. The regimental "hospitals" were mere bell tents, "not fit for treatment of the sick as only one single canvas." Asked about the medicines and medical comforts available, he replied: "I have not been able to obtain for the hospital either the nature or quantity of medicines I have required and I have considered it my duty to make several reports on the subject to the proper authorities."[50] Longmore also had the merit of seeing the value of British–French comparisons on disease and deaths during the Crimean War, later publishing a short book on the subject.[51]

When it came time after Crimea to staff the new Army Medical School, Nightingale wanted Longmore, the "only" person fit to be professor, she told Lord de Grey, then the war secretary.[52] He was indeed named professor of military surgery, a matter pursued in chapter 4.

The defects of the Barrack Hospital, Scutari, would be routinely noted in dispatches from war correspondents, officers' letters, and later reports and memoirs. A French doctor, Michel Lévy, was as critical of the Barrack Hospital as Dr Sutherland: "The most detestable of hospitals is any old Turkish building, but above all a Turkish barrack appropriated to this purpose. Almost always of a quadrilateral form, it has at each angle latrines *a la Turque* which spread their horrible stench to a great distance and envelope the whole edifice in their emanations … sick on every floor breathe the same air … You will understand how the hospital infection had made its preparations in the greater part of our closed establishments."[53]

The Sanitary Commission: Dr John Sutherland

It was the work of the Sanitary Commission sent out in March 1855, as it would later be generally agreed, that did the most to bring down the death rates during the Crimean War, by cleaning up the hospitals and camps. Nightingale's long working relationship with its head, Dr John Sutherland, was so important that he has already been introduced. The second member, Robert (later Sir Robert) Rawlinson (1810–1898), civil engineer, also became a valued colleague, Nightingale's water expert.[54] However, it was another physician, Hector Gavin, who helped arrange for the Sanitary Commission to go out in the first place.[55] He was an expert on public health, secretary of Britain's General Board of Health (set up 1848). He was known to Lord Shaftesbury, who conveniently was a relative by marriage of Lord Palmerston, the prime minister. Both Palmerston and Shaftesbury understood the causal chain from polluted water and air to disease. Shaftesbury made the case to Lord Panmure, the secretary for war, for sending out civilian sanitary experts.[56] Gavin was duly appointed with the other two members. Soon after his arrival, however, he was accidentally shot by his brother, an officer. He was replaced by Dr Gavin Milroy, but the main players on the commission were Dr Sutherland, who stayed on the longest, and Rawlinson.

Dr Sutherland delivered an extraordinary letter to Lord Raglan, commander-in-chief, from the prime minister, Lord Palmerston, who was also a neighbour of the Nightingales in Hampshire. It shows not only Palmerston's understanding of "sanitary science," but also his full awareness of the resistance that the commissioners – none of them military men – would encounter from the army hierarchy:

> This will be given to you by Dr. Sutherland, chief of the Sanitary
> Commission ... whom we have sent out to put the hospitals, the
> port and the camp into a less unhealthy condition than has hitherto
> existed, and I request that you will give them every assistance
> and support in your power. They will, of course, be opposed and
> thwarted by the medical officers, by the men who have charge of
> the port arrangements and by those who have the cleaning of the
> camp. Their mission will be ridiculed and their recommendations
> and directions set aside, unless enforced by the peremptory exercise
> of your authority.

But that authority I must request you to exert in the most peremptory manner for the immediate and exact carrying to execution whatever changes of arrangement they may recommend, for these are matters on which depend the health and lives of many hundreds of men, I may indeed say of thousands. It is scarcely to be expected that officers, whether military or medical, whose time is wholly occupied by the pressing business of each day, should be able to give their attention or their time to the matters to which these commissioners have for many years devoted their action and their thoughts.

But the interposition of men skilled in this way is urgently required. The hospital at Scutari is become a hotbed of pestilence, and if no proper precautions are taken before the sun's rays begin to be felt, your camp will become one vast seat of the most virulent plague. I hope this commission will arrive in time to prevent much evil, but I am very sure that not one hour should be lost after their arrival in carrying into effect the precautionary and remedial measures which they may recommend.[57]

John Sutherland had been the first inspector for a city board of health, in Liverpool, in 1848. He had already published on basic issues that troubled the Crimean War, such as cholera and burial practices, this latter research done for the pope. He took experienced "nuisance inspectors" from Liverpool with him to Scutari and hired local workmen to do the clean-up job. As well as staying on to supervise the work, he wrote the official report after the war and became a member of, and gave evidence to, the royal commission.

On his return from the war, Sutherland was invited to Balmoral Castle to meet the queen, but he was never given any honours. He was never made a fellow of the Royal Society or given an honorary doctorate, honours accorded men with achievements of much less consequence. A pavilion was named after him when the Herbert Hospital, Woolwich, was renovated to become the Royal Herbert Mansions.

The "Supply Commission": McNeill–Tulloch

Of the many commissions appointed to investigate the Crimean disaster, the one Nightingale most praised at the time was the Supply Commission, which was made up of Sir John McNeill (1795–1883), formerly a medical officer for the East India Company in Persia, and Alexander Tulloch (1803–1864), a reform-minded colonel and brilliant statistician, later a major-general. McNeill became a father figure to Nightingale, an older man who, unlike her own father, encouraged her mission. She frequently asked him for advice. He served as a trustee on the original Nightingale Fund. Nightingale became friendly with other members of his family as well, and godmother to a grandson. She stayed with the McNeills twice when in Edinburgh, the first time to consult him and Colonel Tulloch when on route to Balmoral.

While Nightingale's comments, initially, were more complimentary to the Supply than the Sanitary Commission, her charts on death rates mark the "commencement of sanitary improvements" as the point where the British death rates in the war began to fall. With the benefit of hindsight, it seems that the sanitary clean-up work (sewers, drains, cemeteries, hospital wards) was more crucial than improvements in supply (shelter, clothing, and nutrition).

The Supply Commission's two reports, 10 June 1855 and January 1856, set out in chapter and verse the defects in clothing, food, medical supplies, shelter, and transport under the commissariat system. The terms "deficiencies," "very large deficiencies," "most disastrous of the deficiencies," "evil," "failure," "injury to health," "pain," "serious defects," and "sufferings" all appear, some more than once, in the reports. The commissioners named no particular individuals, but their institutions. Perhaps most devastating to the army command, they allowed no excuses: the defects were avoidable mistakes. The Royal Navy prevented scurvy, why not the army? The French Army provided fresh bread and vegetables to its soldiers, why not the British? The report did not blame the doctors, but rather commended them for doing the best they could in the circumstances. The chief culprit was the commissariat, with its rules and regulations, and lassitude when gross defects appeared.

The commissioners described the full horrors of the mismanagement. In some regiments, for example, "hardly a man" was free of scurvy, or scorbutic disease. There was no fresh bread for more than a year, so that the sick complained much, and those with scurvy "from the state of their gums" could not eat the hard biscuit. The commissioners noted that what was needed was sometimes available, such as fresh and preserved vegetables, but not issued. Defective cooking was another source of sickness. The report was firm that the absence of needed medicines cost lives. The usual death rate from cholera, it said, was 1 in 3, but in the Crimea it was 2 in every 3 attacked.[58]

A letter from Nightingale to Sidney Herbert said that their own post mortems had confirmed that the men were suffering from a form of scurvy, "brought on by salt rations, want of vegetables, cold and wet, etc." It was not acute dysentery, but "*scorbutic* [scurvy] dysentery," with extensive ulceration, that was killing the men.[59]

The Supply Commission's description of the filth endured by soldiers in camp was piteous. Soldiers could not wash or change clothes, and thus became "covered with vermin." On account of bowel ailments – diarrhea and dysentery were common – their clothes were laden with excrement; shirts rotted from filth and had to be cut off their backs when they were admitted to hospital.[60] When the need for wooden huts for the winter was realized (the army was in tents), an order was put in, but the wrong sizes and types of wood were sent, so that the pieces could not be fitted together. The Crimean winter was cold, and the men spent it under flimsy tents, with only a blanket or greatcoat for warmth, and that often wet.

The commissioners also noted the cost of *not* providing adequately: "Every soldier has cost a large sum before he is landed in the Crimea fit for duty, and it costs a like sum to replace him. The value of the other considerations [moral and political] cannot be estimated in money, for they are above all price."[61] This human-resource approach was one Nightingale shared. It saves money in the long run, she would explain, to treat soldiers better.

The Supply Commission undoubtedly caused much offence by endorsing the findings of the Sanitary Commission on the causes of the high hospital death rates – bad sanitary conditions – and crediting it with bringing them down. Disease "carried off many men who had entered the hospital with a prospect of speedy recovery," it stated. If the hospitals had been as good as they later became, the result of the Sanitary Commission's clean-up, "there can be little doubt that the mortality would have been perceptibly reduced."[62]

The army command went after McNeill and Tulloch on the publication of their final report. A board of generals was appointed to review it, called the "Chelsea Board" as it met at the army hospital in Chelsea, and found most of its findings unjustified. The Chelsea Board acknowledged only one valid failing, the lack of pressed hay for horse feed – many horses died. McNeill and Tulloch were pilloried in Parliament.

The *Times* then led the attack on the Chelsea Board, just as it had led in exposing mismanagement during the war. McNeill kept his silence, but Tulloch published a rebuttal.[63] Meetings were held in various towns in support of the commissioners, and the tide in public opinion turned. Lord Panmure, who as secretary for war had never thanked the two for their report, offered them each £1,000. They declined it. Sidney Herbert came to their defence in the House of Commons, moving an address to the queen to honour them, which was done. McNeill, who already had a knighthood, was made a privy councillor (Rt Hon. and PC); Tulloch was knighted.

Nightingale had earlier been incensed enough by the treatment of these two men that she considered not taking part in the royal commission that was about to be appointed. As she wrote in January 1857 to Herbert, then about to become chair, if his commission came up with a "faithful" report, "it will draw upon it the enmity of the present government, upon whom several of the members of that commission and almost all those who will be called in evidence are dependent." The members of his royal commission then would either have to sacrifice "their truth and independence" or suffer "for such truth and independence," for her "an equally appalling" result. Or they could issue "an unfaithful report, which would, of course, do the cause we have at heart not good but harm."[64]

The Pathology Commission: Drs Lyons and Aitken

One of the many investigations conducted during the war was the Pathology Commission,[65] led by Drs Robert Dyer Lyons (1826–1886) and his assistant, William (later Sir William) Aitken (1825–1892). Nightingale's general interest in science evidently served her well here. She quoted frequently from the commission's report in her own confidential report, *Notes on Matters Affecting the Health, Efficiency and Hospital Administration of the British Army* (1858). She promoted the study of pathology at the Army Medical School in Chatham when it opened in 1860, with Dr Aitken in the chair.

Lyons was an Irish doctor, chief commissioner of pathology1855–56, but who went back to civilian practice and publication after the war. Nightingale asked him to read her paper "Hospital Statistics and Hospital Plans" to the congress of the National Association for the Promotion of Social Science held in Dublin in 1861, which he was pleased to do.[66]

Lyons sent Nightingale a copy of his book on fever, which was dedicated to Sidney Herbert and Sir James Clark.[67]

However, it remains all too evident that the Pathology Commission did not arrive at any useful results. Numerous post mortems on cholera victims, for example, led to no discovery as to what caused the disease, or indicated any better treatment for it. Cholera victims most often died of heart failure caused by the loss of electrolytes, the result of severe diarrhea but not discernible by autopsy. The cholera bacillus was demonstrated to be the cause of the disease by bacteriologist Robert Koch only in 1883,[68] while it would take until the mid-twentieth century, with the discovery of the sulpha drugs and antibiotics, for an effective remedy to become available.

The Highest Death Rates: Where and Whom to Blame?

Which British army hospital had the highest death rates of the Crimean War became an issue when Hugh Small's *Florence Nightingale: Avenging Angel* (1998) charged that it was Nightingale's, and that her negligence was to blame.[69] Although the author never provided a table or even cited data from the official report, he convinced a number of academic historians.[70] Instead, he relied on rough estimates and then made apples-and-oranges comparisons, for example, that her hospital was "twice" as lethal as the regimental hospitals in the Crimea,[71] perhaps because the latter sent their worst cases to the general hospitals. Small put Nightingale's coloured polar-area chart, based on official returns, on the back cover of his book, but never discussed the data in his text!

Small also failed to specify to which hospitals the rates pertained, and never noticed that there were no separate data for Nightingale's hospital, but only grouped rates for "Scutari hospitals," six or eight, depending on the month, and for some months, "Scutari and Koulali hospitals." He entirely missed the data which showed that, when Koulali results were reported separately, they were higher than Scutari's. The Koulali hospitals were nursed by the Irish Sisters of Mercy, not Nightingale's – not that they should be blamed for the high rates, which were the result of unsanitary conditions beyond their capacity, or Nightingale's, to remedy. The actual data appear in Andrew Smith's two-volume official report – *Medical and Surgical History of the British Army Which Served in Turkey and the Crimea*

(1858) – which Nightingale used in her "Answers to Written Questions" prepared for the royal commission and in her longer *Notes on Matters Affecting the Health, Efficiency and Hospital Administration of the British Army* (1858). Further, she referred to Koulali explicitly as "the worst of all the hospitals" in a letter to medical statistician Dr Balfour.[72]

Small failed as well to note sources, such as Dr Sutherland's Sanitary Commission report, which indicated why Koulali was worse than Scutari, with details about the amount of "filth" removed, measured in tonnes for Koulali, mere cartloads for Scutari. Nightingale presumably first learned of Koulali's problems from Dr Sutherland. The chef, Alexis Soyer, who sailed past Koulali with Nightingale on route to the Crimea, noted: "Miss Nightingale observed that, although the Koulali hospitals were so well situated, it was reported by medical men that they were very unhealthy, more especially the lower one."[73]

Small went on to claim that Nightingale had a nervous breakdown on learning, through Dr Farr, he said – without citing a source – that she was responsible for the highest death rates. However, Farr could hardly have told her that, for he, like Nightingale, used the official data. At the same time as Small has her in complete nervous collapse, she was fully occupied with meetings, briefings, and statistical analysis.[74] A medical historian got the Koulali situation right on the higher death rates in his edition of a memoir of a Crimean War nurse.[75]

A Scottish surgeon's correspondence gives a helpful glimpse at how Scutari and Koulali were viewed at the time. Patrick Heron Watson (1832–1907) was initially assigned to Scutari, but was transferred to Koulali, where he served for five months. On arrival at Scutari he wrote to his mother: "The deaths in the Barrack Hospital amount to fifty a day. They are carted off, sewn up in blankets, in arabas [a primitive vehicle drawn by an ox] and laid in layers in trenches; officers are distinguished only by having a white wood coffin. My first view of this was an araba upset in the mud with the bodies all in a heap. In fact the Barrack Hospital is a lazar house, a dead house. Everything there is bad and I look forward with no very pleasant feeling to being quartered there."[76]

This view of the hospital, he stated, was substantiated by "every published report, official or independent." Hence, he was pleased when he was posted instead to Koulali, "for that hospital was considered to be healthy, comfortable, and delightfully situated between the hills and the sea." War Office returns, however, showed "how little justified" was its reputation for healthiness, showing "that mortality at Koulali was higher than in any other establishment." Heron Watson arrived in February 1855, the month of the highest death rates, 300 out of 1,200 patients, "the majority of fever, dysentery or other infection, much of which originated within the building itself."

The doctor had seen Nightingale at Scutari, albeit only at a distance, he wrote his sister. That was enough to object to the "absurd puff" reports the *Times* gave her "angelic form." She was rather "a very dowdy old maid, about whom the less romance the better." He thought well of her "strong hand" at Scutari, which was needed, but lacking initially at Koulali under Mary Stanley, the "lady volunteer" in charge of a group of Roman Catholic nuns and paid nurses. "The nuns are better than the nurses and if I were ill I would rather have a nun to attend me. Some of the nurses had fever and upon my word they are almost no loss. A bevy of good cooks would be a good deal more useful and not half so troublesome." The paid nurses were "unskilled, disorderly and a number were too fond of the bottle."[77] As to their own working conditions:

> The medical officer's working day began at seven, when a cup of black coffee was brought to his bedside. He then rose and disinfested himself, there being sometimes what is described as "a legion of animals" for the staff was repeatedly reinfested by new batches of patients arriving from the front. The nursing staff had nicknames for the parasites with which they were afflicted, lice being known as "heavy dragoons" in contrast with fleas, which were called "light cavalry," because of their speed and agility. Breakfast, ward at 9 until 4, then 2 hours in evening. Fever horrible, only 1½ feet between beds.[78]

The surgeon reported also on the arrival of the Sanitary Commission on 11 March 1855, that it had "done us good." He considered its practice "sound, which is a mercy as they have much in their power."[79] Conditions in fact greatly improved, not least of all on the vermin front. Rawlinson reported to the commandant at Scutari, Lord William Paulet, on the repairs made to Koulali Hospital, removing the ceiling to clear out "an immense quantity of fleas and other vermin, and of at least diminishing an evil already seriously felt." The repairs, as well, provided more "cubic space."[80] Oddly, not one of the three Irish Sisters of Mercy who published journals on the war ever mentioned the high death rates at the Koulali hospital, or the arrival of and work performed by the Sanitary Commission, although they did write about the vermin.[81]

The lengthy, ongoing dispute as to who was responsible for the reduction of death rates has also been marred by ignorance of the comparative death rates for the French Army. Sutherland, Nightingale, and the Sanitary Commission failed to cover this point, for the simple reason that the French data had not been published when they did their reports. The full data came out only in 1865 in the official report, reprinted as a book in 1870, showing French death rates per army strength at 11 per cent for the first winter of 1854–55, rising to 23 per cent in winter 1855–56. For the British, the first winter was much worse than the French at 20 per cent, but dropped to an astonishing 2.5 per cent in the second.[82]

The British, like everyone else, realized in the second year that the French forces were doing worse than they, by simple observation and informal remarks from their doctors. Nightingale commented to Sidney Herbert in November 1855 that the French losses were greater, "proportionally even," than their own.[83] The following March, she wrote to Harley Street board member Lady Cranworth that the sufferings of the French were now "so frightful" that they had to have peace: "They have lost 16,000 sick, one in eight, 10,000 down here [Scutari]. Typhus alone kills 50–60 per diem in these hospitals alone. The medical men are dying, three in one day. So are the sisters. They themselves tell the same story that we did last year."[84]

What is most remarkable is that the higher French death rates occurred *after* the fighting was over: the last battle (Great Redan, at Sebastopol) took place on 8 September 1855. The deaths over the following autumn, winter, and spring were due to illness, or occasional accidents, not wounds. What then accounts for this great difference between French and British death rates? The case for the Sanitary and Supply Commissions becomes only better when it is understood that the French carried on as usual, while the British made enormous reforms, thanks to their *civilian* commissioners, sent out by the prime minister. Their independence from military authorities – the War Office, army command in the field, the Army Medical Department, and the commissariat – was crucial. The French had pioneered military medicine, but now the British moved ahead of them. Civilian experts made changes that the military failed to see were necessary.

A final point on the high French death rates: Nightingale wrote after the war to sanitary pioneer Edwin Chadwick that she suspected that "the emperor [Napoleon III] *wished* his army to die; it was less expense than bringing them home. And that he was rather displeased than otherwise at whatever was done to prevent this desirable result."[85]

What Nightingale Did and Did Not Do

To complicate matters, Nightingale has always been given undue credit for reducing British deaths during the war. While flattering, this unmerited praise also shows disregard, for she never made such claims, but credited the work of the Sanitary and Supply Commissions. Moreover, exaggerating what dedicated nursing, improved nutrition, and clean bedding and clothing – desirable as they are – could achieve misses the really significant matters. No standard of patient care could have substantially cut mortality without the massive re-engineering of sewers and drains and removal of dead horses from the water supply and cartloads of feces from the drains, all of which involved professional engineers and a well-supervised workforce. Assigning the wrong cause to the improvements not only is bad science, but can lead to mistaken policy in the future.

Some memoirs from the war exaggerate the effect of Nightingale's work. According to that of the American missionary who ran the bakery at Scutari: "Very soon Miss Nightingale transformed that hospital. From the first, she divided her forces into night watches, and there were nurses and assistant nurses walking those corridors and wards all night long. The nights were no longer lonely. Every want was attended to, every pain, if possible, assuaged. The death rate was changed immediately from the moral effect, no doubt, of sympathy and woman's gentle care. I had seen some instances of brutal treatment from surgeons, possibly fuddled with drink, but there was nothing of that after Miss Nightingale came."[86]

This misleading account was repeated years later in an article by the writer's granddaughter, a nurse, in the *American Journal of Nursing*.[87]

The 60 Per Cent Mistake

Nightingale herself exaggerated the initial British death rates in at least three reports, though not in any of the tables published. In her evidence to the royal commission of 1857–58, she stated: "We had, in the first seven months of the Crimean campaign, a mortality among the troops at the rate of 60 percent per annum from disease alone, a rate of mortality which exceeds that of the Great Plague in the population of London, and a higher ratio than the mortality in cholera to the attacks."[88] In the Preface to her long report (*Notes on Matters Affecting* ... [1858]), she presents the "enormous" mortality of the Peninsular War against Napoleon as a "small matter" compared to the 60 per cent over eight months so far in the Crimea.[89] The error appears also in passing in her tribute to Sidney Herbert after his death in August 1861.[90]

The figure of 60 per cent comes from miscalculating one indicator, deaths over "sick population," for one hospital, Koulali, for the worst month of the war, January 1855. The correct figure is 52 per cent, while the rate of deaths per cases was 46.6 per cent.[91] Clearly, mortality was high in all the hospitals, but 60 per cent as an average for all of them over six or more months must look excessive. The army had to send replacements, but to make up 60 per cent of its troops?

Using the official statistics on hospital death rates, and a simple indicator of deaths per admissions, table 2.1 presents the rates for the first seven months and the last six months. A note explains that the deaths are an underestimate, omitting those among commissioned officers, the Land Transport Corps, and others. Table 2.2 shows the percentage deaths over admissions for September 1854, when the first battle took place, and June 1855, when the lower death rates were established. The curmudgeonly commentator might note that the hospital death rate went up *after* the arrival of the nurses in November 1854. Neither Dr Farr nor other statisticians picked up on the exaggeration. The rates continued to go down for the rest of 1855 and 1856. Note that the highest number occurred in January 1855, but the highest rate in February.

The erroneous 60 per cent has been quoted in numerous studies by highly reputable sources, in several fields, adding, as Nightingale had not, a fallacious explanation for the decline: First, Kopf, a statistician, cited Nightingale's "vigorous use" of statistics to bring about reforms that "reduced this terrible rate of mortality." He noted (correctly) the lack of uniformity in death records, to claim that she introduced "an orderly plan of recording the principal sickness and mortality data of the military hospital establishments which came within the sphere of her influence." Nightingale, of course, had no authority over record keeping in any hospital, and hardly had time to keep records herself.[92]

Table 2.1   Percentage deaths over admissions, British Army, early and late in the Crimean War

	Deaths	Admissions	%
Sept. '54–March '55	12,009	56,978	21.1
Jan. '56–June '56	261	20,662	1.3

Table 2.2   Percentage deaths over admissions, British Army, by month, Sept. 1854–June 1855

Date	Deaths	Admissions	%	Note
Sept. 1854	939	6,906	13.6	1st battle
Oct. 1854	763	7,323	10.4	2nd battle
Nov. 1854	1,237	8,314	11.9	3rd battle; nurses arrive
Dec. 1854	1,970	10,675	18.5	
Jan. 1855	3,168	11,328	28.0	
Feb. 1855	2,523	7,119	35.4	
March 1855	1,409	5,313	26.5	San. Comm. arrives
April 1855	582	4,500	12.9	
May 1855	594	5,781	10.6	
June 1855	1,042	11,128	9.3	

Second, I.B. Cohen, founder of the Department of History of Science at Harvard University, followed Kopf, complete with the 60 per cent and the Great Plague, in an article in *Scientific American*. Both authors mistakenly thought that Nightingale had collected the data herself at Scutari. Both articles have much valuable analysis in them, and Cohen later published a book with a full, otherwise excellent chapter on her statistics.[93] Cohen's *Scientific American* article claimed incorrectly that her sanitary reforms began to be implemented in March 1855 – when "mortality among the patients declined precipitously." It was the Sanitary Commission whose work started in March – Nightingale had arrived in November 1854. Cohen was correct when he wrote: "By the end of the war, according to Nightingale, the death rate among sick British soldiers in Turkey was 'not much more' than it was among healthy soldiers in England."[94] It did drop that much, but mainly thanks to the Sanitary and

Supply Commissions. Cohen's later work gives credit to the Sanitary Commission, noting that it had power to act that Nightingale did not – it also had experienced sanitary engineers and budget to hire workmen – and had the latrines cleaned.

Third, a children's book written by the daughter of Nightingale friends Dr Samuel Gridley and Julia Ward Howe used the incorrect death rate of 60 per cent, crediting Nightingale "and her devoted band" with reducing it to 1 per cent "within a few months."[95] A British children's book has her doing the work of the doctors, stating that "no one" but her did anything for the soldiers. "Their wounds even were often not dressed; they were brought there to die. But Florence Nightingale worked so hard that soon the hospitals were sweet and clean, and the men grew well instead of dying."[96]

Fourth, a chapter in a book on women medical pioneers, citing Cohen as the source on the 60 per cent, has Nightingale single-handedly decreasing the death rate and (incorrectly) banning women from the wards.[97]

Other Mistaken Claims

Nightingale also cited 73 per cent as a death rate, but carefully reported it as applying to eight regiments, all "at the front," of a total sixty-eight regiments over a six-month period. She named the regiments.[98] Yet this extreme percentage would be cited in an award-winning biography as if it applied to the whole army.[99]

Hugh Auchincloss (1878–1947), a New York physician who collected Nightingale material, also exaggerated her contribution in a speech, which was subsequently published by bacteriologist Charles-Edward Winslow (1877–1957). The article contains much relevant and apposite material on her work. It presents the correct decline in rates, from 420 per 1,000 to 22 per 1,000, but with too short a period, three months.[100] It correctly credits her with grasping the core relations between "dirt and disease." However, she did not check "all her efforts by statistics, with a scientific caution far ahead of her time."[101] One can agree that Nightingale could be known as "The Lady with the Slide Rule," but she did all her research after Crimea, in collaboration with medical / statistical experts.

A paper in *Epidemiology* has the death rates falling from 32 per cent to 2 per cent in the "first months after her arrival," citing a paper in the *American Journal of Epidemiology* that does not discuss Crimean hospital data at all.[102]

A leading American nursing history, published in fifteen editions, added a claim for "nursing care" in reducing the death rate, along with sanitary improvements, although Nightingale never credited the nursing for the reductions. "In two months, she had transformed the hospital into an efficiently managed institution. In six months she had reduced the death rate to 2 *percent*, and had won the respect of most of the surgeons ... Because of her sanitary improvements and the provision of good nursing care for patients, Miss Nightingale reduced the mortality from 427 per 1,000 in February 1855 to 222 in June 1855. She utilized the scientific method of gathering data and was skilled as a statistician, presenting the factual evidence in a most graphic way."[103] Note the discrepancy in the numbers: 2 per cent would be 22.2 per 1,000. As well, the time it took for the decline to (about) 2 per cent was longer.

The author was then quoted in a later nursing book, with new misinformation; indeed, the points on keeping patient records and nurse training are pure fiction: "Nightingale worked long, hard hours to care for these soldiers. She spent up to twenty hours each day caring for wounds, comforting soldiers, assisting in surgery, directing staff, and keeping records. Nightingale introduced principles of asepsis and infection control, a system for transcribing doctor's orders and a procedure to maintain patient records. By the end of the Crimean War, Nightingale had trained as many as 125 nurses to care for the wounded and ill soldiers."[104]

Numerous nursing books and articles repeat the exaggerated success, usually with other errors added.[105] An American source on community nursing put the 73 per cent in a range, from 42 per cent to 73 per cent, describing a decline in death rates to 2 per cent, in six months, thanks to Nightingale's "radical and well-documented interventions based on sound public health principles." Moreover, she conducted "careful, scientific epidemiological research."[106]

Mistakes appear in other genres as well, such as on women leaders, pioneer medical researchers, and women's history.[107]

Some recent medical sources had the percentage right, but exaggerated Nightingale's role in reducing death rates.[108] Atul Gawande had her "within several months of her arrival" implementing hygiene practices, "use of clean water, clean sheets, and handwashing, that decreased the facility's mortality rate to approximately that of London hospitals at that time."[109]

Post-war reforms by Nightingale and colleagues, to be pursued in chapter 4, continued over many years to make enormous, quantifiable differences, of which Nightingale was mightily proud. But this occurred not because of bedside care but through better nutrition, shelter, and functioning laundries.

What Nightingale actually did can be seen in her reports and the numerous letters she wrote to political leaders, army officers, doctors, nurses, and soldiers' families. The great bulk of them are published in *The Collected Works of Florence Nightingale*; an earlier collection of 100 letters provides excellent context.[110]

A sample letter is given here, written to someone inquiring on behalf of the family – more often Nightingale's letters were to a family member directly. This one shows Nightingale distinguishing between the roles of the doctor and the nurse, neither of whom could save this soldier's life.

Castle Hospital, Balaclava
10 November 1855

Sir, Your letter of the 4th October was forwarded to me at this place, where my hospital duties at present require me. Morris Jones, 13th Light Infantry, died at the Barrack Hospital, Scutari, Ward 8, Corridor F, of fever, 20 August 1855. He was only in hospital three days. He had an abscess in his neck and spoke very little.

At 10 p.m. the night he died, he was sufficiently conscious to express pleasure at having the nurse there, though he always called her "Mother." He would take no food from anyone else. He appeared to rest satisfied in this delusion, which comforted him. He was far too little conscious to send any message to his family.

He was very cold and had hot water tins put round him, which annoyed him, and he insisted upon pushing them away. He was too ill when he entered hospital for any questions to be asked him. The nurse called him her "old man," and when it was ascertained that he was only thirty two years of age, would not believe it. But our men are old at thirty two.

I regret that the anxiety of his family should have been not sooner ended. But I am myself confined to my bed by illness and here I have no one to write for me. I remain, Sir,

your obedient servant
Florence Nightingale

If it is any consolation to his family to know that he was not neglected, but had every care that medical skill and female nursing could give him, they may be certain of this.

Regimental and Land Transport Corps Hospitals

When soldiers were sick, they had to go into hospital, normally their regiment's hospital, run by its doctors, who travelled with the force. At the beginning of the Crimean War, the regimental "hospital" was only a single-layer bell tent, utterly inadequate for sick and wounded men. The War Office sent nurses to Scutari not for regimental hospitals, which were too close to the war zone, but for general hospitals, which received the more serious cases. The Highland Regiment, exceptionally, did hire a nurse. Nightingale agreed generally with regimental hospitals not having women nurses – the men were too healthy, and overly friendly relations were too feasible. This view held also after the war, when again no need for trained women was seen, and the opportunity for mischief too great.

Lack of transport impeded supplies reaching camp or hospital. A railway was built, but until it opened, supplies had to be hauled. A Land Transport Corps (LTC) was sent to the Crimea long after Lord Raglan had asked for one. It had, like a regiment, its own hospital, or two, according to some accounts. Not a "general hospital," the LTC's set-up needed no women nurses, but its PMO, Dr George Taylor (1808–1867), found the orderlies so "drunken, negligent and dishonest" as to be useless, and begged for Nightingale nurses.[III]

The LTC commandant, Colonel William McMurdo, was no less keen, and "gave her every assistance in his power," as Nightingale's messenger recalled:

He sent two of his ambulance cars to convey the nurses from Balaclava; these cars very much resembled the present Irish jaunting car, running on two small wheels. We knew it was quite possible to have an accident, and sure enough, it did come, for on turning off the main road and, close to the destined place, one of the wheels of the car on which Miss Nightingale, Miss Shaw Stewart, two nurses and myself were sitting, rolled over on a large stone and upset the car. I was sitting on the shaft and had nothing to do but to drop on the ground. Miss Nightingale and Miss Stewart were turned up in the air and nearly thrown to the opposite side of the road, and the two nurses were entirely under the whole, and for a time no one knew whether they were hurt or not.[112]

However, there were no lasting injuries.

Nightingale credited Colonel McMurdo for "a most difficult service, that of organizing the Land Transport, with the utmost success."[113] He gave her a captured Russian carriage for her use while in the Crimean camps. After the war, chef Alexis Soyer arranged to have it sent back to England, where it is still periodically put on display.

Colonel McMurdro and Major-General Henry Storks (knighted after the war) "have been and will remain my only friends out here," Nightingale wrote, although she appreciated General Codrington and Colonel Windham for their courtesy (the latter "more than courteous, kind") and Lord Rokeby and General Barnard, "who brought Lord Gough to see me, talk to me as to an old soldier and brother in the field."[114] (Field Marshal Viscount Gough was in the Crimea as the queen's representative to award honours.)

Dr Taylor, of the LTC hospital, became a friend. After his death in 1867, Nightingale went to some trouble to secure a pension for his widow. She recounted his appreciation of the nursing to the mother superior of the Bermondsey Sisters of Mercy: he "expressed to me yesterday, in the strongest words, his feeling of the reform they had worked in his L.T.C. hospital. They do more than medicine he said."[115] She told her family: "He [Dr Taylor] is my present master and a very admirable exception to the general run of my masters. He is strict, but not at all stricter than I like – upright, honest, independent – with the good of his men at heart, for which he has laboured without praise and without reward. He will never be promoted, for the melancholy joke that promotion is in proportion to demerit is here an axiom or a truism. He is a man of very considerable talent. And his hospitals, late the worst, are now the best managed of the Crimea. He is indefatigable, efficient, able."[116]

The Model Hospital at Renkioi: Civilian Doctors

As the Crimean War proceeded, more doctors, nurses, and hospitals were needed. For doctors, the War Office had to resort to sending civilians, who travelled with civilian nurses. More hospitals were established, some of them huts. The finest example was the prefabricated hut hospital for 1,000 men at Renkioi, on the Asiatic side of the Dardanelles. It was designed by engineer Isambard Kingdom Brunel, built in sections in England for assembly after arrival. The huts, which each took fifty patients, followed the pavilion principle, that is, with narrow wards, windows on both sides, facing each other, and a window between every bed, thus minimizing the risk of cross-infection. The pavilions were completely independent of each other, and all had state-of-the-art toilets. However, by the time Renkioi opened, in October 1855, conditions had already improved enormously, thanks to the Sanitary and Supply Commissions, and the fighting was over.

The doctor in charge at Renkioi was Edmund Alexander Parkes (1819–1876), who also selected the site. He had earlier been an army physician. In 1860, when the Army Medical School was opened, he was named its first professor of military hygiene. He, like so many others from the war, became a good colleague of Nightingale's. The nurses at Renkioi were under not Nightingale but Lady Canning, who had assisted in selecting nurses for Scutari, and did so again for Renkioi. The matron consulted Nightingale on particular nurses. Dr Parkes's sister was one of them and deputy matron.

Nightingale was also asked by doctors to send nurses to the Monastery St George, a small hospital situated on the heights of Balaclava, which she did. It was open for only a year, from July 1855 to June 1856.

Nutrition and Scurvy in the British Army

Captain James Cook managed to prevent scurvy on his circumnavigation of the globe beginning in 1768, and the Royal Society awarded him its prestigious Copley Medal for the feat. The ability of citrus juice to prevent scurvy was confirmed in a controlled experiment in 1747 by Royal Navy surgeon James Lind (1716–1794), although it took until 1893 for the Royal Navy to make his recommendations compulsory. Sociologist Herbert Spencer called the delay "the most flagrant example of administrative apathy on record."[117]

Despite all this (available) information, the British Army was utterly unprepared for scurvy when it sent troops to the east in April 1854. When it was clear that the army would have to winter in the Crimea, the troops had been on a salt-meat-and-biscuit diet for eight months. Nightingale ordered lemons and vegetables for the hospital kitchen, as "extra diet" items called for by the doctors, as she reported to Sidney Herbert.[118] However, she, as nursing director, had no say in the regular diet in the field, a matter she, Herbert, and army doctors addressed after the war.

It was only in November 1854, after many cases of scurvy, and dysentery with scurvy, that Dr Andrew Smith ordered lemon and lime juice to be sent, on consultation with the Admiralty. Nightingale queried why he had not ordered potatoes and other fresh vegetables earlier.[119] She also commented on the order for cooking preserved vegetables as an antidote to scurvy: "This is curious – Scutari is opposite a capital [Constantinople] of upward of 600,000 inhabitants who live on vegetables – therefore any quantity is obtainable."[120]

Nightingale thought Dr John Hall all too complacent about this matter, noting his reference in January 1855 to "symptoms of scurvy," that the illness had not "made much progress." For her, "the army was dying, and of scurvy. More than half the infantry were sick in hospital during this month. In January 1855, Smith again urged the sending of lime juice, now 20,000 gallons."[121] The failure to prevent this disease was a major subject of the first report of the Supply Commission. It comes up frequently in Nightingale's *Notes on Matters Affecting ...* (1858).

While soldiers' rations were so severely limited, even in hospital, officers could normally eat well. One officer's memoir records that his daily ration while in hospital consisted of "half a fowl, half a pound of mutton, five eggs, and a due provision of tea, sugar, milk, bread, etc., in addition to which the doctor had unlimited powers to order wine, beer or spirits in any quantity he might think proper." "Medical comforts" such as arrowroot, chocolate, jelly, sago, and sweet biscuits could be obtained "by the mere asking."[122] In camp, officers could purchase meals from the sutlers or *vivandières*. Their servants could prepare food for them or make purchases on their behalf. Scurvy among officers was rare.

Drink: "Stimulants," Drunkenness, Intoxication

Doctors prescribed "stimulants," meaning alcoholic drinks, for their patients as well as medicine and foods. Nurses were responsible for seeing that they were taken, in the case of alcohol, measuring out the amounts. It seems peculiar to people accustomed to a wide variety of prescription drugs, but at the time there were few effective drugs, and different wines were commonly ordered as remedies.

Alcohol was part of the normal "ration" for soldiers and nurses, the prescribed quantity made available every day for free. For soldiers, it was, initially, 1 gill of rum a day, or 5 ounces. On medical review this was reduced to a half-gill per day. Alcohol was also sold by sutlers and *vivandières*, and available also from Turkish soldiers, who were given the same ration as the British but, as Muslims, typically did not drink.

The Supply Commission found out that the army's rum ration made drinkers out of many young soldiers. Men who had previously had no "disposition" for rum, and even found it distasteful, acquired the habit in the Crimea. The commission recommended the substitution of porter, a strong beer favoured by porters. It was "nutritious and antiscorbutic"; in moderate quantities it would even be "beneficial."[123] Nightingale would also (frequently) recommend porter or beer over rum.

The War Office's alcohol allowance for nurses, designed by or at least approved by Nightingale, was healthier. Rule 9 gave each nurse "1 pint of porter or ale at dinner; half a pint of porter, or a wine glass of wine, or 1 oz. of brandy (as she likes best) for supper. In case of constant attendance on cholera or infectious fever, the superintendent may allow an extra quantity at her discretion."[124]

Hospital nurses at the time were notorious for drunkenness, that is, drinking on the wards or before going on duty and passing out. At the Edinburgh Royal Infirmary, the senior house surgeon ensured that drunken night nurses were carried into the wards on a stretcher.[125] Secondary sources sometimes describe Nightingale as opposed to any use of alcohol – a mistake made by Boris Johnson in his *Johnson's Life of London*. According to the Rules, nurses could be dismissed for a single instance of intoxication, but in fact it took repeated violations – the loss of nurses would have been too great. The records show that twelve nurses were dismissed from Scutari for intoxication, one after repeated warnings and being moved to Nightingale's own quarters for a while. Nightingale wrote Lady Cranworth, who had assisted in the selection, that she was "deeply grieved" to have to send home another nurse, after "repeated offences" and warnings over many months.[126]

Comparison of British and French
Hospitals and Doctors

It is not surprising that the French were ahead of the British in preparations for the war. Not only were they its main instigators – under their new emperor, Napoleon III – but they had pioneered both military medicine and military statistics. The British also collected good statistics, while no other army did, but were otherwise behind the French. In the first battles (autumn 1854), the British had no vehicles for carrying their wounded to hospital, which was a mere tent, lacking medical equipment and even bedding. The French helped with transport. Bedding and equipment were improved thanks to the *Times* fund, Nightingale making the purchases. Still, she was on the lookout for such missing items as an apparatus for administering chloroform and splints "like those used in the French hospitals."[127]

Early in 1855, Nightingale pointed out that the French had snapped up the Constantinople hospitals and were preparing for more sick and wounded.[128] However, this all changed with the arrival of the Sanitary and Supply Commissions in March 1855. British death rates had begun to decline and continued to from then on, with one reversal owing to a cholera epidemic, while the French rates rose, and continued to rise, even well after hostilities were over.

In November 1855 (the last battle was on 8 September), it was clear that the French had more dysentery than the British. Nightingale had just visited a field hospital of theirs, with British pathologist Dr Lyons, PMO Dr James Mouat (1815–1899), and other doctors. In amputations, the French acknowledged that they had not saved one in six, while the British saved one quarter.

When Nightingale visited French hospitals in March 1856, it was evident, as her soldier attendant recorded, that "the French were but scantily supplied in comparison to the English; our patients were better accommodated and were much cleaner, happier and far more comfortable than their allies."[129] She commented on the reversal – that they had had to accept French help at the war's start:

> The sufferings of the French are so frightful ... they are suffering
> more than we were last year. They have now 16,000 sick, one in
> eight, 10,000 down here [Scutari], Typhus alone kills fifty-sixty per

diem in these hospitals alone. The medical men are dying, three in one day. So are the sisters. They themselves tell the same story that we did last year, that want of food and clothing sends down the patients in a typhoid state, which is propagated by the overcrowded state of the hospitals ... Their system is worse than ours. I am in a chronic rage ... How little magnanimous they are! We accepted everything from them in our calamity this time last year.[130]

Nightingale had to engage in face-saving measures to help the French at all, by arranging gifts privately.

By June 1856, on a visit to a French tent hospital near Balaclava, she concluded that French bedding, accommodation, and food were far inferior to the British, but the cooking was superior, except for the British extra-diet kitchens, set up to transcend the limits of the standard British diet: salt-meat and hard biscuit.[131] The French themselves were complimentary about the extra-diet kitchens, as they were about British superiority generally, for the second year of the war. Their physicians routinely praised the British, and often Nightingale specifically, in their reports. The official report noted the great improvements made, including Nightingale's influence, during and after the war.[132]

Nightingale noted, from visiting the French hospitals, that they used different methods for treating typhus. All their patients were "under canvas, never more than four, generally not more than two in a tent." The ground was shifted every two weeks. Tent bottoms were regularly turned up to facilitate air flow.[133]

The French Dr Gaspard Scrive, in an early, incomplete report on the Crimean hospitals, related his visits to those of two British divisions. They had been given a terrible lesson at the war's beginning, by the lack of medical means for an army on campaign during the winter, but in the second winter they made a "superb rebound"; their Guards hospital was comprised of huts and large double-strength tents, wood floors, and so on.[134]

Dr Léon Le Fort (1829–1893) was complimentary to Nightingale and the whole "medical corps," which could, in the context, refer only to the Sanitary and Supply Commissions. He noted that the "whole infantry" of the British were "warmly lodged, well-nourished and clothed," passing the winter "sheltered from all the causes of death that had so powerfully and unfortunately acted on them the previous winter." The commissions and Nightingale had greatly improved clothing, hygiene, nutrition, and shelter. He noted especially the Supply Commission's "Crimean huts."[135]

Dr Lucien Baudens (1804–1857), in charge of the French Army's Medical Department in the East, also acknowledged the superiority of the British Army's nourishment, because its doctors could order extra foods, thus providing greater variety, including tea, roast meat, and puddings. They could ask for beer, wines of all sorts, rum, and cognac. Baudens saw even champagne in the supply stores, used in cases of vomiting, he noted. His remarks on Nightingale and her nurses were flattering:

> The attendants discharged their duties with zeal, under the impulse of active and intelligent female hospital assistants, at the head of whom was the celebrated Miss Nightingale. Beautiful, young and wealthy, she sacrificed everything to the noble mission of alleviating suffering. This delicate young woman, mounted on horseback, might be seen passing from one hospital to another, looking after her sick of the three allied armies with a pious solicitude; and at the time of the typhus she sent to the French and Sardinian field hospitals a large present of port wine and preserves of every kind.[136]

The Army Medical Department's Post-war Assessment

Dr Andrew Smith, director-general of Britain's Army Medical Department, prepared a two-volume *Medical and Surgical History of the British Army Which Served in Turkey and the Crimea* (1858), which incorporated reports from doctors on particular diseases and the final data for all regimental and general hospitals: admissions, deaths, type of disease, and so on. Nightingale and Farr used this source for their charts and analysis in all their reports. Smith's study also contained a number of charts of meteorological conditions and disease, prepared by Sir John Hall, evidently reflecting the notion that weather or climate affects illness and death.

Smith's volumes contained a substantial section on cholera, with reports from medical doctors on their attempts at cure. The cause of the disease was not then known, and there was no effective treatment. These reports show that army doctors were more sceptical in their assessment of the treatments they tried than is typical of the period, judging by articles in medical journals. A regimental doctor reported on his use of 2 grains of calomel (mercury chloride) every 10 or 15 minutes, with copious drinks of water, mustard plaster, hot flannels, and friction for cramps, but said that it was a "physical impossibility" to give calomel so frequently and that patients recovered, or not, "entirely irrespective of the remedies administered." He was so convinced of the "perfect uselessness of any medicine," that he took nothing but laudanum when he was attacked with cholera.[137]

Treatment for diarrhea early in the war, in Bulgaria, included calomel, opium, mineral acids, creosote, aromatics, astringents, turpentine, quinine, chloroform, arsenic, hydrocyanic acid, acetate of lead, stimulants, with frictions, liniments, sinapism, and heat. Doctors, however, in reporting later, concluded that they were of "no more than a negative value," even that "all the resources of medicine are of little avail in this disease." Worse, they had gained no experience "of the injury produced by treatment." So, "while asserting that medicine has no power, on account of its non-absorption into the system, it has forgotten to explain in what way pints of brandy, scruples of opium and drachms of calomel are disposed of when the functions are restored and the relation of the secondary fever to the efforts of nature in this critical conjuncture."[138]

In her *Notes on Matters Affecting the Health, Efficiency and Hospital Administration of the British Army* (1858), Nightingale criticized the Army Medical Department for not remarking on "the caution required in prescribing remedies such as calomel."[139] She commented later to Sidney Herbert that people took water cures to remove the mercury from their system.[140] Calomel was available without prescription and was commonly deployed as a home-remedy purgative. A surgeon with the 95th Regiment reported that he and his colleagues used calomel to kill maggots by filling wounds with it, noting that they had it in "plentiful supply."[141]

Smith's *Medical and Surgical History* had one coloured chart that bettered, in one respect, Nightingale and Farr's polar-area charts, by showing deaths per month by five types of disease and total wounds. Cholera was the only disease listed separately; the other categories were bowel diseases, fever, lung diseases, and all other diseases.[142] The large blocks show the great proportion due to fevers and bowel diseases (the general category and cholera). The rectangles decline in size over time. However, since the numbers in the last months were so small, they were grouped together – they would otherwise have disappeared from the chart. Nightingale and Farr's polar-area charts (see figure 2.1), by contrast, conveniently show the continuing decline in deaths, month by month, which they attributed to

Fig 2.1 Medical and surgical history of the British Army, 1858

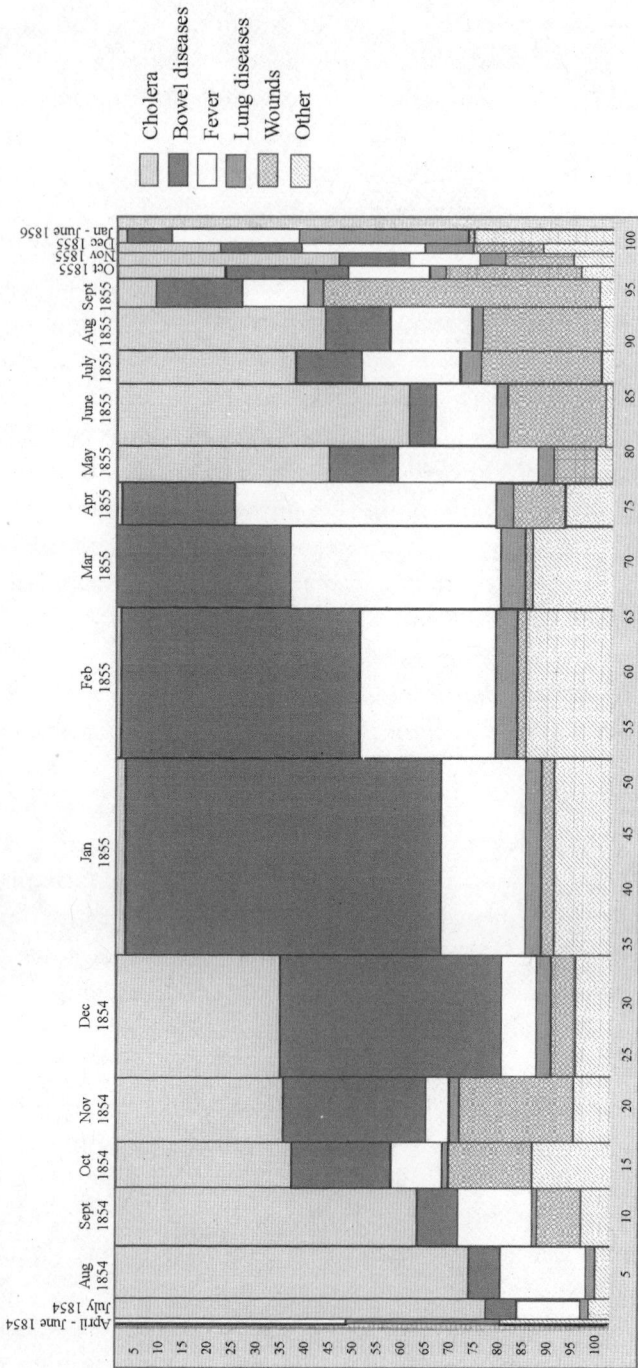

Note: The width of the space allotted to each month represents the proportion which the deaths that occurred during that month bear to the total mortality during the war and the subdivisions of each monthly space show the proportions which the deaths that occurred during the month from the principal classes of disease and the wounds bear to the total mortality of that month. Deaths in action with the enemy are not included in this diagram.

the efforts of the Sanitary and Supply Commissions. Smith, however, did not try to explain the declining death rates, and his only relevant chart effectively omits them from any analysis.

A Royal Commission on the
Crimean War (1857–1858)

After the war, Nightingale agitated behind the scenes for the appointment of a royal commission into the army's administration of sanitation during the Crimean War, influenced the appointment of its members, briefed witnesses before they appeared, and gave her own (written) evidence. She further influenced the commission's positive terms of reference – looking to reform in the future, and drawing on sources on civilian as well as military hospitals. She and the chair, Sidney Herbert, worked together closely while the commission was sitting and through to its formulating of its findings and making of recommendations.[143] While the royal commission was in course, Herbert asked to see everything that she was writing for her report – the précis – "as it goes on."[144] Afterwards, they went on promptly to work on publicizing and implementing the recommendations.

In contrast with all other witnesses, Nightingale gave her (detailed) evidence only in writing, and thus could not be cross-examined. She realized the unfairness of this, but whether or not she ever pressed to be called in person is not clear. Sir John McNeill opposed her giving her evidence "viva voce." Herbert shared that repugnance, but thought that her evidence "would fortify our proceedings and hasten the adoption of our recommendations."[145] But he wanted her to confine her evidence to hospital construction, as Nightingale complained to McNeill.[146] She did not want to be kept to such a narrow subject. When Herbert asked her to write her own questions, she tried, but:

> I have really tried to write questions for my own examination, as you directed. And I cannot. I feel thus: (1) I am quite as well aware as you can be that it is inexpedient and even unprincipled to go back into past delinquencies. (2) What is more, I feel for you who were victimized by a system which you could not possibly understand til you saw its results. It is very easy for me (who lived through them) to be wise after the fact. But it would be equally

untrue and unconscientious for me to give evidence upon an indifferent matter like that of hospital construction, and leave untouched the great matters which will affect the mortality of our sick (and have affected them) far more than any architectural plan could do.[147]

Important as hospital construction was – she was soon to devote much energy to it – the reform of public administration was even more so. Only an effective administrative structure could implement all the reforms needed, including hospital design and site. She explained, "People, government, and sovereign" all thought the problems had been remedied. She thought not: "It would be treachery to the memory of my dead, if I were to allow myself to be examined upon a mere scheme of hospital construction." None of the witnesses stood in the same position as she did: "For none saw so much."[148]

Her evidence was placed at the end of the official report, titled "Answers to Written Questions Addressed to Miss Nightingale by the Commissioners." There were eighty-nine questions and answers, some with notes and tables. The questions, however arrived at, covered the ground well both as to what went wrong and what should be done to avoid such disasters in the future. As in her longer *Notes on Matters Affecting ...* , her points echoed those made earlier by the Sanitary and Supply Commissions.

Nightingale's analysis in "Answers" was highly complimentary to regular, practising army doctors, as opposed to their all-too-complacent superiors. She showed frequently that the physicians knew what was wrong, but lacked the power to act. A note showed the convergence of views of the Sanitary and Supply Commissions, both of them blaming sanitary lacks, not the doctors themselves, for "the loss of an army." She commented to McNeill: "You will have proved that if the M.O.s [medical officers] had the knowledge, they had not the power. I trust that you will not let it drop. For I look upon the sanitary question as even more essential to the life of our army, if possible, than that of supplies. I look upon what you told me yesterday as the most important thing I have heard." The Duke of Wellington, the note continued, "destroyed the army of Masséna by no other means" – a reference to his victory by attrition over the French Marshal Masséna's army at Portugal's Lines of Torres Vedras in winter 1810–11. Nightingale made numerous comparisons of Crimean War losses with those of the Napoleonic period.[149]

Her answers varied enormously in length and complexity. For brevity, question 22 asked: "To what do you mainly ascribe the mortality in the hospitals? Answer: To sanitary defects." On the next question, however, on rates of mortality and their computation, she presented detailed tables and equations from Farr and his office.

Throughout this period of preparation for the royal commission and the taking of evidence, Nightingale was busy behind the scenes suggesting questions and briefing, possibly rehearsing, witnesses. She had recovered from her near-death illness in the Crimea and was full of energy. This would be the last period in her life when she could move around freely. She even contemplated taking a nursing position. When she began to work on starting a nursing school and implementing the royal commission's recommendations, the subjects of the next two, final chapters of part I, she was sick and in pain much of the time.

Epilogue: A Crimean War Soldier Writes to Nightingale Thirty-Two Years Later

Sometimes a letter to Nightingale tells us something about her work not mentioned in any letter of her own. Here is a fine example from 1887, written by a Crimean War soldier about her help of over thirty years earlier. British Army surgeons then did little more than amputate injured limbs; more complicated surgery to reconstruct the limb was still a long way off. The soldier was Samuel Atkins, wounded at the Battle of Inkermann, 5 November 1854. He would thus have been one of the first soldiers Nightingale looked after at the Scutari Barack Hospital.

Birmingham
9 March 1887

Madame
You will doubtless be surprised at receiving a letter from an old Crimean soldier after so many years have passed away, but I have always been anxious to write to you, but could not obtain your address, and have only now quite incidentally, in talking to a friend,

discovered through her the address of your sister to whom I have
addressed this letter for you.

I was one of the soldiers in the 33rd Duke of Wellington
Regiment and was wounded at the Battle of Inkerman, in the head,
muscle of right arm and down the ribs, and taken to the hospital at
Scutari. After being under the doctors treatment for a time, he said
that the next day he must cut my arm off, and I told you what the
doctor had said and you told me that I had not better have it off as
there was no danger and that they could not take it off without my
permission and that my arm would look better in my sleeve. There
the sleeve would tuck in my waistcoat pocket.

A few months after coming home to my native village, when
out one day my arm being still crooked I stooped down, picked
up a stone to throw at a bird and the sudden jerk pulled my arm
straight and I was shortly after this able to take some temporary
employment and have been able to follow my work ever since.

And now you will perhaps ask yourself why I have written
all these particulars to you. It is that I may thank you from the
very bottom of my heart for all your kindness to me and all
other suffering ones while I and they were in the hospital. I often
remember you in my prayers at the throne of grace for thank God
since leaving the Crimea I have found grace in trusting in the
precious blood of Christ.

I trust that you are in the enjoyment of good health and that
the presence of the Master Christ may be always with you. And I
know that you will one day hear him say (Inasmuch as ye have done
it unto one of the least of these my children, ye have done it unto
me). Well done good and faithful servant, enter thou into the joy
of thy Lord. Hoping that you will excuse the liberty I have taken. I
remain, Madame

your obedient servant
Samuel Atkins[150]

WORK WITH CIVILIAN DOCTORS
(1857–1880)

St Thomas' Hospital: Starting the Nightingale School

Nightingale chose St Thomas' Hospital, London, to be the site of her training school, as it had already achieved a higher standard of nursing than was usual, thanks to its matron, Sarah E. Wardroper (1813–1892), and its resident medical officer, Dr Richard G. Whitfield (1801–1877). Wardroper became also the school's superintendent, and Whitfield its first nursing instructor. He had, in 1857, offered to assist Nightingale with hospital information of various types and in those early years assisted her in numerous ways. He commented on her *Subsidiary Notes as to the Introduction of Female Nursing into Military Hospitals* (1858).[1]

Some doctors opposed such a school right from the start. John Flint South (1797–1882), senior surgeon at St Thomas', published a short book on hospital nurses arguing against the need for training. He had been forty-four years at the hospital and saw nothing wrong with the nurses' work or situation – "treated by both surgeons and dressers as if they were old superior family servants," and with tasks easily learned.[2] Moreover, in the large London hospitals, the matrons were generally "fully competent," and the "*hospital nursing is well done.*" South added that nurses deserved pensions. His references to Nightingale were respectful, but he pointedly disagreed with statements about the need for nursing made in creating the Nightingale Fund. He stated that few doctors had subscribed to it.[3] In short, there was no need for a training school. South's professional books, *A Short Description of the Bones* (1825) and *Household Surgery* (1847), both with later editions, were used at the school when it opened, and for years thereafter.

South's "servant" analogy was entirely antithetical to Nightingale's vision of nursing as a profession junior to medicine, but far above the household servant. She did use the expression "handmaiden of the Lord," but mainly in a religious context, from the annunciation of Mary (Luke 1:38). It also appears in some of her late writing, but vis-à-vis commitment to God. She increasingly used "vocation," "profession," and "art" for nursing.

Other St Thomas' doctors would be supportive, agreeing on the need for training. Quaker cardiologist Dr Thomas B. Peacock (1812–1882), for example, wrote Nightingale in 1871 to thank her for a copy of her new *Introductory Notes on Lying-in Institutions*. In his long medical career, he said, "I could not but feel that the great defect in our hospital management was the nursing." From the first, he "thoroughly sympathized" with her efforts to "improve the character of hospital nurses,"[4] which had proved very effective.

St Thomas' authorities and the Nightingale Fund arranged for the nursing school, which opened in June 1860, but always had strained relations, as the hospital tended to regard the pupils as cheap labour and was less concerned than the Fund about training. Nightingale consulted medical officer Whitfield frequently on the running of the training program, such as on rules for the pupils and diet tables, and then on the site for the new building when the hospital had to move (from its original site near Tower Bridge). As interest in nursing at other hospitals grew, he worked with her on ward size and arrangements, furniture, operating space, and hospital plans. She sought his views also on difficulties with their matron in Sydney, New South Wales, and on a replacement for the excellent matron who died on the job in Liverpool.[5] Their correspondence, from 1858 to 1872, shows cordiality, mutual respect, and practicality. His letters include thanks for game she sent him, a frequent gift to obliging correspondents. She, of course, also did favours for him and the hospital, such as arranging for Queen Victoria to lay the cornerstone in 1868 and to open the new building in 1871.

However, after a few years of giving good lectures, Whitfield stopped, began to turn up intoxicated in the wards, flirted, and was overly familiar with nurses and pupils – what we would call sexual harassment – short of sexual assault. This became known all over the hospital, but Nightingale found out about the lack of lectures only by a circuitous route, when a Swedish nurse, back in Sweden, mentioned it in a printed pamphlet, seen by someone in Denmark, who reported it to Nightingale. She was mightily embarrassed, for the school specified lectures by the resident medical officer in its newspaper advertisements. She was also troubled to find out that a nursing sister had no idea that Whitfield had any obligation to teach.[6] In October 1872, she sent Henry Bonham Carter, secretary of the Nightingale Fund Council and her first cousin, to obtain his resignation.[7]

What Nightingale knew about Dr Whitfield's misconduct is not clear. Mrs Wardroper never informed her about either it or his quitting lecturing. From that time on, Nightingale gave much more time to overseeing the school's work and started meeting with pupils at the end of their first year. Most of her letters to Wardroper are missing, but the latter's to her fill five thick volumes in the British Library. The letters give much detail, evidently in response to questions.

In a major repercussion from the fiasco, Nightingale created, contrary to her matron's wishes, the position of "home sister." She would have preferred "under matron" or "mistress of probationers" ("probationer" was the term for student nurse), but the matron objected. The home sister ran the Nightingale Home (the student nurses' residence) and, more important, the tutoring of the pupils (she had been a governess for twenty years). Tutoring had not been provided before. Wardroper did not allow the home sister into the wards, but the latter sat in on the medical instructor's classes, took notes, and coached the pupils for their exams. Mary S. Crossland, the longest-serving home sister, conveniently for us, reported regularly to Nightingale on those classes by letter and occasional meetings.[8]

Whitfield's lectures were probably the first given to nurses in any organized training program. Nuns (both Roman Catholic and Anglican) were given ward training, but no lectures are known of. Kaiserswerth gave deaconess training in pedagogy and the Bible, but not in nursing: not one class. Dr Valentine Seaman (1770–1817) lectured to nurses at New York Hospital as early as 1798, but not as part of a training program, and the practice ended on his death. Dr Susan Dimock began classes for nurses at the New England Hospital for Women and Children, in Roxbury, Massachusetts, in 1872, or twelve years after Whitfield's began.[9]

Surgeon John Croft (1833–1905) succeeded Whitfield as medical instructor to the nurses. He was rated as less able as a lecturer, but solid and steady. He began his appointment by asking for a meeting with Nightingale. He sent her his syllabus for approval – she asked for no changes. She further entirely approved, and more than approved, of his

"Course of Reading" and ordered the books he wanted.[10] His lectures were published, subsidized by the Nightingale Fund, so that what he taught is on record.[11] Among other things, they show rudimentary teaching about germ theory as early as 1873. The tutor's notes from his lectures are another useful source on content. Nightingale flattered Croft, who had been sent them "by Providence," she said, "for surgeons, as well as saints, are made in heaven."[12]

Classes initially were only once every two weeks, with occasional extras, for example, on bones. Increasingly, other doctors were brought in to give additional lectures. Nightingale, in the same (flattering) letter, inquired whether Croft might give a "more advanced" course for ward sisters and potential superintendents of nursing, but apparently this never happened. Croft assigned chapters of Nightingale's *Notes on Nursing* as reading, even though it was never intended as a textbook.

Nightingale took to Croft the problem of the better-educated pupils buying, borrowing, and begging for "disconnected, desultory and untrained medical" reading – she crossed out "dabbling." She worried about their thinking that they knew more than they really did. Their matron in Sydney gave lectures on anatomy! Educated women – "free Britons" – would read, she concluded, so all the school could do was to guide it and examine them on it.[13]

Croft was Nightingale's ally, along with Dr John Sutherland, when sanitary defects became apparent at the new St Thomas'. He updated her on useful information he picked up on visits to other hospitals, and she kept notes on their meetings. In 1874, for example, disinfection procedures for ovariotomies (removal of ovarian cysts) were the subject. In 1878, a meeting concerned a nurse who had succumbed to "finger poisoning," or septicaemia.[14] In 1887, Nightingale passed complaints about the pupils' food on to him. When he dismissed them, she asked for a "dietary," and gave more specifics on the complaints: lack of variety, lack of milk, and lack of sufficient supper.[15] In 1890, when the next matron resigned, Nightingale consulted with Croft on candidates for her successor.[16]

Croft shared Nightingale's vision and general orientation to health and healing. Their correspondence, over twenty years, shows his pleasure in working with her. He was honoured on his retirement, with a gift and a tribute.[17] He wrote Nightingale occasionally after that, sent her lilies of the valley on her birthday in 1897, and made a last visit in 1900. Nightingale left him £100 in her will.[18]

Increasingly, established experts gave lectures to the nurses, including, for many years, chemist Albert J. Bernays (1823–1892), on food, and, after him, neurologist Seymour J.K. Sharkey (1847–1929), physician John Syer Bristowe, FRS (1827–1895), Wyndham Rowland Dunstan, later knighted (1861–1949), on chemistry, Edward Seaton, on hygiene, and Frederick LeGros Clark (1811–1892), surgeon, whose lectures, Nightingale heard, were "far from what he says."[19] An eminent surgeon, Henry Hugh Clutton (1860–1909), gave lectures 1895–1900 that were well liked. C.J. Cullingworth (1841–1908) lectured to staff members and extra nurses at St Thomas' in 1892.[20]

Nightingale recorded comments on the lecturing doctors by the children's ward sister: "Mr Clutton the favourite – he is so thorough – and he likes to pinch and slap and tickle the little patients – and then he likes them to give it him back again. Dr Bristowe very kind, but not playful. Nor Dr Ord – *he* is too dignified."[21]

When Dr Dunstan began teaching chemistry in 1892, Nightingale wrote Henry Bonham Carter that she wished to go over the old material with Miss Crossland, the tutor, before he started. She wanted the classes "to go most simply into elementary chemical principles as regards air: good / foul; water: good / foul; earth, ditto / ditto, food: value of / no value." She was keen on

the practical applications of *Elementary* Chemistry to Hygiene. I would insist upon particularly. P.S. Lord Stanley (Derby) said to me, "you know nothing will be done about foul air in churches, theatres, Exeter Hall, cottage bedrooms, and indeed all bedrooms, till we have invented something, something on the inside walls would be best, which would *change colour of itself* when the *air* was *foul.* I have again and again felt the truth of this – again and again asked a medical officer of health fired by it, but did nothing. Would you ask Mr Dunstan? At all events, it sets them thinking. Everywhere I believe is analysis of *air* now practised.

Would you ask Mr Dunstan about this? simply I mean as regards *foul* air. And there are so many different sorts of foulness. Make him talk about it. Could he teach the probationers in *English,* and not in Latin? I feel, as you do, how risky it is to begin with a new man for us, and a new hospital man, besides, whom we can't oust.[22]

St Thomas' veteran Dr William Miller Ord, her own physician, became an instructor to nurses, replacing J.S. Bristowe, teaching circulation, the lungs, skin, and cholera. When he started, he sent Nightingale a list of the courses offered. In a note of 1892, she stated that he was "of course" to choose his own subjects, following Dr Bristowe, while Dr Sharkey's lectures on anatomy and physiology were to be accommodated to his.[23] In 1893, Dr Ord asked if he could bring his daughter to the nurses' classes; Nightingale agreed.[24]

Florence Haig Brown, when she was "home sister," or tutor, at St Thomas', wanted Ord to write a preface for her planned "handbook on physiology."[25] For whatever reason, this volume did not appear, although her more modest, unprefaced *Probationer's Primer: A Guide for the 1st Year Nurse* came out in 1896.

For many years, at least 1889–98, Dr Ord was also Nightingale's own physician. He ordered more bed rest for her, and particularly that she stop seeing people for a time. Latterly, his son, "young Dr Ord," visited to treat her with a galvanic battery, or, in her words, "he comes every day to galvanize me." That same letter also related that Ord "told me exactly what you did about Baltimore hospitals – told me of another St Thomas' nurse, Venables, who is matron of another hospital at Baltimore. He says there is no nursing worth having in the States but what an Englishwoman is at the head of it, etc. He is going to marry Dr [John Shaw] Billings's daughter – told me what Dr Billings's position is."[26] That was Marie Clare Billings (b. 1863).

Numerous references to Dr Ord senior appear in Nightingale's correspondence and notes. One intriguing item reports him stating: "To 'breathe' a vein is an old quasi-colloquial expression – certainly more than 200 years old. It means blood-letting and 'probably expresses the sense of relief when a much-distended vein is tapped.'"[27] Leeching continued as a treatment, and nurses were routinely taught it.

Alexander Oberlin MacKellar (1845–1904), senior surgeon at St Thomas', offered to give clinical demonstration lectures on bandaging and splints, in his own ward, to probationers, Henry Bonham Carter told Nightingale; he did not consider his motives "ulterior," but did not want to be beholden to him.[28] MacKellar was also an army surgeon, so that Nightingale consulted him on army nursing, related in chapter 4.

John (later Sir John) Simon (1816–1904), was a notable public-health expert and a surgeon at St Thomas'. Nightingale's relationship with him was strained. He opposed her (and Sutherland and Farr's) views on the siting of the Netley army hospital. She thought he was cavalier in his remarks, effectively dismissing the value of strict sanitary conditions. However, he produced an enormous amount of valuable material as medical officer of health, very much in line with their positions. He also brought Semmelweis's breakthrough on reducing maternal deaths in Vienna to the attention of British doctors, as we see in chapter 6. Nightingale could have used the information in 1861 when the midwifery ward was set up at King's College Hospital.

So many of Simon's measures against cholera would also have suppressed other diseases. His holistic, socially conscious stance on many issues of public health makes one wonder about Nightingale's negative opinion of him. For her, his great mistake was accepting deaths from infectious diseases as inevitable in areas with crowded housing and poor ventilation. Public-health authorities, he wrote, "are practically almost powerless against these evils" – scarlatina, smallpox, typhoid, and typhus.[29]

Home Secretary Robert Lowe took Nightingale to task for her view of Simon, who had been his unofficial adviser. He suggested "an undue prejudice in your mind against him" and pointed out that the "medical world has its factions" as much as the political. As "proof that Simon has not overlooked the subject of hospitals," Lowe referred her to several pages in a report of Simon's in 1840 on preventable disease! He then suggested that her *Notes on Hospitals* was flawed in its statistical analysis because it used the proportion of deaths to beds.[30] She had more ambitious goals than did Simon. While he accepted that broader unsanitary conditions would cause unpreventable diseases, she looked to bad housing itself as a problem to be dealt with.

In 1897, at age eighty-one, Simon sought rapprochement with Nightingale. He sent her a copy of his *English Sanitary Institutions* (1890), with a dedication in a frail hand, indicating that it could give her "no new knowledge in its main subject matter, but incidentally it tells the story of what I have tried to do for the interests which you have so signally promoted and, believe me, it is with deep reverence for your devotion of life to the cause you have made your own that I venture, in now preparing to leave the scene, to beg for a little place in your recollection." He thanked her also for agreeing to admit his grandniece to her school, "at my dear old hospital." He hoped that she would find a "permanent place in the surgical service of the hospital," which did not happen, for reasons unknown. He signed off "with truer respect than my crippled handwriting can express, ever your faithful servant, John Simon."[31]

Dr John Bristowe's assessment of nursing, old and reformed, is of interest, as he had trained at St Thomas' and had spent eight years there before the Nightingale School opened, for a total of twenty-eight years. He had early criticized Nightingale's statement on contagion (see chapter 1). Then, in a treatise of 1867, without mentioning her, he gave a brief, but strong statement on hygiene – "the science of health" – echoing her concerns in *Notes on Nursing*.[32] In a later paper, he praised her work, noting the difference trained nurses made. He conceded that the (early) ward sisters were at least "respectable," but the "inferior nurses" "little more than ordinary charwomen," slovenly, dirty, and quite untrustworthy; they received small wages, brought and prepared their own food, and scrubbed the ward floors. Such "unsatisfactory" nursing afflicted "all London hospitals," he stated. He credited the matron, Mrs Wardroper, the treasurer, Richard Baggallay, and the resident medical officer, R.G. Whitfield, for ending the worst practices, then detailed what a difference Nightingale had made.[33]

Further, nursing made "probably the greatest advance in the practice of medicine," he wrote, by tending patients with the most dangerous or critical diseases. This was as important as "the advice and care of well-trained medical practitioners" themselves. The duties of nurse and doctor supplemented each other. On observation, his remarks aligned with Nightingale's: "Without the information which a skilful and observant nurse can always impart with respect to the patient under her charge, and the feeling that any directions he may give will be faithfully and intelligently carried out, the medical man's relation to the patient must always be unsatisfactory."

Bristowe also listed numerous hospitals that had matrons who had trained at the Nightingale School: Sydney, Netley, Edinburgh, St Mary's, Westminster, Putney, Liverpool Royal Infirmary, Liverpool Southern Hospital, Marylebone Workhouse Infirmary, Salisbury Infirmary, Lincoln County Hospital, Leeds Infirmary, Huntingdon County Hospital, Cumberland Infirmary (Carlisle), and several district nursing organizations, including the headquarters. He also suggested that the nursing "home" might be dispensed with in some cases, with nursing students living with friends, not a prospect Nightingale ever contemplated. Demand for skilled nurses would be greater than for physicians, he thought, hence the need for good teaching facilities.

Hospital Forms and St Bartholomew's Hospital

James Paget (1814–1899), made baronet in 1871, was a distinguished surgeon at St Bartholomew's Hospital, London. Nightingale's correspondence with him began in 1859, when she asked him to try out a new form to standardize collection of hospital statistics and allow comparisons in death rates and hospital stays across hospitals:

> I have had a set of new forms prepared (with the Registrar General's sanction) for hospital statistics. I should be very glad if St Bartholomew's would be so good as to fill up a set on trial. But, before presuming to send them one, I should like to ascertain to what extent the information *can* be obtained from the hospital books. The following are the data required to fill up the forms. Of these will be required: the *Remainings* on the last day of any year, say 1857, and of the remains at the end of 1858 (a full year).
> 1. *Age*/ 2. *Sex*/ 3. *Disease*. Also, the *Admissions … Death, Discharged Incurable* and the *Duration of the Cases*. N.B. *Age, Sex* and *Disease* must be shown for each of these headings. St Thomas' Hospital has been so good as to consent to fill up these forms for me for one (past) year. But they have been an immense time about it.[34]

Her letter began with a compliment for Paget's "skill and trouble and time you gave to her [their maid's] poor thumb. I used to think you must feel as if you made a great expenditure of power upon a very little thing. But it was not a little thing to her, and she is now recovering (quite) at my father's place in Derbyshire [Lea Hurst], thanks to you."[35]

Hospitals sent in their statistics, as Nightingale reported later to Paget. Among these, "St Bartholomew has unquestionably the best," although she thought "he [the statistician there] might do still more in improving his statistical forms. And Guy['s Hospital], who used to be the best, is now unquestionably the worst." She wished she could have used Paget's "invaluable materials for the record of 'Causes of Death after Operations.'"[36]

Her work on this project, however, never came to any consequential result. In 1861, she told Paget that St Bart's had produced "the first statistical report which is worth having. The army hospitals are now using similar forms, but they have not yet published any. No one can look at what you have done without seeing what a fund of information for future reduction [analysis] has been collected." However, it would, she felt, need further work by future statisticians.[37] In recognition of Paget's considerable work, she gave him an inkstand, now at the Royal Society of Medicine, "in grateful acknowledgement of most kind assistance."

St Bart's was as old and large as St Thomas', but was slow to accept trained nursing. In 1861, Nightingale sent Paget material about her new school – "an experiment, which has not yet lasted a year," which she hoped would be "much improved upon by you" and others. She asked him to send her "any scheme which may be drawn up by your Apostle [St Bartholomew]," offering to do her best "to revise it, by our experience."[38] However, it was not until 1878 that St Bart's established a training school, with the matron and nurses who returned to England after their dismal experience of nursing at the Montreal General.

Nightingale also, in that 1861 letter, said that she was "transported in pleasure" at the tables Paget had sent her: "I thought they were so good. You may laugh at my enthusiasm. But it is not peculiar to myself. I once heard exactly the same feeling of pleasure expressed by a historian at the sight of a well-made-out column of dates that I feel at a well-compiled table of facts."

In 1862, Paget loaned Nightingale his copy of a book on English surgery by Paul Topinard (1830–1911), *Quelques aperçus sur la chirurgie anglaise* (1860), which stirred up for her memories of its truths and errors, that is, regarding "the old dog's hospital." The book, based on Topinard's visits to English hospitals, esteemed English practices over French. Paget wanted a "Paris medical authority" on an assertion of hers that pyaemia was indigenous in Paris. She had seen it in the wards looked after by the legendary Philippe Joseph Roux, surgeon-in-chief, since dead, at La Charité. Dr Shrimpton, who practised in Paris, then provided an answer, developed from work with the military medical pioneer Baron Larrey (1766–1842).[39]

In 1863, Nightingale sent Paget copies of the operation tables, "completed, in the flower of their perfection," which she considered his achievement. She was sending copies "to our principal London hospitals," but was "not so young" as to expect that they would "be accepted on the face of their obvious usefulness at once." She thought the hospitals would "carp" and alter this and that, but that "in the end a great deal of good will be done, if only by directing attention to the subject, and awakening them to make their own criticisms."[40] She was overly optimistic.

Over the years, Nightingale referred numerous family members to Paget. In 1869, she described him to Sir Harry Verney as "the safest surgeon and soundest authority in England for cancer, and certainly will not 'use the knife' if not expedient or necessary." In the letter, she also discouraged her brother-in-law from consulting "quacks." They made their dishonest reputations by professing to cure cancer, but the tumour they cured was not cancerous.[41]

Her father visited London in 1872 to see Paget about his throat.[42] When he died two years later (of an unrelated cause), she duly informed Paget.[43] In 1873, she wrote him for an appointment for her friend the great classicist Benjamin Jowett, master of Balliol College.[44]

When Sir Harry Verney had an accident in 1876, Nightingale recommended Paget. Moreover, since other surgeons "think it only an honour to meet him in consultation," it would cause no offence to go to him. She was also concerned about the nursing care Verney would receive – for shock, probably frequent feeding in small quantities – but "I am not the least judge and it is most foolish to urge when not on the spot."[45] Paget did look after him, and he did well.[46] Sir Harry's regular physician was Sir Henry Acland, regius professor of medicine at Oxford.

Nightingale and Paget sent each other their books: *Notes on Nursing* and *Introductory Notes on Lying-in Institutions* from her, one from him in 1878, with an apology that he had little to offer her (most of his books were on surgery). In 1885 he praised her work in his Abernethian Lecture to the students at St Bart's, or, as he put it, "I ventured to use your name." In it, he acknowledged how bad the unreformed nursing had long been – contrary to the observations of John Flint South. He thought that the ward sisters were good, but the ordinary nurses not, most of whom "were rough, dull, unobservant, and untaught women; of the best it could only be said that they were kindly and careful and attentive in doing what they were told to do." The change came after the Crimean War, when "Miss Nightingale showed what might be done in hospitals by highly cultivated, courageous, and benevolent gentlewomen." Her "noble example," he further argued, had "more influence than anything else that can be told of in the production of the happy changes" that doctors then at work then enjoyed.[47]

When Isla Stewart, a Nightingale nurse, became the matron at St Bart's in 1887, Paget found it difficult to respond to Nightingale's inquiries – he was "so seldom" there now – but asked former colleagues. They told him that Stewart was "well esteemed" and that the medical staff would help her make the changes she sought. She needed only patience; already the changes made were far more than could have been expected.[48]

Paget's son, in his memoir of his father, described Nightingale as being, with Sir John Simon and Professor Rudolf Virchow, "one of his three oldest living friends."[49] Nightingale's esteem for Paget senior can be seen in a letter she sent him when he was ill in 1881: "Among the many, many thousands to whom your life is precious, none more than Florence Nightingale will pray for your health or rejoice in your recovery. May God grant you to us all!" As well, she thanked him for "two invaluable papers."[50]

Workhouse Doctors

Establishing professional nursing at the dreaded workhouse infirmaries was one of Nightingale's most notable achievements, the one closest to her original "call to service," or serving the sick poor. As for other work, there were doctors who shared her goals, but on this issue she moved further and faster than they could. No one before her introduced trained nurses into the workhouse infirmaries, where "pauper nurses" drank their token wages and stole their patients' liquor. Bed sharing was still common, as numerous official reports show. Reformer Louisa Twining, an ally on the cause, initially went no further than to propose *visiting* workhouse inmates. The idea that these people should receive nursing care as good as that provided at the best hospitals was Nightingale's. In time, both doctors and reformers, like Twining, took courage and raised their goals.

The first doctor to encourage Nightingale in this reform was Henry Bence Jones, FRS (1813–1873), a distinguished chemist, whom she knew before Crimea when he was a physician at her Harley Street hospital. The two corresponded during the Crimean War on what she would take up afterwards. Clearly they had discussed the workhouse possibility earlier at Harley Street.

Bence Jones told Nightingale that there "were at present no means for training nurses in the London hospitals," but mere "permission," which was only "toleration," and that not easily borne. He made some recommendations for how to accommodate nurse training in hospital work, such as through a "superintendent day nurse," with no ward responsibilities, to direct and instruct the pupils. He asked for Nightingale's advice.[51] He wrote her again in February 1856 (letter missing). Her reply was frank and revealing:

> If it please God to give me life and health ... I shall certainly devote that life and health to the one object which we have talked about, and I shall certainly *not* spend any portion of that life in training nurses for *rich* families, except *by parentheses*, but shall begin in the poorest and most neglected institution I can find. This is the only plan I have ... It will be my object to remedy deficiencies among those who can't help themselves and not among those who can. So that you may safely enlist me for any plan of the kind you mention.[52]

For the Poor Law Board, Bence Jones wrote a report on the St Pancras Workhouse Infirmary in London in 1856. It noted overcrowding, smells, patients left on the floor from lack of beds, and sick patients and staffers. His heartfelt report called for government action, which did not materialize.[53] It seems that he did nothing further on the subject.

Bence Jones was named to the original Nightingale Fund Council and served on it until 1863. He was one of the first people to be sent a copy of her *Notes on Nursing*. He published, as well as a great deal on medical work, a biography of chemist Michael Faraday, which Nightingale read avidly. Indeed, when he sent her a copy, she wrote back, "But do you suppose that I had not read it?"[54] Their last contact was in 1872, when she needed a certificate of death for a former patient at Harley Street.[55]

Dr (later Sir) Edward Henry Sieveking (1816–1904) supported Nightingale on workhouse reform, although his own efforts had focused on pauper nurses. He came from a Westphalian family, and Nightingale had visited his philanthropist aunt, Amalie Sieveking, in Hamburg in 1850. The Sievekings' eldest daughter was named Florence Amelia, presumably not a coincidence.

A pamphlet of 1849 by Dr Sieveking urged the use of pauper nurses in the wider community.[56] Nightingale considered it wrong to employ them even in workhouses, let alone to send them out to nurse the sick at home. For Sieveking, however, there were enough, even a "large body of women," who had "proved themselves to be trustworthy" and could be raised from the "able-bodied inmates" of workhouses for the "honourable" occupation of nursing. In Liverpool, this proved not to be the case.

While Nightingale never believed that inmates of workhouses could be relied on to nurse, she wanted the children there to gain work experience through non-nursing jobs at hospitals, such as in the kitchen or cleaning, and then, in their early twenties, apply for admission to a nursing school. (Nurse training did not start until that age, while workhouse children left at age fourteen.) Sieveking's proposal, however, assumed that some inmates, at least, were reliable.

Sieveking's approach was in line with what workhouse authorities liked – and it would cost almost nothing. One stipulation was that the families attended to would pay not the nurses, but the workhouse treasurer. Nursing without pay would lower salary levels generally, or be unfair to the many nurses who needed to earn a living, a point Nightingale made in countering Elizabeth Garrett's espousal of volunteer, "lady" nursing, as noted in chapter 6.

Sieveking developed the subject further in an 1854 paper to the Epidemiological Society that called for raising a "preventive staff of nurses" from workhouses across the country for times of epidemic and other diseases. Lack of nursing, rest, and seclusion, he said, not necessarily bad hygienic conditions, caused a great deal of poverty and destitution. The nurses would work under medical attendants. On average, workhouses had fifteen fit men and twenty-three fit women who could be recruited, an unlikely number, for which he cited the Poor Law Board as a source. Dr Joseph Rogers commented that the paper was "scarcely sufficiently relative to epidemic disease to bring before the Society."[57]

Sieveking wrote Nightingale in 1864 with his views on how to organize district nursing, but whether they had evolved is not clear. He urged her to put his proposal before "people of influence."[58] It seems that no one acted on any of his proposals. Serious workhouse reformers like Louisa Twining shared Nightingale's view that inmates were unsuitable for nursing, especially on account of their drinking. Sieveking's plan "was never carried out," she said, on account of its obvious problems.[59]

Yet medical historian F.B. Smith[60] credited Sieveking with proposing a viable way to train inmates as nurses, both in the workhouse infirmaries and in their local neighbourhoods, but suggested he gave up because he did not want to work with Nightingale. Far from abandoning his project, however, Sieveking told her that his results had been "almost invisible." Further, "to realize the plan completely would demand the devotion of a lifetime and for such a sacrifice I was not qualified." He offered to visit her and give what limited assistance he could.[61] They did not meet then, but he would help her establish trained nursing at St Mary's Hospital, Paddington, as related below.

All but one of the "workhouse doctors" (Nightingale's label for would-be reformers) lacked appointments at such an institution. That exception was Dr Joseph Rogers (1821–1889) of the Strand Union Workhouse (London), who was dismissed, proving how precarious those posts were. He is also the only workhouse medical officer to have left an account of his work.[62] When he joined the staff, there were no paid nurses, and the pauper nurses were typically intoxicated by early afternoon – the master gave out the "stimulants" (alcohol) at 7 a.m., and pauper nurses stole wine and brandy from the patients. An inspection in 1866 found that 446 patients at the Strand Union shared 332 beds; the cubic space per patient was half of that specified for prisoners, and one quarter of that for barracks.[63]

By giving evidence to a select committee of the House of Commons, Rogers succeeded in obtaining a budget for drugs, previously paid for out of the doctor's own remuneration. He argued that the workhouse authorities had the same obligation to pay for drugs as they had to provide food and clothing,[64] but some routinely saved money by cutting the dose or giving a placebo.

Nightingale saw no way to advance workhouse nursing in the immediate post-war period, and took up the cause only in 1864, when Liverpool philanthropist and nursing supporter and patron William Rathbone, soon to be a Liberal MP, gave her the opportunity. One workhouse doctor from that city appears in chapter 6, on midwifery, when he was a useful informant and example for Nightingale. Both the work there and its extension into London have been described in detail elsewhere. Here I note only that the Liverpudlian doctors were impressed with the trained nursing. Dr J.H. Barnes called it "an undoubted success," citing "restoration of health" and the "relief of suffering ... inscribed in the hearts and memories of grateful recipients, of the convalescent, the suffering, the dying."[65] Dr Robert Gee, reporting on the value of the "paid nursing" in its first year, told the workhouse committee of his "earnest desire to see the system introduced into all the parochial hospitals of the kingdom."[66]

Nightingale helped behind the scenes in the extension. C.P. Villiers, president of the Poor Law Board, in effect England's minister of social welfare, sent Poor Law inspector H.B. Farnall to see her in February 1865. She and Farnall devised the "form of inquiry" to collect data from

London workhouses. Villiers ordered a circular to all the boards of guardians suggesting they appoint trained nurses and discontinue the use of untrained inmates, but to little effect.[67]

The attention Nightingale drew to workhouse defects in April 1865 prompted a *Lancet* study of workhouse conditions, by Dr Ernest Hart (1835–1898),[68] then on the journal's staff and later editor of the *British Medical Journal.* This paper was also published in December in the progressive *Fortnightly Review.* It showed only 3,738 beds in eighteen regular London hospitals, compared to 26,555 in workhouse infirmaries, plus 1,683 for the insane. This count included inmates labelled "able-bodied," but who were "sick and infirm," that is, two-thirds of the "able-bodied" were in fact diseased or infirm. Workhouses, in other words, had very few "willfully unemployed" slackers. The vast majority could not work for reasons of illness, age, or a chronic condition. Dr Hart's report was clear: skilled nursing was "deficient" and not easy to remedy; the majority of nurses were paupers, unfitted for the work; and they were unpaid or given a small gratuity.

Nightingale's formulation of the ABCs of workhouse reform in 1865 set out what she considered essential:

A. To insist on the great principle of separating the sick, insane, incurable, and children from the usual pauper population ...

B. To advocate a general metropolitan rate for this purpose and a central administration ...

C. To leave the pauper and casual population ... under the boards of guardians ... Centralize all the sanitary powers at present exercised by the guardians, relieve them from those duties entirely, provide a scheme of suburban hospitals and asylums: 1. For sick; 2. For infirm, aged and invalids; 3. For insane and imbeciles; 4. Industrial schools for children.[69]

Dr Hart's revelations helped force a parliamentary committee to investigate. He told Nightingale that she was the "author" of that investigation, presumably referring to her protest of conditions and success in Liverpool.

In 1856, Dr Rogers founded the Metropolitan Poor Law Medical Officers' Association. In 1867, after Nightingale had both called for more and shown that professional nursing could be taken into a workhouse (in Liverpool), he formed the more ambitious Association for the Improvement of London Workhouse Infirmaries. He, with Drs Francis Edmund Anstie (1833–1874) and Ernest Hart, served as its honorary secretaries. Its initial focus was London metropolitan-area workhouse infirmaries, but it later campaigned for reforms in the whole country.

As for the three "workhouse doctors," Nightingale considered Anstie, physician at Westminster Hospital, the "best": "He knew more than all the College of Physicians put together, and was ever ready to help me in the workhouse work."[70] Anstie was better than Hart, she thought, who had been "muzzled" by Gathorne Hardy, president of the Poor Law Board, during the inquiry on cubic space in workhouse infirmaries.[71] Hart was "a good fellow," but, she told royal engineer Douglas Galton, "very fond of giving me, mysteriously, 'important information.'"[72] Her numerous letters to Anstie have disappeared, but his to her, 1866–68, show how close their views were. Both wanted comprehensive reform of the Poor Law – not just of the workhouse infirmaries. Both paid careful attention to administrative structure.

These points appear also in personal correspondence, for Mrs Anstie came from the Wass family, owners of a lead smelter near the Nightingales' Lea Hurst in Derbyshire. Hence Dr Anstie, when on a family visit, met father William Edward Nightingale "on the green." Anstie wrote him that he was pleased to learn that his younger daughter agreed with his view that decisions on workhouse hospitals should be made by experts, not the "unskilled representatives of ratepayers," who should "only deal with financial matters":[73]

Progress on workhouse reform was set back by the Liberals going out of government and the departure of C.P. Villiers as minister. He had listened to Nightingale, and even sought her out, although her proposed reforms went beyond anything he could contemplate. He was replaced by a Conservative minister, Gathorne Hardy. As Nightingale feared, the bill Hardy brought in fell far short of the comprehensive reform she had hoped for. Dr Anstie was similarly critical. When it appeared, he wrote her that it was not workable. Those who founded the Workhouse Improvement Association, from the first, "altogether distrusted the possibility of working the extremely cumbersome machinery of Mr Hardy's act." For the sake of the sick, and the "whole administration" of the Poor Law in large towns:

I am convinced, and indeed have always believed, that no good will be effected till there is a uniform rating and till the whole executive (as regards the sick) is left to a very small number of highly skilled persons who shall be so remunerated as to be able to give their whole time to the matter. The ordinary (ratepayers') representatives on the committee ought, as you justly observe, to have nothing to do with anything but finances. They should in fact be in the position of the "committee" of an ordinary London hospital.

It will need tremendous pressure on the government [to] make them see the necessity of this. But something surely must be done in next Parliament. The attempts that are being made to put Mr Hardy's act in operation are nothing but helpless floundering. There is no plan, no uniformity of action, and there will be any amount of private jobbery and corruption and waste.[74]

In a later missive, Anstie asked Florence Nightingale to write to the *Times*, which she did not. Nor could she undertake "the coaching of MPs for any Poor Law Parliamentary inquiry next session," which he thought needed doing.[75]

Despite her considerable reservations about Gathorne Hardy's commitment to reform, Nightingale agreed to write a brief for the committee he set up. The request came from the committee chair, Dr Sir Thomas Watson (1792–1882). The terms of reference – cubic space – were far too narrow for her liking, while she wanted the focus to be on the quality of nursing needed; even the requisite superficial space per patient was more significant than cubic space, she thought. As she exclaimed to Douglas Galton, on reading Dr Markham's contribution: "Cubic space be hanged! (excuse swearing – I spend my life in it). It is not the One Thing Needful [Luke 10:42]. It is hardly the first thing needful."[76] Naturally, she turned the subject to the nursing itself, and how the Liverpool example showed it could be done. Cubic space merited but a short paragraph.[77]

Anstie died in 1874 from conditions of his work. He had been called to investigate deaths at an "uninspected" institution, as Nightingale put it, a school run by the Patriotic Fund in Wandsworth. Doing a post mortem there, he suffered a slight wound to his hand, which resulted in septicaemia and acute pleuropneumonia. Nightingale said his death was due to "sewer

WORK WITH CIVILIAN DOCTORS

gas," from exposure to the defective sewers he believed were the cause of the pupils' deaths. She contributed £5 to a memorial fund for him:

> How great is the loss to our country in Dr Anstie. Had he lived, many thousands of deaths would not have died (if I may use such an expression), which now will fall victims to the want of public health measures, of which he was such a devoted supporter … When we were agitating to improve the new Sanitary Acts by giving certain powers of inspection to local boards, we had in view such cases as the place where he laid down his valuable life to serve his country, on what is really the battlefield of this day, both in England and India. They would not follow our advice (though they will some day). And there are many, many, buildings where similar deaths are now taking place, and will continue to take place from want of this inspection.[78]

Nightingale's reforms made a difference. A letter to the *Times* by Dr Hart in 1871 described the nursing at Hampstead Hospital, a workhouse infirmary, as being "in precise accordance with recommendations of Miss Nightingale."[79] She had further contact with Hart on the Franco–Prussian War, related in chapter 4.

The Edinburgh Royal Infirmary, "Beastly Den of Thieves"

The Edinburgh Royal Infirmary that Nightingale was asked to "inspect" in 1857 was the old building of 1729, replaced twice since. The "new," pavilion-style hospital for which she gave advice opened in 1879 – Britain's largest voluntary hospital (i.e., financed by public subscription). In 2003, a new hospital at yet another site was opened. When Nightingale was in Edinburgh in 1857 to meet with Sir John McNeill, she was taken around the city's Royal Infirmary by the distinguished surgeon Sir James Syme (1799–1870), a former Crimea hand. She met his nurse, Janet Porter, a responsible woman he trained to look after his patients – there was no training school anywhere at the time. Syme's assistant in surgery was Joseph Lister (1827–1912), who pioneered antiseptic surgery at his next hospital, the Glasgow Royal Infirmary. Lister (later Lord Lister) married

Syme's daughter and in 1869 succeeded him as chair of clinical surgery at the University of Edinburgh. "Professor Lister" is referred to from time to time in nurse reports back to Nightingale on the school and hospital.

When the medical instructor at St Thomas', Dr R.G. Whitfield, offered to do "anything" for Nightingale while in Edinburgh in 1858, she asked him "to go over the wards, especially the new Surgical and the High School wards, with the particular view of comparing their *construction* with what *we* think ought to be the requirements (in sanitary respects) of the construction of wards." Her recollection of them from her visit was "much too distinct and painful."[80]

Nightingale was pleased to be asked, in 1872, to send a matron and nurses to Edinburgh. St Thomas' was small and tame in comparison, and she always liked a challenge. The Royal Infirmary then was "wretched," a "beastly den of thieves," as she described it to Dr John Sutherland.[81] The invitation to send nurses dates from a few months after the appointment of a new medical superintendent, C.H. Fasson (1857–1892), who had been surgeon-general at the model pavilion hospital at Woolwich – the Herbert Hospital – after serving some years in India.[82] Fasson, in short, was an old army doctor who had seen hospitals without trained women nurses, in India, and then with them, at the Herbert.

As negotiations proceeded, Nightingale told Sutherland that she knew of no hospital, except the Vienna General, that approached Edinburgh in "badness, medical staff in both cases excluded." It was "a lawless place," with "drinking, profligate (old) night nurses," who were being gradually weeded out.[83] They did not like the new no-drinking rules, the hospital manager, James Hope, told Henry Bonham Carter. Yet it was hard to obtain replacements, as they were frightened of the place.[84]

A team of matron and nurses was duly sent, but the first matron, Elizabeth Ann Barclay, a well-qualified nurse, turned out to be a bad choice, for alcohol and opiate abuse. There is considerable correspondence among Dr Fasson, Nightingale, and Bonham Carter on her taking leave for recovery, her (temporary) replacement, then her eventual resignation when the recovery proved inadequate.[85] The delicate investigation of her situation is described elsewhere.[86] Her replacement was Angelique Lucille Pringle, later matron at St Thomas' and a nursing leader.

The Royal Infirmary's nursing school became in effect a second Nightingale school, training and sending out nurses not only to other Scottish hospitals, but elsewhere. Nightingale would often send nurses visiting from abroad to it for experience before they returned home. In 1896, she described the Royal Infirmary as the "best hospital" in Britain for nursing and organization.

The infirmary's head physician, Dr Joseph Bell (1837–1911), who was qualified in both medicine and surgery, had a famous pupil, Arthur Conan Doyle, who modelled his great character Sherlock Holmes on him. Bell famously could tell a patient's occupation and circumstances from small physical cues. For many years he gave lectures on surgery – the first – to the nurses. His wards and Joseph Lister's were side by side. In 1877, Bell published a textbook for nurses from his lecture notes, dedicated to Nightingale, "Chief of the Nursing Staff."[87] The preface describes the material therein as the main points of the lectures he delivered, over a twelve-year period, spoken conversationally. In 1895, Bell revised the volume thoroughly and added a general chapter of advice for a fourth edition.

Dr Bell visited Nightingale when in London in 1881. A.L. Pringle reported back to her that Bell was "much delighted" with seeing her and "would work harder than ever for us."[88] She obviously had a high opinion of him, for she canvassed for him to take the chair in surgery at Edinburgh when it became vacant, but he was not elected. She told Pringle, "I did my best and more than my best."[89] Two drafts of her letter of recommendation are available, which praise his clinical lectures for the nurses as "the best I ever heard of," his connection with the school "invaluable." She thought his "professional claims above those of his principal rival and far above those of the other competitors." While the other candidates had "talent," he had "genius."[90]

Bell's successor at the Royal Infirmary, in 1886, was Dr (later Sir) James Ormiston Affleck (1840–1922). Nightingale never met or corresponded with him, but heard good things of him from the matron. She responded that, while "we can never cease to regret Dr Bell," Dr Affleck "deserves our heartiest thanks."[91] Pringle commented that he was a "real doctor, who consults the sanitary conditions."[92] Nightingale hoped that he would publish his nursing lectures on fevers, which he did not: "I should like to send him my very grateful regards, if I dared. Oh! Make 'a beautiful Edinburgh series of nurses' books' – how invaluable they would be."[93] Affleck did write the entry on fever for the *Encyclopedia Britannica* and would ally with Bell in opposing state registration of nurses.

Nightingale asked Pringle about another Edinburgh doctor, John (later Sir John) Halliday Croom (1847–1923). She wanted him to publish his lectures on midwifery and the nursing required "in the various diseases of women. It would be so valuable. Then I would send that out."[94]

Ups and Downs at St Mary's Hospital, Paddington

St Mary's, Paddington, was the last of London's great voluntary hospitals, posh from its opening in 1851, with the queen as patron. From the start, it had a strong medical school with prominent doctors, including a goodly number of medical knights, baronets, and fellows of the Royal Society. Alexander Fleming discovered penicillin there in 1928. It has had numerous royal patients and royal births, most notably that of Prince George in 2013.

A few months after her return from the Crimean War in 1856, Nightingale was elected a "life governor" at St Mary's. Calling on that connection in 1859, she asked the hospital to use the uniform hospital forms she and Dr Farr had worked out,[95] which it did. In 1864, Dr Farr asked her to use her proxy vote at St Mary's to support Dr Edward Smith, FRS (1819–1874), for appointment. She was often asked for her proxy and gave it when she had a recommendation from someone she trusted. Farr explained that Smith had "coolly" asked him to approach her on his behalf. He thought him the "ablest of the three candidates," although he did not support his dietary, which he sent her.[96] The eventual appointee, however, was William Henry Broadbent (1835–1907), later made a baronet, a distinguished physician who fiercely opposed reformed nursing at St Mary's when it was finally brought in.

The hospital's first matron, Alicia Wright, was untrained, but a doctor's daughter. She made one bid, in 1865, for trained nursing through the Nightingale Fund, by writing to Mrs Wardroper, but for naught. Only in 1876, when Wright retired, did Dr Sieveking, cited above on pauper nurses and by then principal physician at St Mary's, approach Nightingale. He advised her that the hospital was about to advertise for a matron; salary £100. He explained, as she told her candidate, that "anyone" they recommended would get the post, "notwithstanding the necessity for advertising." She added her own opinion: "Nursing arrangement defective."[97]

Her nominee was Rachel Williams (later Norris, 1840–1908), nicknamed "the goddess" for her striking height and good looks, then assistant matron at Edinburgh. She stayed at Nightingale's home for the interviews, and the two conferred frequently, as they would throughout her stormy tenure at St Mary's. Nightingale advised her on her first meeting with Dr Sieveking, that he would be happy to see her "this morning at 10, at 17 Manchester Square [his residence]. I have nothing to suggest: your own wisdom will suggest to you much better than mine." She then gave much advice, beginning with "not to frighten Dr. S. by starting at once any proposal 'to reform the nursing system' or 'to have a training school.' Of course *St. Mary's* is *his* primary object. The proposition of the training school will have to come from us (he is chairman of the Medical Committee of the National Nursing Association and this will be a difficulty). Mrs. Wardroper went over St. Mary's with him yesterday (we wished she could have put it off till today)." Nightingale also mentioned that she had arranged for Williams to confer with both Mrs Wardroper and Henry Bonham Carter.

She also proposed that Williams suggest "that *you* should see *St. Mary's*. He may possibly say 'Now, at once.'"[98] She offered this counsel in a letter of 6 a.m., and another followed at 9: "*Will you particularly ask Dr. Sieveking not only what the matron's duties* will be, but what *assistance* she will have given her, *i.e., about her being allowed one assistant at least* (the *kitchen* is to be under her, as well as the wards and nursing). Mrs. Wardroper did not see the *matron's rooms*. You understand that your fate does not rest at all with Dr. Sieveking alone; there will be other measures to take, and, if he is unfavourable to some exigencies of ours, it does not follow that we shall not get them otherwise."

Nightingale's letter of reference to the governors was lengthy and thorough, reviewing Williams's experience and extolling her ability. She gave her own title as "Foundress of the 'Nightingale' Training Schools for Nurses."[99] Dr Bell wrote a letter of reference as well, from the Edinburgh Royal Infirmary.

Williams's salary at St Mary's was £225 per year, well above the £100 first specified (low for her qualifications). This high salary, however, contributed to her later downfall, when she was accused of having negotiated it by overstating what she had been offered elsewhere. Nightingale thought that this was a misunderstanding and defended her throughout.

On the job, Williams moved quickly to weed out the unqualified nurses, hire trained ones, and begin to give instruction. She brought some staff members with her from Edinburgh, and St Thomas' gave some. Nightingale sent her medical and nursing books.[100]

After only three weeks in the post, Williams wrote Nightingale that the surgeons were to sign a letter on the board's meeting day "recommending the removal and pensioning of Sister Thistlewayte, who has been in office as a sister over twenty years – takes opium [quite legal then] and is otherwise incapacitated. They wanted me to dismiss her discreetly, which would have been rather hard upon me – it was therefore concluded to do it as I have told you, which is a much better plan – and better for the old lady herself."[101] However, some of the doctors objected and went over Williams's head to have the decision reconsidered. A paper reviewing the correspondence commented that "many of the doctors had become used to these 'unreformed' nurses and felt comfortable with them, as they were generally docile."[102]

Dr Broadbent led the opposition, while Sieveking continued to support Williams, who considered resigning, but stayed on. Dr Sieveking wrote Henry Bonham Carter about "the disaster of yesterday," which quite stunned him.[103]

Also in 1877, Williams co-wrote a book on nursing with Alice Fisher. Things calmed down for a while. Nightingale asked to be remembered to the hospital secretary when she sent Williams New Year's greetings, with a pheasant, in 1882. She recalled that the statistics St Mary's provided were the "best of all the London hospitals."[104]

Difficulties about Williams's salary arose in the summer of 1884, as Dr Sieveking advised Nightingale, confirming his "continued support."[105] He kept her updated on the situation, while she devised strategy, calling in prestigious supporters.

Nightingale wanted a fight, not to let it "go by default," not "let the Devil win," as she told Williams. She appealed to Dr Sieveking, stating that "the good nursing" at St Mary's was at stake with "this most unpleasant affair." He had worked for the "good cause," and much had been done thanks to his "great influence." She asked "whether you think that a successful fight be made at your next Friday's board, where your presence will be so essential."[106] Sieveking then arrived at her house to talk, "so exceedingly 'aggravated,'" she told Williams, "(and no wonder) by the malice and injustice that he will not pledge himself to do anything – not even to appear at Friday's meeting – though he does not refuse." She then urged Williams to call in people for the meeting: "to get ten or twelve independent governors, all who will interest themselves in supporting the truth, to attend – but, besides this, to find an independent governor, better *not* a medical officer, who will speak on Friday, put the true view of the case, after having carefully got up the details … If your three friends each brought two independent governors and these six each brought one more, surely that would not be so difficult. But they must find a speaker. Now God defend the right."[107]

Conveniently, the president of the hospital was (Liberal) Lord Privy Seal Lord Carlingford. Nightingale sent brother-in-law Sir Harry Verney the next day to brief him, but he had already left the home of Lord Granville (foreign secretary). The opening of Parliament was that same day, so Nightingale undertook to write a letter, with Williams's input, to Carlingford, which Sir Harry would ask him to read and act on. Delicacy was required, so as not to reveal such "unhappy squabbles" as would alienate their ally, Dr Alfred Meadows (1833–1887), physician-accoucheur at St Mary's and first president of the British Gynaecological Society, founded 1884.

On the anniversary of the "Charge of Balaclava" (15 October 1854), as Nightingale noted on her letter, it seemed that "calamity" was averted, which it was not.[108] She explained to Verney that a "handsome compromise" in Williams's favour had been effected: "Lord Carlingford seems to have done exactly the right thing." He sent for Dr Meadows, showed him "our letters – which perhaps was not quite wise, but Dr Meadows in a very strong speech he made at the meeting said he had seen the letters, but rightly did not mention *from whom*)." Lord Carlingford, Meadows added, "disapproved of the reduction [in salary] as an injustice and recommended, if the whole could not be given, 'certainly a handsome compromise.' A Q.C. followed, showing the illegality of the procedure, of which the enemy's party had been guilty."[109]

However, at a meeting 31 October 1884, "Lord Carlingford's decision was *reversed*. And things are worse than ever," Nightingale told Sir Harry. "I was asked to get Lord Carlingford to attend, but he had a Cabinet and after that went to Balmoral. What is to be done? One can hardly write to Lord C. to Balmoral?"[110]

Nightingale wrote Williams to propose another attempt: "This is most disastrous – most disgraceful, the more reason not to fly before the enemy. It is all important to convince Lord Carlingford that we have been urging that which is right. No one can do that so properly as Dr Meadows. Dr Meadows should write to Lord C., that the two meet on Lord C.'s return to London from Balmoral, that he may convince Lord C. that right is on his side. If he succeeds in doing this, we may expect that Lord C. will take action, defend the right, and make it gain the day." One last point: "God will uphold the cause if we do not despair. St. Mary's shall not be ruined. 'Trust in God and keep your powder dry.'"[111]

Nightingale replied to Williams's next "sad little note" with a letter and a pheasant. She should not resign, but lay the "whole case" before the president, Lord Carlingford, and abide by his decision. She did not want to "waste" eight years of excellent work. "Do not throw up the 'sponge,' and you will not." 'Fight the good fight of faith,' the faith that God is on your side – and you must be on *His* side."[112] Yet another letter went with a pheasant.

The situation only worsened in the new year. The board, at a meeting in January 1885, discontinued the post of assistant to the matron, on the advice of the house and finance committees.[113] Williams told Nightingale that a "majority" on the board was on the "wrong side," a bitter pill to swallow.[114] Her letter the next day urged Williams to continue the fight, but within a week the latter was out. The compromise was that the board "nonconfirmed" its resolution, then accepted her resignation.[115] An advertisement for the vacant post of matron, salary £100 per year, was published in the *Times* on 14 February 1885.

While this last stage was in play, Nightingale was also dealing with a "terrible fright" at St Thomas' Hospital: in late January, eighteen nursing trainees were ill with "a sort of epidemic at the 'Home,' occasioned, as I am certain, by the drainage." They had had to remove one-third of the pupils and hoped to send four into the country.[116]

Williams then took some time off. She was invited to Claydon House, the Verneys' Buckinghamshire residence, for a visit. She offered to go back to the Edinburgh Royal Infirmary, but then volunteered to nurse in the new Egyptian campaign. Nightingale was initially "aghast" at her decision, but soon saw the mission as "magnificent" and did everything she could to facilitate it with the director-general of the Army Medical Department.[117] February was devoted to that task, while the hospital looked for her replacement. Williams would go to Port Said's Gordon Memorial Hospital, named after General Gordon, recently slain defending Khartoum, and given by the Suez Canal Company. The hospital was to be erected "in four months!!!" Nightingale exclaimed.[118] Arrangements were made for a number of nurses to go. Nightingale had her Fund contribute £25 for spiffy, officer-like outfits for Williams and two other nurses.[119] The cost of what she wanted was "beyond" what the War Office would pay, she knew.[120] Williams described the "great excitement" of their send-off at St Mary's: "All the [medical] students turned out and cheered lustily; every window of the hospital had a spectator." Their "scarlet tippets and caps were much admired." They went well with the officers' mess jackets, as intended – Nightingale wanted officer status for her nurses, as doctors in the British Army were officers. She sent flowers to Williams's cabin on ship.[121]

There was further vindication for Williams in the gift of a tea service, from "Friends at St. Mary's" and others, including Drs Sieveking and Joseph Bell in Edinburgh.[122] On her return from her first assignment in Egypt, Williams had a letter on her experiences published in the *Times*,[123] which would have given her friends further satisfaction. Her return in September 1885 from her next assignment received but a brief notice.[124]

Dr Henry Acland, Regius Professor of Medicine, Oxford

Dr Henry Wentworth Dyke Acland (1815–1900), later KCB, FRS, was a friend and valuable ally of Florence Nightingale's on several fronts. He was the fourth son of a tenth baronet, awarded a baronetcy of his own in 1890. He and Nightingale shared a faith, and he was physician to her sister and her family, the Verneys, and also to her good friend Benjamin Jowett, master of Balliol College, Oxford. Not only was Acland a well-published, respected physician, but he and Nightingale saw eye to eye on the basics. Both had had their baptism of fire in 1854, Nightingale at the Crimean War, Acland in heading the response to a cholera epidemic in Oxford. Both did careful assessments after the crisis to understand what went wrong, and what worked.[125] Both used the lessons learned for the rest of their working lives, to stress the broader environmental factors affecting health or disease. Acland is not known for any original contribution to medicine or health care, but his good name, energy, and ability helped move public health forward. He had been one of the five medical members of the Royal Sanitary Commission established in 1869; it recommended systematic measures for sanitation, including each county having its own medical officer of health, and these were enacted. Then followed two years of plodding work that achieved valuable results.

Acland had useful venues from which to promote public health. He was president 1868–69 of the British Medical Association, which formed, with the Social Science Association, a Joint Committee on State Medicine, as discussed in chapter 1. Acland was a member of it, also a member, later chair, of the General Medical Council. He gave opening addresses at the latter's meetings, which often received wide press coverage. These organizations gave occasions for him to call for stronger, state action to prevent disease, and he notably urged recognition of public-health measures. At Oxford University, he helped introduce scientific studies. He caused Nightingale real grief on only one issue, state registration of nurses, which he supported (see chapter 7).

Acland was as holistic as Nightingale, seeing the connection between physical and moral well-being, so that poverty was a determinant of ill health. He worked well with Drs Farr and Sutherland on health promotion and had a worldwide network of physicians, including notably the American Dr John Shaw Billings, plus the Russian–French bacteriologist Waldemar Mordecai Haffkine. Acland also had superb royal connections. He had been mentor of the young Prince of Wales, the future Edward VII, at Christ Church College, Oxford, and accompanied him on his four-month trip to British North America and the United States in summer and autumn 1860.

As was typical of Nightingale's relations with doctors, she also had contacts with other members of Acland's family. When his wife died, the Sarah Acland Memorial Home was established in her honour. Nightingale contributed. When Acland asked for "Miss Nightingale's books" for it, she had Henry Bonham Carter get "all the reports in a tidy heap" to go with the books, remembering "the dear saint, the noble saint who has left us and yet is with us still."[126]

Nightingale corresponded on issues with two Acland sons, one a St Thomas'–trained doctor (Theodore Dyke Acland), the other (Francis Edward Dyke Acland), or "Frank," in the Royal Artillery; also two MP nephews (Charles Thomas Dyke Acland and Arthur Herbert Acland). She was in brief touch with the Aclands' daughter and the admiral son on the return of Acland's letters on his death.[127] Acland appears again in chapter 4 on the cholera epidemic of 1883 in Egypt, where his medical son's practice brought him in contact with Nightingale nurses.

Acland had a broad range of interests, on which he often asked Nightingale for advice, such as the education of doctors for the navy, engineering, and public health, the death of military-hygiene expert Dr Edmund A. Parkes (from Renkioi), the Gordon Boys' Homehealth visitors in Buckinghamshire, the matron at the Devon and Exeter Hospital, and the Empress Frederick (Britain's Princess Victoria). He asked Nightingale to support Dr Nettleship for a position at the Ophthalmic Hospital. She responded that she did not usually do this, but Dr Bowman had already approached her about it and she had sent in a proxy.[128]

Acland was an excellent advocate for nursing and was sometimes of practical help. He took a considerable interest in district (home-visiting) nursing. He assisted district-nursing pioneer Florence Lees by editing her book, *Handbook for Hospital Sisters* (1874). In his speeches, he mentioned nursing (and Nightingale) favourably. He appeared at public meetings in support of such causes as the Countess of Dufferin Fund, which organized female medical care for women in India (where the earl was viceroy) – a letter from Nightingale was read at the same meeting. He attended the public meeting in support of the New Hospital for Women in London, at which, again, a letter of support from Nightingale was read.[129] His opening address to his last meeting as president of the General Medical Council in 1887 included praise of the work of Sidney Herbert and Nightingale.[130]

Acland sometimes raised complex and difficult issues, in 1876 suggesting that women doctors be induced "to take up midwifery and nursing." An exasperated Nightingale pointed out that women physicians were "moving heaven and earth" simply to be able to take the regular men's medical examinations to qualify.[131] However, he not only gave public support to admitting women into medicine, he mentored several young women doctors.

He sometimes needed a speedy response, so that more than one letter of Nightingale's has "6 a.m." added to the date. For example, he needed help for a meeting the next day he had to preside over, of the Zenana Medical Mission to women in India. Nightingale sent him questions to consider, short of denouncing the zenana scheme (*zenana* = "of the women" or "pertaining to women" in the subcontinent's major languages – i.e., the part of the home where women live in seclusion). She acknowledged that "some of the very best Anglo-India women," including the widow of Lord Lawrence, a former viceroy and friend of Nightingale's, were in favour of the mission. She queried the medical background of the women medical missionaries: did they have only the minimum, she wondered, when the maximum was needed? She quoted Dr Mary Ann Scharlieb (later a Dame), a pioneer woman physician whom Acland himself had aided in her career: "It is thought a little is better than nothing for India. *I* say, India is a place where you cannot have enough of medical education, experience, etc., if you want to do *any* good and not much harm." She posed an old question about confusing medicine with nursing. Her own nurse-training schools were constantly asked to admit women for a few months, to "'pick up' *medicine*, by acting as probationer *nurses* for these missions."[132]

While Nightingale approved in general of missions to convert non-Christians, she thought converting Indian women at childbirth would be wrong. "The hour of the native women's pain and danger," she continued, was not the time "to urge upon her the greatest, the most momentous, of all changes to a native woman – one which involves the greatest sacrifice, viz., Christianity." She named no one, but said that "the most devoted Christian, one of the best lady doctors in India, says, it is 'cruel.'"

Nightingale seems to have been happy to humour Acland on his disparate inquiries, perhaps because she knew that she could count on him for support for her causes. When the report of the Royal Commission on the Sanitary State of the Army in India appeared in 1863, good reviews were needed. Acland wrote one for the *Westminster Review*. When a parliamentary committee on cubic space in workhouses was established, he served on it, with royal engineer Douglas Galton. Nightingale wanted to make sure that its report would not be unanimous; Acland and Galton both signed the majority report, but added statements of their own.

Still, she was less than pleased with Acland's contribution on the issue. She told Galton that Acland's letter was "most sensible, but even he does not look at all at the question, whether under workhouse administration, proper hospitals can exist at all. We say not." That is, she insisted that the workhouse infirmaries there be taken out of the Poor Law system and treated as hospitals. Yet the minister concerned, Gathorne Hardy, was determined that the matter not be considered.[133]

In 1876, Nightingale alerted Acland about the "urgent" danger of the abolition of the Army Medical School, and he took up the issue.[134] The school carried on.

When a nasty "row" at the Radcliffe Infirmary in Oxford broke out in 1895, entailing an attack on the matron, Flora Masson, Nightingale tried to enlist Acland's aid: "A word from you would probably have quenched it," she wrote.[135] But by then Acland was at the end of his activist days, and she had to find another intervenor, Viscount Dillon, of Ditchley Park, Charlbury, Oxfordshire.

Her correspondence continued, however, with Acland's son, Theodore, a physician at St Thomas', who wrote her about having a Sinhalese woman trained there. (This did not work out, for circumstances in her home country, then called Ceylon.) Nightingale also exchanged notes with him about a boy dying in a ward in a way similar to that of one of her nurses. She inquired about having the ward purified.[136]

Her letters with the Aclands run from 1863 to just before Sir Henry's death in 1900. Her last letter to him notes her pleasure in hearing of him through Sir Harry's son, Fred Verney, "and almost from him," she said, remembering "when pyemia was almost as common a thing *in* hospitals as any case coming from without. I mean pyemia generated *in* hospital." There had been "an amazing change," thanks "to what you have taught us." Now, they "shout so loud when there is a case that they can hear us all over London ... We do not look upon anything of the kind now as unavoidable."[137]

The Derbyshire Infirmary

Dr William Ogle (1824–1905) helped launch professional nursing in Derbyshire. He first approached Nightingale in 1864, as physician to a "county hospital" in Derby, where he wanted a "better system of nursing" and a training school. She had to start from scratch. They had to form a committee, involve people, agree on a program: "The Training School is of the first importance. The 'Home' of the second. The 'Home' should be attached to the hospital – not the hospital to the 'Home.' The superintendent of nursing and the person in charge of training should be one and the same person, who must have herself the highest knowledge of nursing, be herself resident in the hospital, make the training in nursing her first object, and be herself a trained nurse of the highest order." She sent information from St Thomas' and King's College Hospitals.[138]

Dr Ogle was decidedly Protestant in religion, and Nightingale did not want to become sidelined on the "ecclesiastical differences" he raised in his letter to her. She replied that she had helped "rampant Roman Catholics, rampant Puseyites, rampant nonconformists of all kinds, rampant evangelicals all, as far as I was able, to obtain good nurses." It would be "unsafe" for her to interfere, "unless the entire system, including the nursing, were reconstructed – 'new wine in old bottles.'" She was willing to go over plans of proposed building alterations[139] (see chapter 5). The priority was to get a good "training matron."

The exchange went on for some years, and Derbyshire eventually possessed a matron, trained nurses, and a new building for the Royal Derbyshire Infirmary (now the Nightingale Hospital) in Derby. The last involved much work and numerous complications, although the main

actors were not doctors, but Nightingale's own family, which owned
nearby Lea Hurst, and other local landowning families.[140] Soon after the
opening of the Nightingale Wing in 1869, Dr Ogle gave a speech about
it and the system of nursing. "Ladies are invited [to train] and working
men and their wives."[141] It was only with the opening of the new wing,
Dr Ogle said, that the defects of the old became apparent.[142]

American Doctors and Hospitals

Nightingale liked Americans, especially doctors, and was keen to meet
them when they visited England. We learned in chapter 1 of her connection with the noted Boston doctor Samuel Gridley Howe and his wife,
Julia Ward Howe, and his early encouragement of her career.

In July 1860, at the International Statistical Congress at King's College,
London, a prominent delegate was Dr Edward Jarvis (1803–1884), a psychiatrist and president 1852–82 of the American Statistical Association. He
was invited to all three of Nightingale's breakfast parties for delegates. She
did not sit with her guests, about twenty at each event, but commissioned
her cousin Hilary Bonham Carter to act as hostess, while she herself
listened in from an adjacent room, according to Jarvis.[143] He recorded his
approval of her Crimean War sanitary report, and that "she sent him all
her writings." The two had similar ideas on health and illness.

The first physician to approach her about starting nurse training in the
United States was Walker Gill Wylie (1848–1923), of Bellevue Hospital, a
large public facility in New York City. Prompted by a committee report
that condemned its appalling conditions, he undertook a trip to Europe
to see hospitals. In Paris, he wrote Nightingale to ask for a meeting, but
she was then unable to see him. Instead, she provided a detailed outline
of what was necessary, which he had printed and circulated.[144] Wylie's
views were, as she informed Henry Bonham Carter, "the most undigested
you can well conceive."[145] He visited St Thomas' on the trip and spoke
to at least one of the doctors who gave lectures to the pupil nurses,
Dr LeGros Clark.[146] Nightingale also corresponded with the chair of the
Bellevue committee, philanthropist Elizabeth Hobson, about establishing a
training school.[147] Trained nursing started at Bellevue in 1873, though with
nurses from an Anglican order, not Nightingale nurses. Wylie's *Hospitals:
Their History* (1877) credited Nightingale's *Notes on Hospitals* with doing
"more to bring about reform in hospital construction than any other
work ever written."[148]

Dr Joseph Meredith Toner (1825–1896), president of the American Medical Association in 1873, helped establish nursing in Washington, DC, prior to the Civil War, with the Sisters of Charity. He was an advocate, with Dr John Shaw Billings, in Baltimore, of the plan for a systematic sanitary survey of the United States. In London in 1881 for the International Medical Congress, Toner wanted to meet Nightingale and sent her copies of his books and a photograph of the Nurses' Training School. He was duly invited, and Nightingale took extensive notes on his remarks.[149]

He told her that the Washington Training School for nurses, founded 1878, was situated thirty miles from Baltimore (it was in Washington, DC), its pupils "one third coloured." He commented on the more lucrative positions for nurses in private practice. The doctors initially opposed training nurses, "said we were making women doctors," but had all "come round." On the London gathering, he noted that all the papers on the humanity principle, on progress and civilization, came from English-speaking delegates, not Latin or Teuton. It was "not so much the papers but the bringing people together, has been the good of this congress." Toner was known to be a man of faith, and presumably this was discussed. Nightingale's last note of his remarks is enigmatic: "A great part of Christ's life has been left out till the last fifty years."[150]

Speaking at the opening of the Washington Training School in 1881, he reported his meeting with Nightingale while in London at the above-noted congress. His account frankly relates her weight gain, that she was no longer the "fragile" figure of the Crimean War.

Upon my card being sent to Miss Nightingale, I was immediately conducted to her room on the second floor. Here I found Miss Nightingale reclining upon a lounge, by the side of which stood a small table with writing material upon it and the photographs of the nurses and the pamphlets and china I had sent her. She held my card in her hand and, addressing me by name as I approached, and without rising, extended her hand and made me welcome.

Florence Nightingale, though of English parentage, was born in Florence, Italy, in 1820, and is therefore sixty one years of age, but she looked not a day older than forty five. Miss Nightingale's features are regular, her face is smooth and unwrinkled, she has an English complexion, large brown eyes and a well-nourished body, which would weigh 165 pounds, so that she is not now the slight, fragile person which the engraved portraits taken just after the Crimean War represented her to be. Though she sat upright on the lounge when I entered the room, and again several times during my stay, yet she did not at any time move her lower limbs, which were covered with a shawl. I did not know the character of her invalidness, but whatever it is, it in no way affects her mental energy or sympathy with the work of educating nurses. She has enlarged, clear and distinct views on the subject of nursing and the training of nurses, and expresses them forcibly and fluently.[151]

The president of the New Jersey Training School for Nurses, Dr Henry Genet Taylor, and its secretary, Dr Daniel Strock, in 1893 wrote Nightingale about conferring on her the "honorary degree of Medical and Surgical Nurse." Nightingale was not keen on certificates or diplomas. She complained to Henry Bonham Carter: "For my sins I have this punishment – and a very severe one it is: New Jersey has sent me a diploma!! and a specimen of the diploma it gives in its Training School for Nurses, a non nursendo after a 'course of study.' No hospital appears from the programme ... What is to be done?" He evidently mollified her, for she accepted.[152] Her letter of thanks made points about nursing, including warnings against relying on written qualifications without "the most essential characteristics of a nurse," which were moral, an old theme.[153] The honorary degree is an early indication of American leadership in linking nursing with academe.

Dr Alfred Worcester (1855–1951), a surgeon and later the first professor of hygiene at Harvard University, approached Nightingale in 1895 about nursing at Waltham (near Boston), where he had founded both a hospital and the Waltham Training School for Nurses. The school, however, as he described it in a book he sent Nightingale, A New Way of Training Nurses, was entirely contrary to her methods. Only one trained nurse was needed, and they were "easy to procure," he thought, and no trained matron or nurse tutor was required.[154] Arrangements were made for Canadian-born Charlotte Macleod, the superintendent, to gain experience at St Thomas' and at Liverpool.[155] When Dr Worcester visited London in 1895, Nightingale set up meetings for him with appropriate people, and met with him herself.[156]

Dr Worcester came to the rescue in 1897 when Lady Aberdeen, wife of the governor general of Canada, sought to establish district nursing in Toronto and Ottawa, under the auspices of the Queen's Diamond Jubilee Fund. Canadian doctors opposed what they called the Aberdeens' project, which in due course became the Victorian Order of Nurses, still in operation. Lady Aberdeen visited the Waltham School and met with Dr Worcester, who volunteered to go to Ottawa to try to persuade the doctors. As Macleod reported back to Nightingale, he gave two weeks of his time and strength to convince the men (medical doctors) "of the great benefit the district nurse would be to the country and to themselves. He has returned victorious."[157] Lady Aberdeen's letter to Nightingale about his help called it a "splendid crusade," which "converted the leading doctors of Ottawa and Toronto." He also did the favour of persuading the Waltham authorities to let Macleod go to Ottawa to set it up.[158] The doctors were a tough sell. Lady Aberdeen won them over by writing each a personal invitation to a grand event at Rideau Hall to meet Worcester. Many came. Lord Aberdeen then funded the first two years of district nursing.

A new association with the Waltham school occurred in 1905 when A.L. Pringle, who had been matron both at Edinburgh and St Thomas', became superintendent at Waltham for two years. Dr Worcester asked her to remember him to Nightingale with this renewed contact.[159] His later *Nurses and Nursing* (1927) has a chapter on Nightingale. It is also a fine source on overcoming medical opposition to trained nursing in Canada.

The Sydney Infirmary and the Doctor-as-Matron Problem

One of the great achievements of the Nightingale School was the introduction of professional nursing into Australia, followed by the building of a fine new hospital and the best nurses' home then in existence. Sydney was the first place outside Britain to receive Nightingale School graduates, in 1868. Most of the correspondence on these matters was with Henry (later Sir Henry) Parkes, colonial secretary of New South Wales and eventually premier, and Deas (later Sir Deas) Thomson, president of the hospital board. The initiative came from Lady Harriet Dowling, widow of the late chief justice, who reminded Nightingale, in 1863, of her obligation to the Australia colonies for their enormous contribution to the fund that financed her schools.

New South Wales surgeon Alfred (later Sir Alfred) Roberts (1823–1898) played a key role in launching the new nursing. He soon, however, became the antagonist of the matron sent, Lucy Osburn. It was a classic case of a doctor interfering with nursing, acting as matron himself.[160] Describing himself as "a hospital surgeon," Roberts told Nightingale that he was "a strong advocate for good nursing and trained staff," who had "year after year ... met with disappointment."[161] He wrote her detailed letters about the Sydney Infirmary and its arrangements. His wife, Susan E. Roberts, also provided information. Surviving documents are only his eleven letters to Nightingale and her, Dr Sutherland's, and others' notes and letters.

Early on, Nightingale turned the material over to St Thomas' Hospital matron Sarah Wardroper for her advice. The matron replied with a detailed layout of how many nurses, scrubbers, night nurses, porters, and bathmen would be needed at Sydney. She was the first to recognize the problem Roberts posed, telling Nightingale plainly that a "trained matron or superintendent is the missing link in Dr Roberts's plan."[162] He acceded, or at least appeared to, on the inclusion of a matron with the nurses to be sent. His correspondence with Nightingale was cordial throughout, although he clearly never accepted the independence of the nursing profession.

An early letter he wrote her called her previous missive "kind and valuable," the advice arriving "just in time to be of material assistance" to them. He sent her a photograph of Australian aboriginal women, with his comments – a subject on which Nightingale had earlier worked.[163] She sent him printed reports as well, notably her brief to the Poor Law Board (which outlined her views on nursing), *Notes on Hospitals*, and material on the Liverpool Workhouse Infirmary.

Roberts initially approved of Osburn's selection as matron – "most valuable for the post she is to occupy."[164] Her first comments on him pointed out that he was unpopular, adding that she got along with both him and his wife; it was an advantage that they were "gentle folks."[165] However, troubles soon appeared, and numerous letters would recount the distress he caused her.[166]

In 1870, Osburn complained that he "gives orders," although he had no position at the hospital. She herself made mistakes as matron, so that both Nightingale and Henry Bonham Carter regretted having sent her, although they had no one else available.[167] Nightingale saved Osburn's job for the first time after she passed on confidential information about a Sydney patient, Prince Alfred, Duke of Edinburgh, son of Queen Victoria, to a relative of hers in England. The fact that the new trained nurses successfully nursed the prince, after an assassination attempt in Sydney in March 1868, naturally attracted wide attention to them. The queen sent her appreciation to Nightingale through a distinguished physician, Sir William Jenner (1815–1898),[168] who discovered the distinction between typhus and typhoid fever. In 1870, Osburn was investigated for "Bible burning," in fact disposing of rat-infested Bibles left in a storage room, but offensive to evangelical Sydney. Nightingale's support of Osburn was cited in her defence.[169]

Both Henry Bonham Carter and Sarah Wardroper considered Osburn a failure, and he told Dr Roberts so when the latter visited London.[170] However, Osburn largely coped with the challenge. Professional-level nursing was established and spread to other hospitals in Australian colonies.

When New South Wales set up a royal commission in 1873, under William C. Windeyer,[171] to investigate Osburn's management, and other matters, Nightingale again defended her. Both Henry Parkes, then premier, and the infirmary's president, Deas Thomson, did not want Osburn driven out. Roberts gave evidence against her.[172] Windeyer, not incidentally, was a strong liberal, a supporter of women's education and suffrage; both he and his wife were English born, his wife indeed from Buckinghamshire, with Verney connections.

Nightingale took time to respond to Windeyer's request for her views.[173] She eventually produced a lengthy letter (four printed pages). It did not mention Roberts but strongly defended the matron's leadership: "The experiment of the matron and her nurses being virtually under the medical officer has been tried since hospitals began, and has always ended ill either for the moral or the efficient element. A medical officer has quite other things to do than to be head of the nurses." If the lady superintendent is not the best judge of nursing, she asked, how can she be the head of it? She pointed out the need for an appeal system. The matron and the medical officer must both be under the committee of management, administratively equal. The matron and her nurses must obey the "*professional* instructions" of doctors.[174] Nightingale's letter arrived too late for the commission's first report (the letter was kept in the Windeyer family until 1922, when it was given to the Sydney Infirmary[175]).

In his inquiry's final report, Windeyer quoted Nightingale's views extensively from a published source, her *Method of Improving the Nursing Service of Hospitals* (1868), a short paper she had sent Osburn in 1869. The paper outlined the core specifications for organizing nursing and nurse training, under the matron. It also covered "structural arrangements" of hospital buildings, which Windeyer also used to find fault with the Sydney building. He also quoted Nightingale on Osburn's suitability for the position. Press coverage included lengthy quotations of Nightingale's views on all three points: nursing organization, Osburn's qualifications, and defects in the Sydney building.[176]

Oddly, Roberts's cordial letters to Nightingale continued even while the investigation was going on. He told her that the hospital was finally, in 1873, on a secure basis; he was beginning to feel ashamed of the "abominations" at it.[177] Yet he continued to say "bitter and damaging things" against the matron.[178] In 1880, fifty-three nurses at Sydney's new Prince Alfred Hospital, still a-building, sent Nightingale thanks for all she had done "for their comfort and accommodation." The message was conveyed through Roberts, by then Sir Alfred.[179]

Osburn was not reappointed in 1884, and returned to England, where she worked as a district nurse and superintendent of district nursing in Newington and Walworth, London. In Sydney, she was replaced by an Australian she had trained. In her will, she left a legacy of £100 to royal commissioner William Windeyer's daughter.

In 1889, Roberts reported back to Nightingale on the training school: many applicants, a three-year program, with three examinations each year; he calculated that the colony had 150–200 trained nurses. The school was still struggling, however, to raise money to erect a nurses' home on the grounds. He also asked for a bust of Nightingale to display.[180] She commented to Captain Edmund Verney, her sister's stepson, that "she knew Sir Alfred Roberts personally, and his training of nurses. Two of his home-trained nurses have won the 'Gold Medal' against nurses trained in any part of the world, upon a competitive examination!! ... The mania for public exams has spread to nurses!"[181] Nightingale never relented in her disapproval of judging nurses by examination results.

German Doctors

Nightingale's first hospital experience was at the Deaconess Hospital at Kaiserswerth, near Düsseldorf, in 1851. However, the small hospital and the associated deaconess institute were both run by the pastor. A doctor visited the hospital daily, as noted in Nightingale's journal,[182] but he gave no training. Indeed, there is no mention of his ever speaking with her (she spoke and read German well, but could not write it).

During the Franco–Prussian War of 1870–71, she was in contact with the renowned Rudolf Virchow (1821–1902), a brilliant Prussian / German pathologist and statesman known as the founder of "social medicine." There is no extant correspondence of hers with him, but she called him "an old acquaintance," through the Crown Princess of Prussia (later the Empress Frederick), an advocate of reformed nursing and Queen Victoria's oldest child. They corresponded initially about the mundane matter of sending lint to a hospital at his request[183] This led to collaboration on the building of the City Hospital, Friedrichshain, Berlin, opened in 1874 (see chapter 5).

For Virchow, politics was "medicine writ large," the place to work to reduce disease by improving social conditions. He held many political offices, but Nightingale was appalled to learn how little influence he had. The crown princess, her friend and a liberal in conservative Prussia, explained: "If they want to build a hospital, they ask a pastor and a count – and such a man as Virchow is absolutely in disgrace, because he is neither Tory nor High Church."[184] In 1871, when her *Introductory Notes on Lying-in Institutions* was published, Nightingale wanted to find out where Virchow was to send him a copy.[185]

When bacteriologist Robert Koch returned to Germany from Calcutta, after making his great breakthrough in early 1884 on the identification of cholera, Nightingale speculated that there would be an outcry, merely if he described the appalling conditions he had seen there. Virchow in fact declared "that the English Government of India was a perpetual menace to the world." Nightingale had some sympathy with this, because Koch had demonstrated that cholera was spread not by contagion (hand contact), "but by overflow,"[186] meaning sewage.

Some nurses passed on examples of better German practice to Nightingale. Fraulein von Cornberg told her in 1881 than antiseptic practice was better in Heidelberg than at St Thomas', that "doctors make nurses dip their hands in carbolic before them before touching patient."[187] Osburn visited hospitals in Berlin in 1885 and wrote Nightingale about the nursing and hospital conditions there. She reported also that a German nurse, Luise Fuhrmann, who had been at St Thomas', considered that the antiseptic procedures in Berlin were more rigorous than at St Thomas', but acknowledged that Fuhrmann had not been at St Thomas' for two years.[188]

French Doctors

Nightingale had seen French medicine in practice in 1853 when she worked in several Paris hospitals along with the Sisters of Charity and (possibly) several other orders. She observed the distinguished M. Roux conduct surgery in Paris. She saw dedicated nuns serving as nurses, but later came to consider their standards of hygiene poor. She visited French hospitals in the Crimea late in the war. French Army doctors made positive comments about her in their publications. However, none of this amounted to any protracted association.

France had pioneered the pavilion principle in hospital construction, so that Nightingale was keen to show French doctors and administrators the progress England had made since Crimea. She wanted to acquaint herself especially with Armand Husson, the director of the Assistance publique, which ran the public hospitals of Paris (he was an administrator, not a doctor). He sent her his 1862 report, which she used in *Notes on Hospitals*.[189]

When Husson visited London in 1865, she went to some trouble to arrange visits for him at top hospitals, but she did not meet with him herself. She told her sister that "no one in the world knew so much about poor relief" in France. She sent Husson Douglas Galton's book on the Herbert Hospital (which Galton designed), the model army-pavilion hospital. It would, she told the author, "do a great deal of good," so that she wanted many copies, as she wanted to "instruct *all* the hospital builders in England!!"[190] In London, Husson called on Nightingale without an appointment. She wrote him in French, offering to prepare for him an introduction to the person who could most help him, Poor Law inspector H.B. Farnall. Naturally, she wanted him to meet Dr John Sutherland, who would arrange for him to visit the Herbert Hospital and would be an admirable guide for him also in the civil hospitals of London.[191]

When "that dreadful M. Husson" made a second trip to London to see English hospitals, Nightingale asked Galton to see him. Husson intended to see all the workhouses and hospitals in five days. Nightingale commented: "He really terrifies me like a whirlwind or cyclone." She asked Galton for an introduction for him for the Herbert Hospital again, and asked what other hospitals he should visit.[192]

Public Health and the Social Science Congresses

The National Association for the Promotion of Social Science (NAPSS), or Social Science Association, which we met above, was founded in 1857, thanks largely to the efforts of Dr George Woodyat Hastings (1825–1917), himself the son of the physician Sir Charles Hastings, who founded the British Medical Association (BMA). The model for the new body, however, was the British Association for the Advancement of Science (BAAS), whose meetings Nightingale had attended at Oxford with her father in 1847. Dr Hastings persuaded Lord Brougham, FRS, to be the medical body's patron, while he himself did the behind-the-scenes work.

The Social Science Association gathered for a week each year in fine venues, with dinners and social life, attended typically by over a thousand people, sometimes by over two thousand. Women belonged in large numbers, and read papers. The meetings received extensive coverage in leading newspapers. Articles in the *Times* were then often picked up by Australian and New Zealand newspapers. Nightingale's contributions, in particular, were widely reported.

One of the association's five sections was on public health, where Nightingale's colleague medical statistician Dr William Farr was a leading member, and so the Social Science Congress, as it was called, proved an excellent venue for her ideas. She sent seven papers to its meetings, beginning in 1858 in Liverpool. The papers were published in the association's *Transactions* the following year. Nightingale usually had hers also published separately for convenient distribution.

Her first contribution consisted of two papers read on consecutive days at Liverpool in October 1858 by Dr Holland. Lord Shaftesbury, chair of the section, urged her to send the (handwritten) paper to the mayor of Liverpool, which she did. The two papers were the first version of what became her book-length *Notes on Hospitals* (1863). The *Times*, as well as covering her papers' chief points, shows how her team supported her, noting comments by former sanitary commissioner Robert Rawlinson, CE, Douglas Galton, Sir Harry Verney, and C.H. Bracebridge, who with his wife stayed nearly a year with Nightingale at her hospital at Scutari.[193]

Her paper to the 1861 meetings, in Dublin, was "Hospital Statistics and Hospital Plans," read by pathologist Dr Lyons, whom she knew from the Crimean War.

She did not send a paper to the 1862 congress proper in London, but Joshua Jebb, chair of the Nightingale Fund, reported on the progress of the new training school. That congress was followed immediately by the Congrès de Bienfaisance, also in London, to which Nightingale sent her tribute to Sidney Herbert, who had died the previous year. It showed, by statistics, the effects of his / their reforms in hygiene in reducing mortality rates.[194]

For Edinburgh, in 1863, she sent papers on two subjects: "Sanitary Statistics of Native Colonial Schools and Hospitals" and "How People May Live and Not Die in India." The second was the first publication for the general public from the vast amount of work done for the Royal Commission on the Sanitary State of the Army in India, whose report had just appeared.

"Sanitary Statistics of Native Colonial Schools and Hospitals" was a report of Nightingale's findings from a questionnaire sent out by the Colonial Office. After discussion, the congress's section on public health unanimously adopted a motion, proposed by statistician James Heywood, "to represent to the Colonial Office the importance of considering the valuable reports of Miss Nightingale on native colonial schools, native colonial hospitals and the causes of the disappearance of native races in British colonies, and that they also represent the desirableness of endeavouring to obtain additional information respecting native races."[195] The session was notable also for the attendance of Prince Alfred. The paper itself was widely covered both in the British press[196] and in Australia.[197] However, the Colonial Office took no further action on its recommendations.

Nightingale sent a short follow-up paper to the 1864 congress in York, "Note on the Aboriginal Races of Australia." She produced three further papers for congresses: in 1870 at Newcastle, "On Indian Sanitation"; in 1873 at Norwich, "How Some People Have Lived and Not Died in India"; and in 1874 at Glasgow, "Life or Death in India," with an appendix on irrigation. The progression of ideas is obvious in the titles.

Homerton Fever Hospital

The London fever hospitals were created under the Poor Law legislation, but run by a new body, the Metropolitan Asylums Board, and physically separate from the old workhouses. They were an intermediate body and, in a sense, the forerunners of NHS hospitals. The need was great, for the regular, civil hospitals typically did not take fever cases.

Nightingale was familiar with the problems at the fever hospital at Homerton, east London, as she had been sending nurses and matrons from her school there for years. In 1881, she explained to a workhouse nurse, "Vast experience in fever is to be gained at these places, of course, and a certain amount of good nursing is no doubt to be seen at all of them. But systematic 'training,' or 'training' at all, in the sense in which you and we understand 'training,' is certainly not to be had at any of them."[198] Supervision, also, was lacking.

There was a minor crisis at Homerton in 1890, when the matron, a Nightingale nurse, reported to Nightingale that there could be no "hope for reform" while Dr Colley, the medical superintendent, was there.[199] The matron left, for Gibraltar, and an inquiry followed. The appointment of Miss H. Mackenzie, who had been trained with Elizabeth Vincent, matron at the St Marylebone Workhouse Infirmary, evidently brought peace and improvements. However, on her marriage to the medical superintendent at Homerton, Dr E.W. Goodall, she had to leave that post. Dr Goodall seems to have been the one physician who terrified Nightingale, as we see below.

A junior, woman doctor at Homerton in 1890 made a difference in the care given, Nightingale thought. This was "Miss Webb, M.B.," third assistant medical officer, "a very great safeguard." Children with hip-joint and other diseases, who contracted scarlet fever in a regular civil hospital, were sent to Homerton. "The *fever nurses* do not know how to handle these most suffering cases ... The children get worse," and the matron was not allowed to interfere. Dr Webb's presence, said Nightingale, "appears absolutely essential for these poor children." She made at least one nightly round and insisted on the night nurse sending for her, if needed. "She understands nursing as no man can do. She is motherly and devoted, and her appointment in the hospital seems the only real guarantee for supervision at night."[200]

The lack of nurse training at fever hospitals came up again in 1893, a thorny problem, for such facilities would not be suitable for training general nurses. Medical students were trained at the regular hospitals, then sent to the fever hospitals for several days a week to gain experience. The untrained nurses were a danger to themselves and to patients, as Henry Bonham Carter pointed out.[201]

Nightingale had an ally in the Hon. Maude Stanley (1833–1915), who was manager of the Metropolitan Asylums Board. Stanley visited her and wrote her frequently, to be converted to the need for better training. However, that too posed a problem, as Nightingale told Henry Bonham Carter: "*Miss Stanley* turned up again on Sunday night. And now I am frightened at the rapidity of her conversion. She has tried a good many provincial hospital places including St. Marylebone, and none of them will take *Homerton probationers* for a year's training ... She did not see that a year's training in another, a provincial hospital, ends in nothing but technical knowledge." Stanley was "an admirable woman, full of energy and hard working." But she was on four boards and did not see the "necessity of *training herself* in the knowledge of things," while her ideal hospital was "disastrously like a Woman's Club room."[202]

Nightingale asked Douglas Galton, also a member of the Metropolitan Asylums Board, for help in preparing to meet Medical Superintendent Dr Goodall: "Apparently we have to begin again at the A.B.C." She did not have a copy left of her very practical brief to the Cubic Space Committee and needed material to give him.[203]

Dr Goodall wanted a recipe, a "receipt," from Nightingale for the best way to train nurses, for all the hospitals of the Metropolitan Asylums Board. Her idea of their interview was to obtain information from him before prescribing anything. After the "dreaded" interview, she reported back to Bonham Carter that she had spent 3¼ hours with Goodall. He "thawed in the latter half," and she had a "strong impression of his honesty. But he is astoundingly ignorant of all progress."[204] Clearly there was no meeting of minds. Nightingale called him a "medical a non-medicando." He was "never in the wards," he told her, as he had no time, except when he had to show a case clinically to his medical students. He was a "Guy's [Hospital] man," but knew nothing about their training.[205]

Early in 1894, Maude Stanley was to take a motion to the board to start a training school at Homerton, but Nightingale considered that, given the state of the current nurses, "a training school *now* would lead to certain failure, which later must succeed."[206] It is not clear if the meeting with Dr Goodall led to any changes. Nightingale continued to assist Homerton with appointments, including referral of the highly esteemed Flora Masson in 1897. Correspondence is lacking as to any concrete results from these endeavours. The hospital is now Homerton University Hospital NHS Trust, linked with City University for training.

Dr Goodall published his own account of his meeting with Nightingale many years after her death. The "almost plump little woman," was "not conversant with … the attitude of the nursing profession at that time," but looked back to women taking up nursing as a "sacred duty towards suffering humanity." She gave "excellent counsel" on the general question of hospital nursing, but "did not help much in respect of the feasibility" of his scheme.[207]

Books on Nursing (Mainly by Doctors)

Physicians' books on nursing were a mixed blessing for Nightingale. On the one hand, no one but a doctor could instruct nurses, for no one else had the requisite academic education. But doctors were not nurses, and got things wrong, or were overly medical, trying to make doctors out of nurses. She complained about James W. Anderson's *Lectures on Medical Nursing* for recommending teaching physiology to nurses, which was "nothing without dissection," which apparently was not intended for nurses. She thought it would be as useful as learning about the "structure of the gun" without ever firing a shot, "what would that profit you?" If you taught the structure of the body, and the actions of certain organs, "what would that profit you if you had never seen a sick person?"[208]

Some doctors sent Nightingale a copy of their books for nurses, and others she heard of and purchased. Mary Crossland kept her up to date with what was available. Some nursing texts were widely used, as is evident in the number of reprints and revisions. Humphry's *Manual of Nursing: Medical and Surgical*, for example, had its twenty-eighth edition in 1905, and J. Watson's *Handbook for Nurses* its tenth in 1934, up to 1,159 pages from 415 in 1899. A list of books for nurses by both physicians and nurses available in Nightingale's working lifetime is in print.[209]

Some doctors discussed Nightingale favourably in their books, for example, Cullingworth in *Nurse's Companion*. His introduction ended with the advice that "every nurse" should have a copy of Nightingale's *Notes on Nursing*, which was "clearly and pleasantly written," with an "immense number of hints as to the management of the sick, which can be found nowhere else, and are of the utmost value."[210] Cullingworth was an obstetrician and expert on puerperal fever, firm on antiseptic use. Nightingale was pleased when he sent her "his flyleaf of the rules as to antiseptics and cleanliness for *midwives* with mother and infant."[211]

She quoted him, that the "lying-in woman is not a sick woman." She approved his teaching "antiseptics: washing hands between each case, keeping patients and all instruments and utensils antiseptically."[212] Also in 1892, she inquired about Cullingworth's *Short Manual of Monthly Nursing* (about the first month after childbirth), which Crossland told her had not a word of its title matter in it. Crossland thought that she would like *A Manual of Nursing, Medical and Surgical* by Laurence Humphry, of Addenbrooke's Hospital, and Percy George Lewis's *Theory and Practice of Nursing.*[213]

Dr Croft, and other physicians, recommended books for the nurses' library, many of them written for medical students; Nightingale saw that they were ordered. Matrons asked for medical books for their library; for example, Flora Masson wanted the second edition of Fagge's *Principles and Practice of Medicine.*[214] Nightingale frequently asked nurses visiting her what book they would like as a gift. Many wanted medical books, and she obliged. Gray's *Anatomy* was a favourite choice. Often it is clear that it is the only textbook they owned.

There were frequent orders for such classics as Druitt's *Vade Mecum*; Garrod's *Materia Medica*; Heath's *Dictionary of Practical Surgery*; Hill's *Essentials of Bandaging*; Hooper's *The Anatomist's Vade Mecum*; Huxley's *Elementary Lessons in Physiology*; Swayne's *Obstetric Aphorisms*; Tanner's *An Index of Diseases and Their Treatment*; Watson's *Lectures on the Principles and Practice of Physic*; and Spencer Wells's *On Ovarian and Uterine Tumours.*

Nightingale promoted books on hygiene, especially for use in India, some with qualification. For example, Dr Dhanakoti Raju's *Easy Lessons on the Laws of Health*, published at Madras, was "valuable," but the "reverse of 'easy,'" plus "too English – a compilation from English books and *not* easy English books." Except for some material on food grains, "it otherwise almost ignores the poor."[215] Also in 1886, Nightingale was seeking advice on obstetrics books for India.[216]

The 1889 article by Dr John Lindsay Steven on nurse training in the *Glasgow Medical Journal*, cited in chapter 1, on "intelligent obedience," ended with a recommendation for four nursing books, three by doctors (Allan, Anderson, and Bell) and Nightingale's *Notes on Nursing*. The wry comment on her book aptly reflects opinion thirty years after she wrote it:

I would like you all carefully to read Miss Nightingale's book, partly from its historical value and the associations it recalls, and partly because of the sound common sense which pervades its every page. Never mind, although you may feel inclined sometimes to resent the assertiveness of the writer, every feeling of this kind is soon lost in the memory of the noble devoted life of one whose name was a household word in our land in a time of great national sorrow and trial, and whose influence is still felt in every hospital of the country. You will find in the book things to make you smile, and things to excite your pity and indignation, and withal, I believe, you will rise from the perusal better and wiser than before.[217]

Nightingale and doctors assisted nurses on their books. We saw above Acland's assistance on Florence Lees's *Handbook for Hospital Sisters* (editing and a preface). *Hints for Hospital Nurses* (1877) was the joint work of two Nightingale nurses, Rachel Williams and Alice Fisher. On Fisher's death, Williams, under her married name, Norris, thoroughly revised the book, as *Norris's Nursing Notes*. Two doctors (one a leading surgeon at St Mary's) and a nurse are acknowledged for their assistance. The Nightingale School is used as an example, and the nursing lecturer, surgeon John Croft, is substantially quoted. There are several chapters on medical matters, a subject Nightingale never attempted to write on.

Nightingale's *Notes on Nursing* stood unrivalled for decades. It would not be until the 1890s that nursing books, by nurses other than her, began to appear that went beyond the founder's. The best example, discussed in chapter 8, is Isabel Hampton Robb's *Nursing: Its Principles and Practice* (1893).

4

MILITARY MEDICINE
IN PEACETIME AND LATER WARS

Appointing the Right Doctors to Ensure Reforms

The reforms needed to reduce mortality were carefully set out in the 1858 report of the Royal Commission on the Crimean War. The next task then was to ensure that the appointments made to key positions were adequate to make the reforms happen. When Sir Andrew Smith retired as director-general of the Army Medical Department in 1858, Nightingale went to some trouble to see that he was not succeeded by Sir John Hall, her nemesis as principal medical officer in the Crimea. Her choice was Dr Thomas Alexander, for his courage and vigour in reporting defects during the war. He took the post, and the two worked together effectively on the Army Medical School, statistics, and nutrition. When he died, after only two years into the job, she called his loss "irreparable," one that would undo "a great part of the work I have done.[1] She wrote a eulogy for the *Lancet*.[2] She called a later director-general, Sir William Mure Muir (1818–1885), not only "by far the best man in the department," but "a second Dr Alexander."[3]

Early on after her return from the Crimean War, when she was still able to move around, Nightingale visited military hospitals, navy as well as army. She told Sir John McNeill that she found the army hospitals at Chatham in Kent "disgraceful."[4] She had been taken there by the director-general of the Navy Medical Department, Sir John Liddell (1794–1868), who wanted her advice. She was pleased to be courted by the navy – hoping that "that would 'shame the *army* hospitals into doing what they require so much more,'" as she told Sidney Herbert. She assured him of her fidelity: "I cannot forget my first love, nor marry another department again so soon."[5] The navy was pleased to receive publicity about her visit, telling the press that she had "pronounced the Melville Hospital [renamed the Royal Naval Hospital, Chatham] to be in every respect the best of the national hospitals in this kingdom."[6]

Nightingale kept in touch with her favourite Crimean War doctors. Peter Pincoffs (1816–1872), who had sett up cafés for the men in the Crimea, consulted her on his manuscript: he would "willingly make any addition or change you may think desirable."[7] Her response was favourable, especially vis-à-vis his French material. His book duly came out as *Experiences of a Civilian in Eastern Military Hospitals* (1857). She sent Pincoffs her comments on her visits to "most of the military and naval hospitals" that she had done "by order of Lord Panmure": "The naval hospitals are very good in point of organization (much like the French), tolerably good in point of sanitary precaution, ventilation, and *not* good in points of nursing. But what will you say when I tell you that I have not seen one military hospital to compare with those of Scutari in May 1855, in point of excellence?"[8]

The many reforms in army hospitals and barracks can be seen in later statistics. Nightingale told Harriet Martineau that the effect of the new Army Regulations, in force for two years, could be seen in China, that only 6 per cent died of disease, instead of 60 per 100 "as we had in the first winter of the Crimean War."[9] The next year she reported to Edwin Chadwick that zymotic diseases were less frequent in the army than in civil life: "I send you our numbers, after three years sanitary work."[10] Much later, in her obituary of Dr John Sutherland, she again called on statistics to illuminate his work, which was most clear when comparing "the vital statistics of the Army prior to the time of the Crimea War and those of the present date."[11]

Nightingale did face frustration: she told Sir John McNeill, "The War Office is always planning and never doing." There were "four heads of departments – all to a certain extent independent in money matters": the commissariat, stores, barracks, and purveyor. The work, after Sidney Herbert's death, was "heartbreaking."[12]

An early concern was the defective design of the massive army hospital at Netley, the Royal Victoria. Construction of the facility, on Southampton Water, began in 1856. Nightingale and Dr Sutherland succeeded, with much agitation, in having the design significantly adjusted, to improve ventilation. But the sheer size and length of corridors frequently raised problems. To publicize defects, Nightingale published several articles in the architects' journal, the *Builder*, and sent letters to the editor of major newspapers.

Nightingale told Dr Longmore at the Army Medical School, in response to a memo of his, that her fears had been realized, "that the miles of work at Netley" would seriously interfere with proper training of orderlies. They, the orderlies, would be doing much of the nursing there, under trained nurses.[13] She thought that Dr Longmore was sacrificing himself, and the War Office should not have accepted it, and they "were not men if they were men. But we have hardly a man now in the government."[14]

In 1880, Mrs Wardroper advised her that, when nurses for war hospitals or field service were needed, the large London hospitals, especially St Thomas', were better sources than Netley.[15] That year, also, Nightingale consulted the senior surgeon at St Thomas', Alexander Oberlin MacKellar (1845–1904), on nurse training at Netley. After meeting with him, she wrote Sir Harry Verney, her brother-in-law and a vice-president of the National Aid Society: "He told me even more than I knew before, of the unfitness of Netley for training nurses. (The patients are almost all out of bed and generally do their own dressings!) as well as of the *large proportion* of dressings, etc., done by our nurses and probationers at St Thomas' (not by dressers!)."[16] Nightingale took note of MacKellar's description of Netley nursing, apparently from another meeting, comparing it to that of civil hospitals: "St T.'s nurses do three out of the four dressings daily, compressing hemorrhage, extemporizing splints, antiseptic … English behind every other country."[17]

Nightingale was always concerned with how well training worked in practice, which is why she preferred apprenticeship-type training with an experienced supervisor to hand. An army doctor in 1882 told her of the various defects in the training of orderlies at British Army headquarters at Aldershot, in Hampshire – the four months was "purely useless."

A well man is labelled "tibia and fibula broken," well, what the orderly does for him won't do for a real compound fracture. When he comes to deal with a real compound fracture, it's another sort of thing. *He never* sees a sick or wounded man at Aldershot. He bandages on a dummy and the general puts on his spectacles and looks close and says "beautiful." When there's real blood and wounds, he's quite at sea … They bandage like a picture, as I could not do it myself, but on the real patient it's so tight that it will kill him. Aldershot has nothing but the patients of a remarkably healthy division."[18]

The Army Medical School

To make health promotion, or hygiene, a key goal of army medicine required that the new medical school deliver a different kind of medical education. Nightingale was greatly involved in the appointment of the first chairs, and kept a watching brief thereafter. The school was based initially in Chatham, to move to Netley when the massive Royal Victoria Hospital there opened in 1863. Nightingale would have preferred it to go to the architecturally better Herbert Hospital at Woolwich, but she lost that battle. The school remained at Netley until 1902, when it moved to Millbank and was incorporated into a larger, joint medical school.

Dr Edmund A. Parkes (from Renkioi), the first professor of military hygiene, proved highly able. He had not been Nightingale's choice – she preferred Dr S.B.F. de Chaumont (1833–1888)[19] – but worked closely and effectively with Parkes. (De Chaumont succeeded him.) When Parkes drew up his syllabus, he sent it to Nightingale and asked her to review it and comment: "If you have time to make any alterations and suggestions, I shall be very grateful."[20] She suggested only that he add "Soils" after "Air, Food, Clothing" in Lecture 22: "At the scientific arrangement of the subject, I am worth nothing, and could, I am quite sure, suggest nothing to *you*." However, as for "some of your *practical* lectures, and to any of my own peculiar subjects, such as ward construction and nursing hygiene (those things which an old nurse like me has had most experience in), I could give you any, the least, practical assistance, I should be happy and grateful to have the opportunity."[21] In 1861, Dr Parkes told her that he was using her material in his lectures.[22] He also delicately raised differences of opinion on contagion with her.[23]

Dr William Aitken, who had been the assistant to Dr Lyons on the Pathology Commission during the Crimean War, was the school's first professor of pathology, and proved a good ally, soon sending to Nightingale for data.[24] She recommended Topinard's book on English surgery to him.[25]

The school was in a shambles when its first students arrived. Basic equipment and instruments were missing, a terrible embarrassment. However, the appointments were good, and the school soon gained an international reputation and became a model for other countries, such as

Saxony. Parkes's *Manual of Practical Hygiene*, which covered such basics as water purification and sewage treatment, came out in numerous editions. Nightingale's correspondence with and about him[26] reveals him as a fellow believer in health promotion as a divine mission.

On his death in 1876, the school's existence was threatened. Nightingale rallied her friends to save it. Dr Acland, at Oxford, was sympathetic; Dr Longmore, at the school itself, was a helpful informant. When writing Acland about the school's survival, Nightingale said that Parkes "died like a true Christian hero 'at his post' … His death was like a resurrection. When he was dying, he dictated letters or gave messages to everybody, *all* about what ought to be done for the School for the spread of hygienic knowledge, for other useful and Army purposes, *none* about himself."[27] She told Longmore that Parkes's dictated note was the "most touching" she ever saw, and that he "went to the sacrifice of himself with joy and praise like the heroes of old."[28]

Parkes's last letter to her stated frankly that he wrote (dictated) it from "what must be, I believe, my deathbed. Perhaps before you receive this I shall be summoned to my account." He then gave his account to her, noting that his last, short work, *The Personal Care of Health*, only twenty-six pages, was to be published in two months by the Society for Promoting Christian Knowledge. He would have a copy sent to her. "I put in as much sanitary information as I could, of a very simple kind. I hope it may be a little useful to you. It is addressed entirely to the poor." He signed off with his blessing and thanks for all the support she had always given him.

Parkes's death also caused a vacancy in the examination of candidates for the army, navy, and Indian services. Acland's help was especially useful now, as he had the clout to meet with the minister on the subject.[29] Aitken, the pathologist, was called on again. Nightingale was pleased when Dr de Chaumont was appointed to the chair in 1876. He edited later versions of Parkes's *Practical Hygiene*. His own publications show much common ground with Nightingale.[30]

The school was threatened again in 1881, and Nightingale had again to rally her crew. The institution had particular meaning for her thanks to its link with Sidney Herbert. As she told Acland, who shared her high view of Sidney Herbert, it was "founded on Herbert's intentions." That letter ends with "God speed your Artillery son in S. Africa,"[31] a reference to his son, Frank, on whom more below. Nightingale corresponded on the school with Acland yet again in 1887, when their main subject was state registration.

The Army Statistics Branch

Nightingale had a gut feeling for statistics – numbers to her meant real people. She told Sir John McNeill that it was "criminal to have a mortality of 17, 19, and 20 per 1000 in the army in England, when in civil life it is only 11 per 1000." It was like taking 1,100 men out to Salisbury Plain and shooting them.[32] In 1869, after improved sanitary conditions had reduced army mortality in peacetime, she could say: "We have 729 men alive who would have been dead ... and 5184 men ... on active duty who would have been 'constantly sick' in bed."[33]

Her serious statistical work began soon after her return from the Crimean War, as we saw in chapter 2. By early January 1857, she was receiving statistical material on army- and civil-hospital stays and death rates from Major George Graham, the head of the General Register Office. He sent her, with the printed tables, a memorandum by William Farr on English hospital mortality. Farr then took over the processing and sending of material. By May 1857, she wanted his feedback on her analysis. A letter of his began: "I have read with much profit your admirable observations. It is like light shining in a dark place. You might, when you have completed your task, give some preliminary explanation for the sake of the *ignorant* reader."[34] Another instalment shared Farr's anxiety "to see the mortality of our brave army reduced to half its present amount. It is a thing beyond all doubt to be done."[35]

Surgeon-General Thomas Graham Balfour (1813–1891) served as secretary of the Royal Commission on the Crimean War and then headed the new Statistics Branch of the Army Medical Department. Nightingale called him, with Alexander Tulloch, the "real founders of military vital statistics." "Dr Balfour has all the experience of statistical problems which exists anywhere. There is no second to him, either in the army or elsewhere. His Army Statistical reports are models," and they improved every year.[36] One reason they did so is that he sent drafts to Nightingale for comment. She sent detailed advice, with praise when he got it right. She compared him favourably with Dr Longmore. Not only did he have greater statistical experience than anyone, but he produced a comparison between French and English army syphilis and was "perhaps the most scientific man in the A.M.D."[37] She assisted him later in his voluntary work for the Royal Hospital for Incurables in Putney, London.

Timely statistics were needed, Nightingale thought. Tulloch's annual Blue Books (statistical compendia) appeared too late to be of use; the men reported on were either already dead or discharged. Speedier reporting was required, every month, to turn into daily reporting as soon as an epidemic appeared. Data should normally be available for each regiment, on mean strength, with the mean number of sick from fever, consumption, and other causes. These figures could then be aggregated to the whole army. The secretary of state for war should be able to judge health status for the army "as clearly as the movements of time on the face of a clock,"[38] Nightingale insisted to Dr Balfour. "Not until we have a complete system of sanitary statistics in the army shall we be able to administer the laws of health with that certainty with which we know they are capable of being administered."[39]

Later Dr Alexander informed her that Balfour was "founding a house," which she called "a strong and bright pillar worthy of Solomon's temple."[40] In 1873, she complimented Balfour on his "capital report," praising it for including "facts only, leaving discussions and opinions to the medical journals." It was important not to support anybody's peculiar views. She cited Robert Burns that "'facts are chils that downa ding,' You can't knock them over. Opinions, on the contrary, are the scriptural 'fowls of the air'" (Matthew 6:26).[41]

Nutrition

Nutrition was a new discipline, emerging just as Nightingale was seeking a firm basis for reforming food in the British Army. A leading expert was a civilian doctor, Robert Christison (1797–1882), later made a baronet, an expert on poisons. (He was also an opponent of women in medicine.) Nightingale quoted him both on needed nutrients, for soldiers' health, and on what form the sick could take them. When Christison provided her with his advice on diet, she asked Alexander to read it, "to see whether you would make any modification in consequence of your own draft," which she conveniently enclosed.[42]

New "diet tables" had to be incorporated into the Regulations, with menus for breakfast, lunch, and dinner.[43] If the Regulations were not adequate, Nightingale realized, decent food would not be produced, and men's health would suffer. She was a stickler for detail, noting, for example, that if lime juice is ordered, sugar must be added.

Dr Sutherland gave Nightingale sound advice on improving army nutrition, a subject she pursued assiduously, and with success. The army needed, for all general and regimental hospitals, at home and in the temperate colonies, a scale of diets, based on the army scale, but more subdivided, and containing the medical comforts and extras needed. For India and tropical stations, it would have to be modified by the medical officer, to order diets lower in the scale than he would give at home. Said Sutherland:

> We want for field service a dietary based on the nutritive power
> of preserved provisions, with the equivalent in nutritious value
> stated of fresh provisions (so much essence of beef equivalent to so
> much fresh beef or mutton) … Let Dr Alexander be requested to
> draw up a hospital dietary of preserved provisions such as they had
> during the second winter at the Crimea. Ask Christison to review
> this dietary. Ask Christison also to frame a scale of, say, nine diets
> based on the existing scale in the army for general and regimental
> hospitals and then to collate with the Alexander dietary of preserved
> provisions. Ask Alexander to improve the scheme of hospital diets
> so as to include extras.[44]

Sutherland's letter, which summarized Christison's position, shows how close it was to Nightingale's (and his) in insisting on administrative efficiency. This meant an end to the cumbersome system of inadequate meals, which had to be supplemented supplanted by "extras" prescribed for each patient: "We want to prevent the absurdity of medical officers being purveyors, storekeepers, etc.; (2) we want to abolish the requisition system in general hospitals; (3) we want a field dietary."[45]

The American Civil War

Nightingale was involved in numerous later wars, sending nurses and advising on hospitals and amenities for soldiers. The first after the Crimean was the US Civil War (1861–65), when her advice on hospitals was used on both sides.[46] She was already well known to people there for her Crimea work, which was widely covered by the American press. Jefferson Davis, then US war secretary, sent a three-man delegation to the Crimea and Scutari to see the hospitals and camps. All three officials met Nightingale, and one was briefly in her hospital.[47] Davis was subsequently president of the Confederacy.

It was the Union army, however, that was sent her useful forms and reports. The Confederate army had to rely on her publications, and clearly used them. Its largest hospital, a hut hospital at Richmond, Virginia, was built on her principles. The Confederate army also used her advice on nutrition.[48]

In 1861, Nightingale sent all the War Office forms it had available to Dr Edward Jarvis, president of the American Statistical Association and a member of the United States Sanitary Commission. He had been a guest at her home in London during the meetings of the International Statistical Congress in 1860 and subsequently asked for them.[49] Dr Farr later asked for Crimean War material from her to send to the founder of the Western Sanitary Commission, William Greenleaf Eliot; she sent the "coxcombs" or charts of mortality rates.[50] The US Sanitary Commission, like the Western Sanitary Commission, was a voluntary agency, unlike the British namesake. It is known that the US Sanitary Commission used Nightingale's material, although she thought not as well as it could have. The death rates in that war were enormous. A history of the Sanitary Commission, however, expressed appreciation of her material for its clarity; it enabled solutions to be arrived at "with the exactness of a scientific demonstration."[51]

Nightingale's name was used, without her knowledge, in the cause of finding nurses and raising aid for the Union cause. In Pennsylvania, a "Nightingale Association for the Relief of our Soldiers" was formed to furnish nurses and to supply lint and bandages.[52] New Jersey's similar "Florence Nightingale Relief Association" promoted sanitary work.[53]

Dr Sutherland later pointed out the negatives of forces having to rely on a voluntary sanitary commission during the Civil War. The American example was "the most splendid and costly example" of this mistake. In "no case" had the result been "satisfactory." Rather, he wrote:

> When governments go to war, they do not calculate the chances
> of the battlefield, although they ought to be considered as closely
> as those of army subsistence. When 100,000 or 150,000 men are

sent on a great military service in which great battles are most likely to follow, it is always possible to arrive at some estimate of their contingencies and every effort should be made to provide for them. Governments are the only parties who should be held responsible for the wounded and sick in war. This should be one of their highest responsibilities. But to fulfil it there should be an organization in peace which could be easily expanded to meet the necessities of the field.[54]

A footnote: as a voluntary agency, the US Sanitary Commission had to raise its own money. English novelist Elizabeth Gaskell contributed a letter of Nightingale's to be sold for its benefit.[55]

During the Civil War, the possibility of an American invasion of Canada emerged after Union forces seized a British mail ship, the *Trent*, which was carrying Confederate diplomats to Britain to promote their side. In the end, nothing came of the "Trent Affair," but Nightingale was consulted on preparations for a winter campaign in the Canadian colonies. Mindful of the terrible frostbite suffered in the Crimea, she examined distances to be covered by sleds and the comparative weight and warmth of blankets and buffalo robes. Buffalo coats would be best, she asserted, but a letter from Lord de Grey informed her that there would be "great difficulty in obtaining an adequate supply of buffalo robes in this country for the whole force." Each man would have "two good blankets" in addition to other "warm clothing."[56]

Nightingale gave advice also on sanitary preparations and a possible medical officer for New Brunswick.[57] She considered the director-general's instructions adequate for short sledging, as between Fredericton (New Brunswick) and Rivière-du-Loup (Canada East / Quebec), but not more. She proposed that buffalo robes could be taken, and moved back and forth for sledging operations.[58]

She was asked also to advise on the setting up of general hospitals, possibly for Quebec City, Montreal, and Ottawa. An average sick of 3 per cent of troops in Canada, or 3½ per cent with contingencies, meant 420 beds for 1,200 men.[59] Reinforcements were sent, but in the end the Americans did not invade.

The Army in India

Sir John Lawrence became viceroy of India in January 1864, soon after the Royal Commission on the Sanitary State of the Army in India released its report. Nightingale briefed him on its recommendations before his departure, and he wrote her soon after arrival to outline the prompt actions he had taken: the establishment of sanitary commissions in Bombay (now Mumbai), Calcutta (Kolkata), and Madras (Chennai).[60] Their doctor members, in effect medical officers of health for large regions, became her allies. This section gives details of five of them.

Nightingale had a high opinion of the work of Thomas Crawford (1824–1895), who was principal medical officer in India when the station hospitals were introduced. In 1882, he became director-general of Britain's Army Medical Department, serving until 1889. In his retirement, he was appointed to the Nightingale Fund Council, but died soon afterwards.

James McNabb Cuningham (1829–1905) was surgeon-general and chief sanitary commissioner in India, a member of the Army Sanitary Commission and the Bengal Sanitary Commission. When Robert Koch published his identification of the bacillus for Asiatic cholera, Cuningham gave a paper critical of his findings, later worked into a book, published by the government of India.[61]

Nightingale also was in touch with Dr Charles Hathaway (1817–1903), assistant to the viceroy, who told her, "Nothing you have ever written or conceived of the horrible state of practices pursued at Calcutta comes up to the reality."[62]

Perhaps Nightingale's favourite "Indian" doctor was Thomas Gillham Hewlett (1831–1889), the first sanitary commissioner for Bombay, and her best source generally. Her papers on a "missionary health officer" concerned his work combatting famine. He reminded her of General Gordon (of Khartoum) for his "righteous indignation."[63] When he was writing his last annual report, she urged him, at Douglas Galton's request, to make it – as his last – "as full as possible." He could not, he told her, but assured her that his final remarks would be part of the next one.[64] Naturally, he asked her for "the points" that should go into that "posthumous report," as she told Galton.[65] She next noted that she had better answer Hewlett's letter, "or he will be doing something we don't like." She wanted him to take another appointment: "We have no one at all to compare with him in practical knowledge and keen interest ... It would be a sin to let Mr *Hewlett* fall out of our ranks. We have no one like him."[66] She tried to have him succeed Dr Sutherland on the Army Sanitary Commission, but his failing health precluded that.

Another greatly esteemed doctor was Surgeon-General George (later Sir George) J.H. Evatt (1843–1921), who had a long career in India, plus other appointments, including Afghanistan. He was a valued source on the Army Hospital Corps (orderlies) and nurse training. Early on in their work together, Nightingale remonstrated with him for more facts, to support reform. He sought to give her "some particulars as to the *actual condition* of the 'nursing' for the European soldier when sick," but there was nothing on the "*actual facts* of the present case," only recommendations. What she needed was "what they want and *don't* have – what you have observed as to actual neglects, and the sufferings, slow recoveries, or *no* recoveries, and death caused by such total absence of nursing." It would "be quite impossible to arouse the interest necessary to get *anything done* without making out a detailed case (which I know to be a very strong one) of the evils the patients suffer, first, with chapter and verse of some type cases."[67]

In 1885, for the (second) Egyptian campaign, Nightingale was "grieved" that England would lose Evatt for a time, but exulted in the prospect of his ideas being put into practice: "Now we shall see all your conclusions carried out in wartime." She looked forward, when that was done, to their becoming the "system" for peace and war, "to forward the true cause."[68] On his retirement, Evatt sought a political career, and asked for Nightingale's help. She wrote a campaign letter for him in 1886, read out at an election meeting of 3,000 people.[69]

Strenuously desiring, as we all of us must, that *administration*, as well as politics, should be well represented in Parliament, and that vital matters of social, sanitary and general interest should find there their voice, we could desire no better representative and advocate of these essential matters – matters of life and death – than a man who, like yourself, unites with almost exhaustless energy and public spirit, sympathy with the wronged and enthusiasm for the right – a persevering acuteness in unravelling the causes of the evil and the good, large and varied experience, and practical power limited only by the nature of the objects for which it is exerted.

It is important beyond measure that such a man's thoughtful and
well-considered opinions and energetic voice should be heard in the
House of Commons.

Nightingale hoped that he would win, less for his own sake than for
England's,[70] but he lost. She later arranged for him to meet the Liberal
leader, Lord Rosebery.

Cholera Inquiry in India

Cholera was endemic in India, and a concern throughout Nightingale's
working life. She was a strong advocate of the cholera inquiry conducted
in that country in 1870. When a doctor, W.C. MacLean (1811–1898),
criticized her publicly for *opposing* such an inquiry, she protested forcefully.
Her letter to the *Lancet* refers to recent research on possible causes of
the disease, mentioning negative results on fungoid causes and evidence
that a dry-earth system for treating excreta had not "stayed the ravages
of cholera." She cited published reports on these points, stressing the
differences between theory and fact: "These statements are not theories,
but facts. If they are facts, they cease to be theories. The theories remain
just where they were. Of course, if the theories were found no longer on
inquiry to be true, they too would be no longer theories, but facts, and as
such would afford good ground for expending public money in applying
the *facts* to save life."

She went on to rebut a point made by her medical critic on Edward
Jenner (1749–1823) and vaccination: "Jenner first started a theory, but the
Vaccination Acts, with the costs and penalties, were not enacted until
Jenner's theory had become a fact by long experience." The object for all
was "saving human life." It could not be done without expenditure: "And
as theories are many and uncertain, all we ask is that the public should
know what we are spending their money for. This the said cholera inquiry
will, perhaps more than anything else, help to tell us."[71]

The Geneva Convention and the Red Cross

Nightingale did the briefing note for the British delegation to the
first Geneva Convention, held in 1864. The two delegates were both
Crimean War surgeons, Thomas Longmore, already introduced above for

his immediate post-war work, and William Rutherford (1817–1887), an excellent surgeon, Nightingale thought, but without knowledge of sanitary measures. He also did not know "a blessed word of French," as he admitted in his diary while on route to Geneva. To Nightingale, he described the new Red Cross, founded by Henri Dunant the previous year, as "a kind of international amateur society to assist the sick and wounded."[72] Rutherford's opposition was noted at the conclave: "Welfare societies appeared to him to be a bad remedy for the evil which they were seeking to cure. Care of the wounded was the responsibility of governments and of governments alone. If the medical corps was insufficient, it must be reinforced, but there should be no question of calling on civilians."[73]

Dr John Sutherland's caution about the use of voluntary help in war appeared above, vis-à-vis the American Civil War. A note of his for Nightingale explained his objection to Henri Dunant's proposal, that it "amounted to the introduction of voluntary lay agency as a supplement to or as a substitute for government action, because my own experience was all against this." However, "when the conference at Geneva limited its recommendations to the neutralization of the field medical service, I joined heartily in its principles."[74]

Nightingale and Sutherland saw eye to eye on the need for armies to assume full responsibility for the care of their sick and wounded in war. She was forceful in declaring to her brother-in-law, Sir Harry Verney, vice-chair of the National Aid Society:

The Prussian government makes war cheap by throwing all its duties and responsibilities with regard to its *sick* men overboard, and leaving us and others to pick them up *if we please. If not, not.* It is exactly what we told our own government in 1864 with regard to the Geneva Convention: "Take care that it in no way diminishes the responsibilities of each belligerent government for its own sick and wounded, and for making preparations in time of peace for its sick and wounded in time of war." *We* are *in fact* paying a large quota to the expenses of the Prussians making war.[75]

They had support on this point from other doctors, such as surgeon William MacCormac, who shared her view that the Red Cross would "militarize charity."[76] In fact, as is well known, the Red Cross idea took hold and was not challenged on this issue.

Dunant had erred also, Nightingale thought, in "supposing that a voluntary agency of any value could be extemporized." It could not, because it needed training and discipline. Sutherland had been in touch with Dunant "long before the Geneva Conference."[77]

The Franco–Prussian War

The United Kingdom was not a belligerent in the Franco–Prussian War of 1870–71, but its National Aid Society sent doctors, supplies, and "ambulances," or field hospitals, to it. Nightingale was involved in organizing supplies, for both sides. Neither the French nor the Germans wanted nurses from other countries – both had nuns, the Germans also Protestant deaconesses. The Crown Princess of Prussia eventually wanted one nurse from Nightingale, Florence Lees, who spoke French and German fluently and was already in France when her services were asked for.

Nightingale's first instinct on the outbreak of the war was to "be off this afternoon to the seat of war to organize something."[78] However, she could not, and instead was confined to assisting the National Aid Society, the forerunner of the British Red Cross. It was headed by Colonel Robert Loyd-Lindsay, who had a Victoria Cross from the Crimean War, with Sir Harry Verney, as vice-chair. Serving both sides, or "neutralization," was a desideratum from the outset.

"Franco–Prussian" is the term used here for the war, which is also known as the Franco–German War. Prussia was the instigator, but increasingly other German states joined in, to arrive at the formation of a German empire by war's end. Nightingale herself normally used "Prussian" for the state, so that it could be pejorative, reserving "German" for the language and culture, for which she had highly positive feelings. The war is noteworthy for the great increase in army size and fire-power, with no commensurate improvement in medical or nursing assistance or hospital administration. Nightingale made numerous comparisons with the mistakes and deficiencies of the Crimean War fifteen years earlier.

The struggle soon became for Nightingale "this awful war ... this lamentable, this deadly war." She regretted that it had found concerned observers "without any organization wherewith to proceed at once to the assistance of our suffering brothers and sisters across the channel."[79] To a German friend then living in Paris, she called the guillotine "merciful" in comparison to the "unutterable woe and horror of this misery": "acres of wounded, especially French, even after they had been removed under some kind of shelter and received some kind of first dressing, appear to have been left with nothing under nor over them, no food, water or wine, cleanliness or attendance. From the proportion of dead to wounded, which is unspeakably larger than anything I ever heard of before, thousands must have died of sheer want, after having been wounded."[80]

Joseph Lister, who had published his pioneering work in antiseptic surgery in 1867, released a practical two-page account in September 1870 on applying antiseptic principles in the field.[81] This was late for the war, however, since the first battles took place in July and August and the French surrendered the very day his letter appeared. Then the war resumed in the autumn, with uprisings in Paris, a new government, the Commune, and a siege. In short, conditions worsened and casualties mounted. Lister's complicated and time-consuming advice was only "sporadically" applied, more by the Germans than the French.[82] Conditions in the hospitals, not only in the field, were grim.

Reports came to Nightingale that soldiers were left untreated for days. A letter has her questioning the competence of the French Red Cross, based on information she received from Mme Canrobert, widow of the second French commander-in-chief in the Crimea. She noted high death rates from typhus and dysentery, among amputation cases held in old hospitals, not the field hospitals. She hoped to receive a report from Douglas Galton on "the methods in use in the two armies for supplying the hospitals – where the weak points were – and in what way we could avoid these. Also the weak points in the 'Red Cross societies' work.'" She asked what direction they could give, "What kind of temporary hospital accommodation" should they be using?"[83]

Nightingale had letters "from surgeons on the spot" who reported losing "all" their amputation cases. She thought the proportion of deaths to amputations was "terrible enough at Scutari, but this, it appears, is more terrible still." Surgeons attributed it partly to "the want and exposure endured by the men in the time, two–five days before they were removed from the field ... partly to the state of things in hospitals."[84]

Correspondence from the Crown Princess of Prussia during the war reported as much difficulty in dealing with Prussia's Medical Department, "with some noble exceptions," Nightingale noted, "as we had in the Crimea." She wondered if "the most likely way to undo these stupid doctors would be, just as our government issued a commission (Sutherland

and Rawlinson) with powers under which they acted, quite new and unprecedented in all armies, for Von Roon, the war minister, to have an inspector of his own. (The crown princess would be the only person who could select him, and I believe she could lay her hand on an efficient Prussian inspector) and give him power to deal with such cases."[85] In the same letter, she recalled a nurse telling her of seeing both incompetence and cruelty. "They don't learn," Nightingale commented, "and the poor men suffer." Another source told her that "the most ordinary essential and sanitary necessities are not provided for" in the Prussian camps around Paris. Clementina Rumpff, a German nurse who had been at St Thomas', told her that, even near Prussian headquarters:

> Where we must suppose supplies to be most plentiful, in the very Palace of Versailles itself, e.g., there were only 36 flannel jackets for 600 patients, and at Brie-en-Robert 256 typhus cases!!! without beef-tea or the commonest hospital provisions, actually "dying for want"! If these things are done or rather left undone at Prussian headquarters round Paris, and at the typhus "stations" round Metz (as described by Miss Lees[86]), if the German camps are in such an insanitary state round Paris, too – *if* these things could occur in mid-autumn on what is really Prussian ground – what will happen in mid-winter if the Prussians are still at war? I shall be all anxiety to hear of your ambulance, the giant, where it goes.[87]

Florence Lees had nothing but praise for the crown princess's own small hospital, where she served, but found much to fault in the regular lazareths in which she also (briefly) served and those she visited. She was chief nurse at the typhus station for the *10e corps d'armée*, where the doctor – luckily he arrived only the day before she left – was "obstinate and prejudiced in favour of *closed* windows!" It was always difficult getting fresh air in "a French or German 'village house,'" she said, but he insisted on shutting all the windows. When she protested about the intolerable smell, he would allow one window if the door was shut: "I will have no English ways here," he told her, and he also "forbade any wine, quinine, cognac or bouillon to be given to *any* of the sick," allowing only a "little extract of milk and as much cold water as they pleased." She fairly cried with vexation.[88]

Nightingale was invited both to attend and to send a "communication" to a meeting at which Ernest Hart was speaking in November 1870.

She declined both, graciously, on grounds of illness.[89] She was evidently concerned, however, about what he would say. She told Harry Verney that he was "clever but unsound."[90] Verney thought that she could point out to Dr Hart in what he had been "mistaken in the formation of the Red Cross Society, and how it may be rendered useful in future."[91]

Early in 1871, when the fighting was over, Nightingale reported such unhappy facts as the "beautiful French military hospitals (in time of peace) at Metz, Strasburg, etc.," when in German possession had "floor and bedsteads going to ruin from uncleanliness; typhus cases gasping for air – windows all bunged up; patients who ought to have been fed every hour sinking for want." Meals were late, the bedding dirty, the smell sickening, patients lay around "in saturated bedclothes." There was "no *polishing* of the floors and lockers (only wiped)," which did not leave them clean. The Red Cross stores at Versailles went "almost entirely" to the Germans. The German aid society grabbed "wholesale at the English and French stores." The mortality among amputation cases was "frightful," attributed to "the crowding, without beds or cleanliness, in closed buildings."[92]

Some British doctors gave their services through the Anglo–American Ambulance, founded by an American doctor, James Marion Sims (1813–1883), who had been in Paris when the war started. His assistant was William MacCormac (1836–1901), later a surgeon at St Thomas' and first baronet. He was one whose "brave doings" Nightingale had heard about. He sent her a copy of his *Notes and Recollections of an Ambulance Surgeon* (1871), about his Franco–Prussian War experiences; she responded with a copy of her *Introductory Notes on Lying-in Institutions*, "though not much in his line," as her dedication put it.[93]

MacCormac, who served with the French Army, reported that it did not generally employ antiseptic measures, and he was indeed critical of it. The French used non-sterile lint to pack wounds and had a higher incidence of gas gangrene among their troops than the Prussians. According to a history of the period, the Prussians made "some use" of Lister's methods of antisepsis,[94] a finding generally held.

Nightingale throughout was inundated with information on the course of the war, the field hospitals, and related problems. The crown princess wrote her, as well as nurses (Lees and Rumpff), doctors, National Aid Society officials, and volunteer aid workers.

Death Rates French and German

Available estimates suggest lower death rates in the French Army, even though the Germans were the winners, from the earliest battles on. Nightingale wrote Sir Harry Verney:

> I hear (I will not say, "on the highest authority" like a newspaper, since there *can* be no "authority" for this, as the Germans cannot have made up their statistics and the French still less), I hear that, whereas the mortality in the French ambulances has only been 1 in 8½, that in the Prussian has been 1 in 5. This is enormous – 20 percent. (My informant very modestly adds that he cannot account for the difference.) *We* can account for it very well, since the Prussian ambulances have had every essential to make them a manufactory of typhus, gangrene, and erysipelas. And I very much fear that the mortality will prove something still higher than this, though they, being the conquerors, have had a far greater command of supplies than the French.[95]

The French Army's rates, though lower, were similar to those it incurred during the first winter of the Crimean War. Its death rates had then risen in the second winter, when the British rates declined. Nor had the French done better during their next war, the Italian War of Independence in 1859.

The estimated death rate of 1 in 5, or 20 per cent, reached Nightingale also from the head of the National Aid Society, Loyd-Lindsay, about the hospitals it was funding. This revealed rates of Prussian sickness of 20 per cent, with a 20 per cent estimated rate of death of the sick. From private accounts she had heard worse: the typhus stations in particular had cases "lying or rather dying on straw," so that she thought 20 per cent "far below the truth." Again, a comparison with Crimean War: "I do not hesitate to say that the state of the Scutari hospitals, which roused the horror of all England, and, at its worst time, was not so bad as that of the Prussian ambulances at its best time." The Prussian hospital system "was an utter sham ... They are just where the French were in the early part of Louis XIV. They have beaten the French in soldiering. But their hospitals have still to march a century and a half (or ever since Frederic the Great) to keep up to our present standard."[96]

After the Crimean War, Nightingale had given some thought as to better care after battle, to avoid moving men into hospital. She took this up again during the Franco–Prussian War: "All Europe, ourselves included, have taken *the hospital idea* as the fundamental one for the Red Cross. This appears to be the error." Hospitals, if properly conducted, were "most essential ... But we must not forget (1) the *immediate* want of help after the battle to the wounded; (2) that nearly every kind of wound can be better dealt with separately, in the open air, than by removal to the finest hospitals." She thought that the wounded did better in farmhouses, or without medical equipment, than in the "large crowded old buildings and churches" then used, which were "destructive." Speed of supply was crucial.[97]

While Nightingale soon saw the Franco–Prussian War as that "horrid" war, as she told a German correspondent, it would worsen, especially in Paris with the siege.[98] She also understood how the peace treaty's punitive terms for France would breed further violence. The war had fostered the German Empire, out of the confederation that came together to fight it. Looking back on it years later, Nightingale said, "I hate war."[99] In a letter to the editor much later, she quoted "a great writer," not named, that "we hate war, we admire discipline as an aid to duty."[100]

The Transvaal War

Nightingale's involvement in the Anglo–Zulu War of 1879 and the Transvaal War of 1880–81 (First Boer War) was minimal, but enough for her to see old defects reappear, especially the inadequacy and often drunkenness of the orderlies. An inquiry had to be launched, and witnesses found who would speak up, as before, risking their own career advancement by so doing.

When nurses were being sent to the Transvaal War, Nightingale asked a favour of surgeon Alexander MacKellar, to order a *"dresser's case* for Mrs Fellowes, who is going to nurse the wounded in the Transvaal War, also for hints as to *lint,* linen, etc., whether these will be properly supplied by the Cape Town people, *or how?"* Further, she asked him for advice on *outfit* for the nurses.[101] Mrs Fellowes would be a prime informant on problems.

Nightingale was appalled, yet again, at the lack of preparation. Three battles resulted in an average of 500 "severely wounded" in hospital, where the only equipment was that planned for a "peace footing." The principal medical officer managed to send up some chloroform by a cart. "There were wounded who were four days unattended to." Yet the medical officer in charge of Fort Amiel, near Newcastle, Natal, wrote home to Dr Longmore "a flaming letter of praise of the arrangements, and of self-congratulation on '*everything so good*' (which I saw). Orderlies atrocious." Colonel Loyd-Lindsay "again" wrote her that everything was provided. She remarked on the parallels with the Crimean War: though on a smaller scale, it was Balaclava, the front, and the Crimean War "over again."[102]

Another informant in Natal on hospital defects was Amy Hawthorn, wife of Colonel Robert Hawthorn, Royal Engineers, and a cousin of General Gordon. At the same fever hospital, Hawthorn saw another Acland son, Frank, an artillery officer, who wrote his father about the unsatisfactory orderlies. Hawthorn described them as "careless and cruel" young men, "often drunk."[103] Nightingale wanted young Dr Acland to pursue this, to ask "*how the men in hospital are nursed*, whether he hears any complaints about orderly nursing, or the diets and drinks – and you might tell Dr Acland [senior] what we have heard."[104] When an inquiry, finally, started, Nightingale was back to her old trade of formulating questions for doctors, to coax out their evidence to best effect.

She continued to be moved by individual cases she was told about. To Amy Hawthorn, who wrote her from Natal, she expressed her feelings for her "*and* for them. The blood of that poor man, Dunn, who died of dysentery and could not get a drink, cries to God from the ground. I do not mean for vengeance, but for reform, that future comrades may not suffer as he did."[105]

The Egyptian Campaigns, 1882 and 1885

The Egyptian campaign of 1882 began as the Transvaal War was winding down. The commander was the same for the two, Garnet Wolseley, and many of the same personnel served in both. Dr Thomas Crawford, director-general of the Army Medical Department, asked Nightingale to advise him on sending nurses to Egypt. He also, in a departure from earlier practice, asked Mrs Fellowes, then at Portsmouth, for her views. Crawford reported back to Nightingale on the deployment of her nurses.[106]

The Egyptian campaign of 1882 was notable for a cholera epidemic (1882–83) that prompted the sending of three teams of investigators and led, by a circuitous route, to the definitive identification of the cause of cholera, related in chapter 7. The epidemic, of course, meant an enormous amount of work for doctors and nurses, and questions about local sanitary conditions. Nurses were sent back to London and then back again to Egypt. They served both on a hospital ship, the *Carthage,* and in hospitals in Alexandria and Cairo.

On the return of the troops to London in November 1882, Prime Minister William Ewart Gladstone invited Nightingale to Victoria Station to join in the official welcome. She sat between him and Mrs Gladstone. The queen, in attendance, sent her a message of greeting.[107]

Nightingale was concerned – shades of the Crimean War – after learning that a Dr Ferguson was shown a list and asked if he wanted anything more, but replied that nothing was needed, "though everything was wanting" (her words). There was "bad, coarse meat from Malta and Alexandria on board ... Dr Pennington applied for meat, and could not get it ... Orderlies' drunkenness .... [An] orderly six years at Herbert in charge of two critical cases, found drunk in bed by Mrs Fellowes." The same note indicated that there was carbolic oil, a disinfectant, and plenty of gauze, but no spray.[108]

Nightingale inquired of Dr Sutherland about Dr (J.A.) Marston (1831–1911), the sanitary officer, who was spoken of as the "coming man" but who entirely ignored the sanitary subject, to dwell on there "having been *no wants* of stores." At his station at Ismailia, "the *ground was polluted* to such an extent *round the hospital* that tents could not be pitched. The *barracks* were in such a state when our troops were put into them at *Cairo* that the men had to be turned out in twenty four hours (not by sanitary but by commanding officer) ... *Where was the sanitary officer?*"[109]

Nightingale was soon drawing up questions for Dr Marston to be asked at an inquiry.[110] Subsequent notes on his evidence report "admission of and defence of failures, failure in every way as to system, *not* as to men. They say the system has broken down. The system has never been tried. No workable system, *no real sanitary appreciation of problems at stake.*" Nightingale disagreed with Marston's claim that civil hospitals were efficient because the medical staff had supreme power. It was "just the reverse," for her. Civil hospitals had three distinct elements: medical, administration, and nursing, "each with its distinct duties, not doing one another's work, but each working to keep the whole machine in order." Her comments became more and more scathing on the faults of administration: "A.M.D. [Army Medical Department] at a dead level of inefficiency." Naturally, she asked about the principal medical officer, Sir James Hanbury (1832–1908), the doctors' superior (he had been head at Netley).[111]

Nightingale discussed the inquiry with Dr Evatt and took notes of his comments, which were more positive than her own: "Our interest is not to hush up, not to deny everything. I only hope that Dr Hanbury will not deny everything. Let him say: this is what was wanting; this is what we want. England will give it. England wants the hospital to be the home of the sick soldier. She wants it not to be prison cells but a home. You have the ball of progress at your feet. You have only to kick it. The wave is coming in: You have only to come in on the wave."[112]

Nightingale, as well as receiving letters from her nurses, met with them on their return to England and took extensive notes of the defects they reported. For example, from Mrs Fellowes, she recorded:

> No organization. No nursing. Orderlies will pull a dying man
> out of a bed to put him on the night stool or a fractured thigh
> groin wound vomiting into a bedpan lid soaked in hemorrhage ...
> *Carthage* doctors always in wards ... Much work done by the
> patients. Wounds came to us ... Patients with sandbags extensions,
> no clean sheets were put on; he and his comrades put them on
> themselves; he got out of bed with his fractured knee and put the
> sandbags under the bed and untied all the bandages to please
> the doctor ... *Carthage* badly fitted up. No washing of helpless
> patients ... I did the dressings generally alone, 5 a.m. to breakfast,
> then dinner, then till 5, then from 6 to anytime – midnight.
> Dr Pennington said, Ah, we see the civil training wanted to make a
> good nurse. He said Netley [a] nest of jobbery [bribe taking].[113]

Nightingale nurse Sybil Airy served at the Cholera Hospital in Cairo in 1883 and sent Nightingale detailed letters about the work. She noted the "surprise visit by young Dr Acland of St Thomas', who has come to work among the Egyptian Army." He was Henry Acland's medical son, Theodore Dyke Acland (1851–1931), sent by the Foreign Office to the Egyptian army hospitals. A new level of collegial relations is apparent with his visit. In October, the "young Dr Acland" asked Airy over to his hospital to show his people "how to pad splints properly." Another problem – the Egyptian cooks could not make beef tea – so Acland asked Airy for a recipe, which he had translated into Arabic. The cook, proud of his results, had them taste it. Airy and Acland were both keen to replicate St Thomas' standards in their hospitals.

Airy was highly complimentary about Acland's management. She and other nurses had seen his "Bed Hospital" six weeks earlier and were impressed with how "beautifully" he had transformed it, in such a short time and under so many difficulties. Earlier, it "scarcely looked like a hospital, *now* the wards, kitchen, dispensary, laundry, etc., are in beautiful working order, with quite a tone of '*St Thomas'* about everything, quite delightful to see in *Egypt!*" Further, she said, the "khedive" (king) had visited it the previous day "and had expressed great approbation with all the arrangements." He promised to send them a quantity of orange trees and so on from his own grounds to plant in their garden: "Dr Acland must have worked very hard to have completed so much in such a short time."[114]

Dr Acland senior asked Nightingale to forward a book to his son at his hospital at Cairo. She added a note of her own, "with earnest good wishes for his highest success in every way and warmest admiration of his devotion."[115]

Airy's matter-of-fact letters to Nightingale on their work mentioned the cholera crisis frequently, but not its outcome. The nurses had been moved from their quarters for sanitary improvements to be made, and were temporarily housed in the Officers' Mess. A Dr Lewis they had worked with had died of cholera.[116] By her next letter, cholera was subsiding where they were – only four deaths the previous day – but increasing in Alexandria. A sunstroke patient had died, which prompted the doctor to comment that "had there been a night sister on, he might have been saved." She thought that army doctors would "in time get converted to sisters!"[117]

The cholera epidemic of 1882–83 in Egypt was brought to an end with improved sanitary measures, and Dr William Guyer Hunter (1827–1902), who headed the response team, wrote a detailed report. Yet, as Dr Acland senior pointed out in a letter to the editor of the *Times* in 1886, nothing had been done since. Filth was a chronic condition. Cities could become uninhabitable from pestilential conditions, not just war. Acland then praised the work done by Englishwomen in the Citadel of Cairo, showing how they perpetuated "Miss Nightingale's example in the East."[118]

The 1885 Egyptian campaign was sparked by events in Sudan, where General Gordon was held for months in Khartoum, only to be assassinated shortly before the arrival of British troops to rescue him. The Suez Canal Company established a fund for a "Gordon Memorial Hospital," 100 beds, to be built in "four months!!!," as Nightingale commented.[119]

The 1885 campaign was noted in chapter 3, on matron Rachel Williams's volunteering. The director-general of the Army Medical Department asked Nightingale's assistance in recruitment, and the nurses were given further support by the National Aid Society and a new Ladies' Committee organized by Lady Rosebery, wife of the prime minister. They were all concerned now to have "*educated women.*"[120] Nightingale nurses served in Cairo, Suakim, the Suez, on hospital ships, at base hospitals at Aswan and Wady Halfa, and in a dahabiah on the Nile.

Crimea-like botch-ups occurred, now thirty years later. When Rachel Williams and other nurses arrived in Egypt, they found that they were unexpected. Put out in the desert, they had to make their way in the dark to the hospital, where the nurse who answered the door would not let them in, even to stay overnight. They went to the Hotel Suez, found the doctor in charge, who assisted them, but he could not put them to work until proper orders came through. This took some time, so that Williams was about to return to England when they were assigned.[121] They would soon – some of them – be overworked, while some were sent where they were not needed. All this Williams reported back to Nightingale, who would pass on the concerns to the Army Medical Department. She would soon caution Williams, who had telegraphed her with one problem: "It is always better to be as quiet as possible and 'appeal' little to headquarters."[122]

Much correspondence dealt with supplying missing food items and inquiring about fresh fruit. In a refreshing change, medical officers called for more nurses. Nightingale would point out that more were available – seven had been sent home![123]

Correspondence in 1888 shows further developments in professional expectations for international work. English (missionary) nurses in Cairo were given daily Arabic lessons and had to pass an examination in it after six months.[124] Nightingale sent them several books on modern Arabic, after consulting with her "pundits" and Oxford and London publishers.[125]

Last Work with Military Doctors

An American surgeon-general, J.B. Hamilton, later editor of the *Journal of the American Medical Association.* approached Nightingale in 1893 about the lack of practical training in the care of army patients, on which he had written to the *Times*. The two corresponded; he paid her a visit and left her a paper. He told her that no assistance could be expected from the British commander, Sir Redvers Buller, whom he blamed, with Lord [Garnet] Wolseley, for the poor "state of affairs."[126] He saw political action, in the House of Commons, as essential. Nightingale got him together with Douglas Galton on the matter, and a question was raised in the House, although she noted that a "mere question in the House is proverbially ineffective." "It is awful to think what, if our army had to fight *in Europe* the day after landing, as at the Alma, what would become of our wounded."[127] The Hon. Horace Plunkett asked the question about practical experience "in field duties," the "weak point" in the system, as he pointed out to the secretary for war, Henry Campbell-Bannerman. The feeble reply was that steps would be taken for a two-week course the next summer.[128]

Nightingale's work in 1897 sending nurses to a plague hospital in India appears in chapter 7, as part of a discussion on bacteriology. Here note is made of the plague outbreak in Hong Kong in 1896, which spread through army ranks. The matter could only be "tackled by Mr Chamberlain and Lord Lansdowne," colonial secretary and secretary for war, respectively. Nightingale did not know Joseph Chamberlain, and she had to tackle Lansdowne on another matter, as she told Douglas Galton.[129] She complained to Galton that "MPs have no idea but of asking questions in the House, which government resents."[130] She wrote Chamberlain, she told Galton, with extracts from Dr Evatt, who had to remain anonymous in the matter.[131]

Also in 1896, Nightingale was told about an outbreak of enteric fever in Dublin, by a nurse she mentored who was head of nursing at the Royal Military Infirmary there. Sister E.M.M. Snodgrass (former night superintendent at St Thomas') explained: "The cause is not far to seek. They are at a *lower* level than the Liffey, which is a tidal river, and the sewage comes back into the barracks. (It is supposed that the whole of the sub-soil of Dublin is impregnated, which accounts for the prevalence of enteric among the civil population.)"[132] Again, the connections between military and civilian environmental conditions and their impact on disease come out, obvious to Nightingale and her nurse, but still, apparently, not to the authorities, civil or military, in 1896.

PART TWO

Reimagining Hospitals and Women's Medicine

SAFER HOSPITALS BY DESIGN

Applying the Lessons of the Crimean War

How unsafe hospitals were was little understood at the time Nightingale took on the issue after Crimea. Hospitals in Britain were then, except for military hospitals and workhouse infirmaries, run by voluntary boards, as charities. They had elite patrons, often members of the royal family. Their numerous "governors" included members of the nobility. Nightingale herself was "life governor" of several. These voluntary hospitals varied greatly in size and shape, site and amenities, all of which would add to the complications for reformers.

Paris led the move to the new pavilion design. Most notably, in the years 1837–44, the Beaujon Hospital, on the legendary rue du Faubourg Saint-Honoré (no. 208), down the street from the Elysée Palace (no. 55, which namesake Nicolas Beaujon also owned), added four pavilions on the grounds of an older hospital.[1] Then, in 1854, the exemplary Lariboisière Hospital, near the Gare du Nord, was opened.

The British had, in fact, built pavilion hospitals in the late eighteenth century, at Greenwich, Plymouth, and Portsmouth, but these were for purposes of style – grand, military edifices – not for health. A French doctor, Jacques-René Tenon (1724–1816), was the first, in 1788, to advocate the new, pavilion style, for reasons of health;[2] a British Army doctor, John Pringle (1707–1782), in 1752, had set out the defects of military hospitals, but without this leading to new construction. Superiority in design, however, must not be assumed to ensure improved safety. Nightingale frequently pointed out that the "artificial ventilation" installed at the Lariboisière undid the benefits of the pavilion model, so that its death rates were high.

In 1866, when "that dreadful M. Husson," director of the public hospitals of Paris, travelled to London to see English hospitals (a second trip), Nightingale asked Douglas Galton to see him. Husson intended to visit all the workhouses and hospitals in five days. Nightingale commented: "He really terrifies me like a whirlwind or cyclone." She asked Galton for an introduction for Husson to see the Herbert Hospital again, and inquired what other facilities he should go to.[3]

Dr John Roberton and Pavilions

When Nightingale returned to England in summer 1856, after the Crimean War, Dr John Roberton (1797–1876) had just begun to raise the issue of bad hospital design. He was a Scottish-born surgeon, then practising in Manchester, who had earlier published on midwifery. In March 1856, he gave a paper to the Manchester Statistical Society, of which he was vice-president, on hospital defects. In it, he reported his visits to the Beaujon Hospital in Paris, St John's (Saint-Jean) in Brussels, and the Lariboisière in Paris, which last he called "a palace for the sick."

He gave details of the "totally different," "novel" St André Hospital in Bordeaux, points Nightingale would repeatedly make herself. The structure was set in open ground, with a "beautiful court," plants, an arcade, and gardens on both sides of the pavilions. Each pavilion / ward was 140 feet long, 30 feet wide, and 19 or 20 feet high, with tall, narrow windows directly facing each other, and thirty-eight beds, nineteen on each side. The room for nurses or sisters was at the entrance, and the lavatories were at the other end. Each ward had only one door – people entered and left through fresh air. "It follows, of course, that each ward is itself *a separate hospital*, having no communication with the other wards, so that, if we were to suppose one of these to be crowded with the worst kind of surgical maladies for causing foulness, the foul air could not find a passage into any other ward – a hospital atmosphere would be impossible."[4]

The meetings of the Manchester Statistical Society would prove to be a good venue for advancing ideas on hospital reform, and its *Transactions* circulated them. George Godwin, architect and editor of the influential architecture journal, the *Builder*, used Roberton's examples of the pavilion model in an issue in September 1856.[5]

Nightingale acknowledged Roberton in her first paper on hospital defects.[6] She had a copy of her massive report on the Crimean War hospitals sent to him with a warm letter. No one, except him, Whitfield at St Thomas', and the officers of the Middlesex, had "taken up the question of hospitals on the large sanitary ground. Your two pamphlets were read by us all with the greatest interest." She added that she differed with his views on nursing, "but of that anon." Most of the (1858) letter sets out the administrative arrangements that she considered essential for good nursing.[7] Roberton's 1860 paper quoted her at length.[8]

She wrote him in 1861 with her regrets that the Manchester Infirmary was being enlarged: "I thought it was agreed among you that the ill-placed, ill-constructed, ill-ventilated Manchester Infirmary was not a place to give the sick a fair chance – however improved – and that, if added to, it would be fatal. Sold, it would make an admirable warehouse, being indeed fit for nothing else. And the price would be available for a new building out of the town."[9]

Clearly the two saw eye to eye on hospital design. She was pleased to be able to quote an established doctor, and he was at least as happy to be able to quote her. Their views were so similar that a doctor in the Royal Artillery credited him with three (anonymous) papers by her that appeared in the *Builder*.[10]

The pavilion came into wide use, and British instances proved exemplary. As soon as it opened, in 1871, St Thomas' became the civil model, as the Herbert Hospital, opened in 1865, would be for the army. Nightingale continued to send visiting doctors to see the French and Belgian examples, but made sure they saw these top British ones too. The French as well visited England to see them.

Simpson's Attack on "Hospitalism"

A major force working for safer hospitals was James Y. Simpson (1811–1870), an obstetrician and professor of midwifery at Edinburgh University, who was knighted and made a baronet. His daughter's biography of him has Nightingale heading the list of famous women who visited their home in Edinburgh, along with the novelist Mrs Gaskell and notorious divorcée, Mrs Norton, but giving no details or dates.[11] He was a pioneer user of chloroform, as we saw in chapter 2. Here, "hospitalism," his term, is the focus. He and Nightingale were in full agreement on hospital reform.

Simpson did a study of post-operative mortality from limb amputations in 1869, a reply to an article by surgeon Holmes Coote of St Bart's, who had served at Renkioi and Smyrna.[12] He used that material also in an argument with James Syme regarding the design of the new Edinburgh Infirmary, published first in the *Scotsman*, later in the *British Medical Journal*. Syme was in favour of large hospital buildings, to rely on disinfectants, especially carbolic acid, to prevent the spread of disease. Simpson wanted a totally different design, using temporary or moveable buildings of iron or wood. He called for "non-storeyed blocks," covering as much ground as could be obtained, in line with Nightingale's preference for one-storey pavilions, two at most. He stated that about three times as many patients died after limb amputations in large hospitals as in private and country practice. After giving the relevant statistics, he added that "hospitals seem generally to be much more healthy when built than after they become used for a few years." The existing Edinburgh maternity hospital was "wretched" and discreditable; he trusted that "an obstetric hospital would be added to the proposed new Infirmary" and suggested a cheap structure, with temporary rooms and wards, and separated from the other hospital buildings.[13]

Simpson was uncompromising in his language in comparing mortality from London teaching hospitals – St Bart's no less – and provincial hospitals. Our ancestors had committed "hygienic blunders of the gravest and most disastrous kind," he said. In many hospitals in Britain and on the Continent, patients were placed in four rows, betwixt the side walls of each ward. Instead, independent and separate ventilation was required.

Elsewhere, he argued forcefully for a change in public opinion. There was no necessity for "the needless sacrifice of human health and life connected with our present hospital system," which would change when it was "sufficiently impressed upon the mind of the public and of the profession" that the system itself needed altering. "Money could be saved by shorter hospital stays," he added.[14]

Someone sent Nightingale Simpson's *Scotsman* letter, which she forwarded to Dr John Sutherland, adding that the public ought to be "wakened up" to hospital statistics. She asked if these should not be part of Dr Farr's returns. "Practical remedies" should be proposed, she said, as it was a "difficult thing to retract an error" on such a great scale.[15]

An article in *Scientific American* endorsed Simpson's views; the administration should be in a central, separate building, and patients in "hospital villages or wards."[16] There is further reference to Simpson in the next chapter, on maternity hospitals.

Nightingale's Advice on New Hospitals

Nightingale was frequently asked to advise on new hospital building, usually by a major landowner, a philanthropist, or the mayor or chair of a hospital committee. She was pleased when, exceptionally, a doctor made the contact, as is clear in the examples below. Sometimes she was approached both by a doctor and by another person, each of whom contributed to the final result. Too often there were warring local factions, which she avoided like the plague. She wanted an invitation from the hospital committee itself, not from an individual or faction. In some cases, notably the first example here, there were complications resulting from the involvement of her own father and family friends. Nightingale also gave considerable time to ensuring construction of better workhouse infirmaries and fever hospitals. These, however, apart from the usual input from Dr John Sutherland, required political negotiations, not medical, and I discuss these are discussed elsewhere.[17]

We begin with examples of Nightingale's short involvement on a variety of hospitals before longer sections on hospitals on which she did considerable work. In 1860, she consulted surgeon Sir James Paget on the vexing matter of the Winchester Infirmary, near Embley Park, her family's Hampshire home, which she was advising. She needed allies to convince the hospital authorities to build on a new site:

> Here is an indictment, to which the verdict must be "wilful murder." Here are, in nine months, in a country hospital (of only 100 patients), and by no means the worst of its class – twenty four poor creatures brought together to run the gauntlet of their lives – through erysipelas contracted in the hospital, of whom eight perish and sixteen just escape with life from this fatal building.
>
> Depend upon it, other hospitals, if as well inquired into, would give as disastrous or *more* disastrous results. It is not the cubic space, but the ward construction (and other causes which make foul the ward air) which produces the result in *this* case. We are trying to get this hospital removed and rebuilt. And I think I have a fine handle in my hands with this table.[18]

Nightingale's work with Dr Thomas Williams (c. 1819–1864), physician to the Swansea Infirmary, in Wales, is an unusually strife-free success story.

Williams, a naturalist interested in sanitary issues, contacted her in 1864 to ask for help on building a new hospital. She recommended an architect, Alexander Graham (1831–1912), met with him on the plans, which were initially faulty on drainage, she thought. She gave detailed advice, on which the principals acted. There were the usual points about cutting off out-patients from the hospital, separate buildings for the deadhouse and post-mortem room, risk of drainage from nearby houses – for a possible "fatal objection to the site" – and more unusual items such as the placement of the Turkish bath. She concluded: "When these matters are satisfactorily arranged, Swansea will have one of the finest hospitals in the kingdom. I only wish the site had been as good as the plan."[19]

Dr Williams died in 1864, but the work proceeded, very much in the direction she had urged. A 120-bed hospital, of native sandstone, pavilion style, and only two floors, was duly opened. A local guidebook reported her approval: "Your enlightened committee has rendered a real service to the cause of humanity in adopting these beautiful plans; when completed you will have, perhaps, the finest and most perfect small hospital in the kingdom."[20]

Also of interest in 1864 is an article sent to Nightingale praising the Norfolk and Norwich Hospital for its low post-surgery mortality rates. It gave credit for adequate cubic space, natural ventilation, and lack of crowding to the hospital, not to the "Norwich air." Good practices by doctors and dressers while leaving the dissecting room were noted.[21] A surgeon / medical director at the hospital, Charles Williams, sent Nightingale their statistics.[22] She sent him a copy of St Bartholomew's statistics as a better example. Theirs afforded "a number of points of comparison," but were not sufficient "for many practical purposes." She encouraged him: "It is a pity that yours should not be perfect – especially now when the comparative mortality of different hospitals and of the hospitals of different countries is daily becoming a more pressing question. And Norwich has already done so much towards its solution." She commented also on its night nurses, and the need for adequate space for them to get "*eight hours*" sleep in bed "*every day*."[23]

In 1875, Nightingale and Douglas Galton were consulted about a new building for the Norfolk and Norwich Hospital. Rising mortality rates were of concern. In 1876, plans were prepared by a local architect and later mayor, Edward Boardman, with T.H. Wyatt, an architect Nightingale favoured. A new two-storey structure, with wards of twenty-two beds, clearly followed Nightingale and Galton's advice.[24] It remained in operation until 2003.

In 1867, Dr Duncan Macdonald Forbes (1837–1912) wrote Nightingale about a Nottinghamshire colliery proprietor who would cooperate with the workmen to build a hospital for accidents, size eight to twelve beds. The proprietor was his father-in-law, Thomas Barber (1805–1874), of Barber Walker & Co., at Eastwood, Notts. However, Forbes was not clear "about the best kind of building" and asked her opinion; he had read her book on hospitals but saw nothing in it that quite suited him. John Sutherland drafted a reply for her, proposing "a long cottage raised on a basement about two or three feet above ground. The patients might be placed at one end of the building, the offices at the other. Or the cottage might be in two floors, the patients being above the offices and stores below ... The latter arrangement would be the best. If you could have a plan sketched to show this, adopting the arrangements as to wards, W.C.s., etc, as showed in my *Notes on Hospitals*, I should be glad to look it over."[25]

Sometimes doctors contacted Nightingale with ideas on hospital design she considered thoroughly wrong. Dr Henry Greenway in Plymouth sent her a copy of a paper of his on hospital construction. It was a response to proposals made by Douglas Galton at the meetings of the British Medical Association at Leeds in 1869. Greenway's object was to "secure the advantages of a large hospital without its dangers, and the safety of the hut system without its inconveniences." Glass walls, he thought, would serve to separate patients and allow them to observe each other. His proposal was for a long room, 30 feet wide and 14 feet high, with floor and ceiling of glass and iron, a double row of cells back to back, made of glass with iron framework, each cell 10 feet square, ventilated by a tube passing through the wall.[26] Sutherland reviewed Greenway's letter and paper, telling Nightingale that she need not answer, unless she meant "to battle a man out of opinions to which he has already committed himself." He sketched out a hypothetical reply for her.[27]

Greenway, however, was not dissuaded. He revised his paper, and had it published in the *British Medical Journal*, a copy of which he sent Nightingale,[28] which she annotated with her opposing views.[29] He did not help matters by referring to her in his introduction, at which she commented: "And who disapproved this plan." All her annotations were negative. Particularly objectionable was the "back-to-back" ward construction, "condemned by all experience." It was the great fault of Netley and other large army hospitals, with pathogen-laden air passing over four rows of patients before reaching an outlet. The pavilion design, by contrast, featured narrow wards, with windows facing each other to speed up the outflow of air and minimize cross-infection.

Nightingale was horrified by the plan to employ patients to monitor each other. Moreover, she thought, observation through glass walls (and ceilings) would be especially disturbing for those with fevers – "an intolerable nuisance" to have the best light at the foot of the bed and somebody else behind one: "It would send a fever patient delirious." As well, nurses would "patrol" those left in the corridors. Nightingale commented: "!!! !!! !!! Then am I to train not nurses, but patrols? a patrol training school!"[30]

In some cases, the approach to Nightingale for assistance on hospitals came from a doctor's wife. Thus Mrs Lewis, wife of a surgeon and medical officer of health for Glamorganshire, wrote her about their plans for a convalescent hospital. Nightingale was impressed by the "quiet, persevering" manner in which the two had proceeded. While other people began with "a prospectus and great names, a secretary, public meeting and a castle in the air," they had begun with "personal exertions and wise practical benevolence." Nightingale was willing to look at any "sketch plans" sent, to which should be added any "inconveniences to be provided against in a new building." "Mere ornament" should be avoided; all that was needed for a seaside building was "substantial wood and stone work."[31]

It was several years before the Lewises' full plans arrived, which Nightingale passed on to Dr Sutherland. She had nothing good to say about them:

> I have never seen so much *complication* with so little
> *accommodation* … It has all high-wrought accessories of a *hospital*,
> without its means of *supervision* … The wards are like the famous
> goose, *too much* (for a *home*), *too little* (for a *hospital*) … Every
> arrangement seems to be made for something else; The blocks are
> like *pavilions* seen through the wrong end of a telescope, and called
> *cottages* … The matron's rooms must not be in the *offices* and the
> *manager's* room must not be by the sick … There is *no supervision*
> *whatever* for *ground* floors of *side pavilions*.[32]

Leeds General Infirmary

In 1862, Nightingale was asked to advise on enlarging or establishing a new building for the Leeds General Infirmary. The approach came from William Beckett Denison, later a Conservative MP. The chief physician of the hospital, Charles Chadwick (1815–1886), was much involved in the planning. The architect selected, George Gilbert Scott, was a "fortunate" choice, Nightingale told them. Both Dr Chadwick and Scott travelled extensively, on Nightingale's advice, to visit "all the best continental hospitals." They succeeded in producing "a hospital second to none in existence."[33]

There was lengthy public consultation on whether to enlarge only or to put up something new, which latter was agreed on and the money raised. Nightingale's *Notes on Hospitals* and her evidence on hospital design to the royal commission on the Crimean War were used, as was Douglas Galton's model of a small military hospital.

The foundation stone was laid in 1864, and the hospital opened to patients in 1868. The design incorporated the core elements of the pavilion model: "perfect freedom of ventilation … abundance of light … cheerfulness of appearance" and all the necessary "adjuncts" for nursing on the floor, though not accommodation for nurses. Gothic revival in design – a George Gilbert Scott specialty – it was ornamented by coloured brick and stone, embellished by polished granite.[34]

The British Medical Association held its 1869 meetings in Leeds, when Dr Acland handed over as president to Dr Chadwick. Acland's final address, characteristically, gave a positive nod to the committee on "state medicine." Tours of the new facility were arranged. Chadwick's inaugural address explained the pavilion model, showing how Leeds fitted it so admirably, and commented on his travels to see the European examples. He praised Bordeaux as "the most exact specimen," except for its too small space between pavilions – a defect also of the Edinburgh Royal Infirmary. Leeds had five pavilions, the preferred north–south orientation (to permit in light from east and west), two storeys, correct placement of toilet facilities, separate space for administration, and "perfect ventilation." Chadwick claimed that it, and the Herbert Hospital, were "the first complete hospitals built in England on the pavilion principle." While he would not call it "an exact and perfect adoption of the pavilion plan," it "very nearly" approached it, "for all essential purposes." He took exception, however, to Nightingale's acceptance of lower standards on ventilation for convalescent hospitals.[35] Douglas Galton gave a paper later at the meetings, again with details of the pavilion principle, all in line with Nightingale's.[36]

A "pictorial picture" of the Leeds Infirmary shows it alongside the famous Lariboisière and the grand Plymouth Naval Hospital of 1758.[37] The original buildings are still standing, the pavilions modified for use other than as wards. Leeds, however, lost its top billing as a pavilion hospital in 1871 when the "new" St Thomas' opened in London.

Derbyshire General Infirmary

When Dr Ogle approached Nightingale in 1864 about nursing for the "county hospital" in Derby (see chapter 3), he raised also the need for a new hospital building. He sent her a brief description of their plans to date and asked for her opinion. She replied – a standard response – that she could not comment given so little information. She had to have the detailed plans.[38] Later, she explained that she did not want her name used as "an authority." She was willing to help their committees (note the plural), but "to do this effectually," they had to "ask my advice." "Painful experience" of "endless trouble" occurred otherwise, from jealousy of one member acting separately: "I am used to being skinned alive every day."[39]

Ogle sent her "a sheet," and Nightingale set to work on it warily, "under protestation." "Such criticism generally only succeeds in alienating those who ask for it." She wanted "architects's plans," but there was enough wrong for her to start: "The fever wing is a nest of holes and corners – equally destructive to health and to nursing. Nothing can be done with it but sweep it from end to end, in the way of improvement." She acknowledged that "the architect knows his business," and she thought well of the "alterations and additions" done. Comments moved on to such specifics as the need for two wings: the proposed one and the rebuilt fever wing. The central block should be only for administration. She was willing to have another go at the plans when the committee had decided on the points before it.

Nightingale needed further information, evidently unsupplied so far: the number of operations per year, men and women (typically, there were many more for men), the number of surgical cases and medical cases, again for men and women separately. "It is impossible to arrange the wards and the nursing without knowing these and an infinity of other details."

Nightingale had more to say about the fever wards and their corridor, which "ought to be cleared away altogether, with as little delay as possible." The best place for the operating theatre was "where it can have a large skylight sloping to the north, as well as a window under the skylight to the north wall. It is better not to be in the attic."[40]

Dr Ogle apparently raised concerns about religious differences, again, as a problem, and Nightingale, again, protested. She had given her services "to any Christian denomination (and even to Jews and Muhammedans)." She would not support one party against another, and regretted it when she had been "fool enough to do it."[41]

After many vexed exchanges, Nightingale was finally satisfied with the plans and agreed to have the infirmary's new "wing," in fact a new building, named after her. It was opened on 11 November 1869 by the hospital president, Lord Vernon, of Sudbury Hall, Derbyshire. Accounts were lavish in praise, for its "spacious, airy wards ... every accommodation for nurses – sculleries, baths, and lavatories." The wards held thirty-two beds. There was a "separation ward" as well as men's and women's.[42]

The local newspaper story on the opening of the Nightingale Wing said that it embodied "every improvement modern science and experience have suggested for the treatment of the sick."[43] Subsequent articles on annual meetings of the hospital continued to flag the great improvements in ventilation and consistency in temperature between the new wing and the old hospital. It seems that problems in nursing continued, but improvements were noted.[44]

The Sydney Infirmary and the Royal Prince Alfred Hospital

Nightingale's great debt to the people of Australia was noted in chapter 3 on the sending of nurses to Sydney – the colonies' residents had contributed generously to the Nightingale Fund that made her school possible. When the matron, Lucy Osburn, and five nurses arrived in Sydney in March 1868, they were housed at the old infirmary, where Osburn soon fell ill. By May, she was writing Nightingale about the bad conditions, notably the drains. "Sister Miller" was "miserable" on account of the conditions.[45] In July, she reported a nurse had fever, and "difficulties" of the ward included "lack of water (no sink, no tap)."[46]

Nightingale had sent Dr Alfred Roberts her *Notes on Hospitals* early on. He related a problem with the size and place of the infirmary building.[47] Dr Sutherland drafted material on what was needed to accommodate a matron and nurses.[48]

In 1868, the hospital's annual meeting adopted a resolution acknowledging Nightingale's assistance on the "improvement of the hospital buildings and treatment," as well as the sending of nursing staff.[49] Roberts used her material extensively in a paper on hospitals he gave to the Royal Society later that year.[50] In 1879, Roberts advised her that the hospital wanted to name a ward after her, which was done.[51]

When the nurses' home was opened in 1881, its superiority to those elsewhere was cited in the newspapers: "The noble structure has been arranged and fitted up with every consideration for the comfort and convenience and the plan was submitted to Miss Nightingale and obtained her unqualified approval. She has observed, indeed, that she knows of no similar institution that has equally well provided for the accommodation of its nursing and training staff and domestics."[52]

In 1890, Lady Carrington, wife of the governor of New South Wales, laid the foundation stone for the new nurses' home at the Royal Prince Alfred Hospital. It opened in 1892.

The Vladimir Children's Hospital, Moscow

Nightingale was approached in 1874 by paediatrician Karl Andreyevich Rauchfuss (1835–1915). Then director of the St Petersburg Children's Hospital, Dr Rauchfuss was in London to confer about the building of the Vladimir Children's Hospital in Moscow. Two nurses approached Nightingale on his behalf, the first, Emily Gregory, a Nightingale nurse who later became a missionary.[53] Nightingale evidently commented on the plans sent to her without seeing Dr Rauchfuss. He thanked her for her criticisms, but explained to the next intervenor, Canadian-born Maria Machin, then the "home sister" or tutor at the Nightingale School, that he wanted to see Nightingale in person with the plans, to explain them. He seemed to have "unbounded confidence in your judgement and opinion," Machin told her, and said about her *Notes on Hospitals*, "There is no such other valuable book on hospitals existing."[54] Nightingale met him, when he provided information on winter conditions useful to her in advising on the Montreal General Hospital. She recounted their meeting to Dr John Sutherland:

One of my criticisms to the most intelligent projector (Dr Rauchfuss) was that *all* the nurses' rooms were away from the wards. He concludes from this that I wish *all* the nurses' rooms to adjoin wards. Like a man, he does not see (all the nurses, it appears, are under him at St Petersburg, as under a direct*or* at Moscow) the absolute necessity, rather *more* in a *children's* hospital than anywhere else, rather more where *mothers* are admitted to nurse their own children in *one*-bed wards than under any other circumstances – of having a *head nurse* or sister *sleeping off her own ward* in command of her own ward or division day *and night*, and of having a matron. (It is rather disheartening to be having always to repeat this self-evident axiom.)[55]

The 180-bed hospital was opened in 1876 on St Vladimir's Day, 15 July. It was built on the pavilion principle, on a large plot of land. In 1897, it was awarded a gold medal at the World Exhibition in Brussels for the best children's hospital in Europe.[56]

Johns Hopkins University Hospital and Dr John Shaw Billings

Dr John Shaw Billings (1833–1913), a Union army doctor during the Civil War, was given the task by the trustees of philanthropist Johns Hopkins (1795–1873) of designing a new hospital for Baltimore. Not an architect, Billings took on the task and eventually produced the plans, with considerable help from Nightingale and numerous others. However, during the Panic of 1873 and its aftermath, the value of Hopkins's bequest declined greatly with the fall in value of his railway shares in the B&O (Baltimore and Ohio Railroad). After many delays, a model pavilion-style hospital was built. The prestigious medical school followed, and, soon after it, a nursing school.[57]

The correspondence on the university hospital began in October 1876, when Billings, visiting in London, sent Nightingale, through the

St Thomas' matron, Mrs Wardroper, several proposals under consideration and asked for a critique. At that point, there was only a "rough sketch" of the proposed hospital, with mention of the intention to build a training school for nurses, a convalescent hospital, an orphan asylum, and other projects. Billings was on route to the Continent to see hospitals, hoping to be back in London in two months. He asked Nightingale to examine the plans, with two accompanying pamphlets: "They are only sketch plans, and I desire criticism before going further."[58] In December, he thanked her for her letter and twelve sheets of notes, which unhappily have not survived. He told her that her remarks would be taken to the trustees, who, he felt sure, would be greatly influenced by her criticism. He agreed with it.[59]

Dr Billings's plans took isolation precautions further than any other hospital designer of the time. There is no surviving correspondence with Nightingale on the point, but it is evident that infectious cases were isolated in single rooms in a separate building – an innovation then. Further, each room was separately ventilated through the roof, and there was a vestibule between the room and the central corridor. The nurse slept in a room at the corridor's end, and did not return to the nurses' residence after her shift. However, there are no data on the results.

The nursing school opened in 1889, with very substantial input from Nightingale.

Billings made a further contribution when, late in life, he became the founding director of the Office of the (U.S.) Surgeon General. Its collection, which he began to amass, formed the basis of the National Library of Medicine. In this capacity, he sought out information on the Nightingale School, its books, forms, regulations, and so on.[60]

City Hospital, Friedrichshain, Berlin

Nightingale advised on numerous other hospitals, although little information on the process survives. When a new, pavilion hospital was being planned in Berlin, Nightingale was consulted c. 1868. This was the City Hospital, Friedrichshain, designed by two leading architects and opened in 1874. There are positive comments about Nightingale in the description of the hospital.[61]

A major proponent was Professor Rudolf Virchow, a leading German doctor and statesman known as the founder of "social medicine."

Nightingale never met him, but both she and John Sutherland assisted in the hospital's design.[62] She and Virchow must have corresponded on the plans, notably on the midwifery space, but no letters remain. The intermediary was the Crown Princess of Prussia, Queen Victoria and Prince Albert's oldest child, Victoria. For Nightingale, Virchow was an "old acquaintance" from the Franco–Prussian War – she had sent him supplies of lint. Notes by Sutherland indicate that he agreed with Virchow's views (typically, Nightingale asked him for his comments on plans after she had made hers).[63] She arranged for Virchow to be sent a copy of her *Introductory Notes on Lying-in Institutions*.[64]

When Florence Lees visited the Friedrichshain in 1879, she reported it as "admirable" in construction, with tiled floors and iron bedsteads, indicating proper attention to materials. But the most severe cases were put in a room that received the "foulest air in the building." There was a school for nurses, but "with no matron or superintendent and no head nurses or sisters."[65] Achieving low death rates required a great complex of improvements, of which design was essential, but no guarantee.

Nightingale continued to believe that the quality of a country's public hospitals was "a standard of the knowledge and care of the governing body, or of civilization amongst a people."[66] Better hospitals were a reasonable expectation.

The Montreal General Hospital

Nightingale's letters on sending a matron and nurses to Montreal, as discussed in chapter 3, flagged from the beginning the need for a new building. One had indeed been intimated when she was first approached. She told Sutherland that "two Canadian gentlemen" had visited her when she was dealing with the Moscow hospital in August 1874, to ask her "to send a Canadian lady we have in training (an admirable one [presumably Maria Machin]) and nurses to their *old* hospital – *improvements* to be made, at Montreal." "The collision was in the nick of time," she said, "since the *Russian* declared that what the *Canadians* said was *impossible* was *perfectly easy*, viz., ventilation by *windows* open – open fireplaces – W.C.s in outside wall, apparatus to prevent water and soil pipes from freezing."[67]

Nightingale urged great caution before agreeing to the Montreal request for personnel. She wrote Maria Machin: "I do most solemnly say, don't commit yourself to Montreal on any such understanding as this:

'that, if your demands are within reason, they are ready to do everything, etc.' Have the *plans* of what they consent to do sent here to you (I will show them to the War Office). If they are what we think 'within reason,' then, and not till then, consider their proposal for yourself and nurses." Further, she advised, adding "written at 5 a.m.": "When I see what sanitary arrangements they propose as feasible in a much severer climate like Russia, I think it simply impossible to let nurses go to that Montreal hospital till we know what they will do to improve it."[68] Machin, however, had already accepted the offer, and plans for going proceeded. The nurses visited Nightingale at Lea Hurst in Derbyshire for a last briefing before embarking for Montreal at Liverpool. They arrived in October 1875.

The English architect selected for the would-be new Montreal General, Alexander Graham, whom we met above re the Swansea Infirmary, was one Nightingale liked, particularly for his design of the Lincoln Hospital (completed 1878). He wrote her for an appointment to confer on plans "for a proposed new hospital at Montreal."[69] By April 1876, she had reason to call the new facility a "definite prospect," with the site purchased and Graham's plans adopted.[70] An economic downturn in Montreal, however, made it impossible to raise the funds for the new hospital and nurses' home. Neither was ever built.[71]

Nightingale greatly influenced the design of the later, magnificent Royal Victoria Hospital, a pavilion-style building and a notable landmark, perched on the "mountain" and opened in 1893. On this, however, while she worked with the English architect Henry Saxon Snell (1830–1904), renowned for his hospital designs, she was not involved with any doctors.

The New Women's Hospital, Euston Road, London

The New Hospital for Women in London's Euston Road was a modest answer to the need for a place for women doctors to be able to practise, a small hospital created out of several houses. Nightingale advised on the design. It could not be the favoured pavilion model, but she did succeed in making it more manageable for nursing and improved its hygiene. She was appalled to see defective ventilation in the original plans for a medical school for women doctors. She asked royal engineer Douglas Galton for his advice, "Do you think the great *staircase* with single window sufficient to air and light this most intricate hospital – which requires Fortunio's [Liceti] telescope which could see round angles?" She asked him also if he approved of their choice of sanitary engineer. She sent him her eleven pages of notes on the plans for his comments.

Her "chief anxiety": the ward floors were like a "rabbit warren, one-bedded wards without direct inspection – hardly anywhere for anyone to sit down, nowhere for anyone to sleep besides the poor patients." This would be both inefficient and unhealthy, for staff as well as patients. "I am afraid the air will be always losing its way through these intricate rooms and corridors."[72] Galton provided advice, and the building committee agreed to remodel accordingly. It was evidently more difficult to design a small hospital for ventilation and sanitary conditions than a larger one. The placement of the out-patients' department, "underneath!!," generated another complaint.[73]

Since this was a women's hospital, obstetrics was a priority. Nightingale found the design faulty for not making convenient space for "minor operations." Inadequate space was given for a "ward kitchen," for heating up food, drinks, and fomentations. Space for nurses was inadequate, and the servants' accommodation was "almost better than the nurses'."[74]

Evidently these defects were taken care of sufficiently to pass muster. Nightingale gave a financial contribution herself and wrote a letter for a fund-raising meeting at the Mansion House in the City. The letter is short and punchy: "You want efficient women doctors, for India most of all, whose native women are now our sisters, our charge. (There are at least 40 millions who will only have women doctors, and who have none.) But for England, too, you want them. Give them, then, besides a women's school of medicine, a practical school in a women's hospital. Life and death depend on the training."[75]

The Women's Hospital in the late twentieth century became the headquarters of a large nursing union, Unison. In 1999, in a unanimous resolution, it denounced Nightingale as the founder of nursing.[76]

MIDWIFERY AND
WOMEN IN MEDICINE

Midwifery and Safer Childbirth

For Nightingale, safer childbirth was a lifelong concern, to be achieved with better training of nurse midwives and safer (better designed and managed) midwifery hospitals and wards. She was not successful in either endeavour. In the course of investigating the failure of the midwifery ward at King's College Hospital, she produced a substantial book, *Introductory Notes on Lying-in Institutions* (1871), with much useful comparative data on death rates in other institutions and home deliveries. However, she never could see her way to a resumption of training midwifery nurses, or even a second edition of the book.

The obstacle was the highly contagious "puerperal fever," a term used for post-partum fever, now known to be caused by several different staphylococcal bacilli. A major form – Streptococcus pyogenes, or Group A streptococcus – was not identified until about 1902. Death rates did decline with improved antiseptic procedures, brought in gradually in the late nineteenth century, but an effective cure emerged only in the mid-twentieth, with antibiotics.

Midwifery training formed the Nightingale Fund's second project, for King's College Hospital, which opened in September 1861. The matron was Anglican nun Mary Jones, who had first proposed the idea to Nightingale, and a nurse whom she greatly respected. The ward's history, with its unhappy end, has been written up in detail.[1] Here we explore the rise of obstetrics as a medical specialty, often described as the "male medicalization" of childbirth, and the entry of women into medicine, very often with midwifery as their prime concern.

In nineteenth-century Britain, most births took place at home. The workhouse infirmaries took in destitute women, often prostitutes, but few women gave birth at a regular hospital – British doctors were well aware of its risks. "Lying-in" or maternity hospitals varied greatly in quality. Some (regular, civil) hospitals arranged to send out doctors to women's homes to attend their deliveries. The ward at King's College Hospital, a general hospital, was an innovation, later to be called "a dangerous experiment."

Obstetrics (from Latin *obstetrix*, midwife) emerged as a specialization in Britain in the mid- to late nineteenth century. The term "man midwife" was used earlier. Such "accoucheurs" had long been common in France and in other parts of Europe. Britain's Medical Act of 1858 did not mention midwifery. The London Obstetric Society held its first meeting in 1859.

British doctors were (wisely) cautious about supervising hospital births. Few hospitals had midwifery wards, so that autopsies on women who died in childbirth were rare. By contrast, it was "the rule in virtually all European institutions" for doctors to practise autopsies on women who died that way.[2]

The greatest cause of these fatalities when Nightingale took on midwifery training was "accidents" of childbirth, such as breech births, for which better training would seem a good remedy. Puerperal fever was the other major factor, sometimes killing the baby as well. That it was transmitted by the hands of a doctor or midwife was well known by this time, although the relative importance of hands (of doctor, medical student, or midwife) as opposed to another birthing mother, or the walls, bedding, or other surfaces, was not known. Dr Edward Rigby (1804–1860), later the first president of the London Obstetrical Society, wrote in 1841 that it would be "unsafe" for a practitioner, after a post-mortem examination of a puerperal-fever case, "to attend a case of labour for some days." Disease could be conveyed by using the same sponge in washing.[3] Rigby's book, however, includes climate as a cause of puerperal fever, and recommends bloodletting, the lancet, and purging as treatments.

The American physician Oliver Wendell Holmes senior (1809–1894), though using only anecdotal evidence, gave examples in 1843 of doctors going home from an autopsy and, summoned to a new confinement, transmitting the disease. He ended his paper by recommending that a physician expecting to be summoned to a birth "never" take any active part in a puerperal post mortem, and that anyone present at such autopsies should wash thoroughly, change "every article of clothing," and wait 24 hours or more before attending another case.[4]

The initial plan for the midwifery ward at King's College was characteristically modest, the training of only six midwifery nurses. The ward seemed to have been set up well. Arrangements were made for a leading obstetrician, Dr Arthur Farre (1811–1887), whom Nightingale knew from her Harley Street hospital, to conduct deliveries. He soon left, however, for reasons unknown. Her confidant Dr William Bowman considered Farre's involvement "useful," and Farre himself saw the space and judged it to be "perfect."[5]

There were no deaths in the first (partial) year at King's, and never any deaths of infants. However, three birthing mothers died in 1862, to rise to ten in 1867. Jones never advised Nightingale of the deaths and was greatly occupied on other matters. In 1866, she was preparing for new work at Charing Cross Hospital and went, with other Anglican nuns, to the city's east end to assist in a cholera epidemic. In 1867, she was busy withdrawing the order's services at a British hospital in Paris.[6] For much of 1866–67, she was preoccupied with a dispute with the men who governed her order, St John's House, and resigned for those reasons, with no mention of the high death rates. Throughout this period, King's continued to admit pupils for regular training, plus some nurses visiting from other countries for British experience.

Correspondence from Jones shows no indication that she was even aware of problems in the ward until Nightingale wrote her with questions. Jones's regrets, in 1863, were not about the death rates, but "the blindness, pig-headed faults in the construction of this hospital." It was an "inconvenient costly mistake" relative to "nursing arrangements.'[7]

Nightingale began her search for causes of the deaths only in January 1867. Jones then raised a concern with her about space per bed, but more of her letter concerned differences with the bishop.[8] In June, Jones wrote to her with a list of admissions, deaths, and causes of death, and suggested that the post-mortem theatre might be the problem.[9] Another letter had her regretting that she had not insisted more strongly about the "evil" of the post-mortem room, "which has always haunted me, instead of hoping I might be mistaken."[10] She next advised Nightingale that the hospital authorities were trying to neutralize "the mischief from the post-mortem." "All necessary regulations as to students and patients admitted are to be strictly enforced," which suggests that they had previously not been. Jones was ready to "try again" after more precautions were taken, in hope of "a much less mortality under God's blessing."[11]

Nightingale continued to have confidence in the good judgment of Jones, who disagreed with the assessment of W.O. (later Sir William)

Priestley (1829–1900), the doctor in charge. Moreover, she thought that he had "introduced erysipelas" at the ward. She told Nightingale that she was "positive" that the increase in illness came "mainly from the post-mortem theatre and its proximity" to the ward. Priestley thought it was because of having a midwifery ward in a general hospital at all. Jones argued that there were "no other patients on the floor or near them." She thought that Priestley considered the school "beneath him" and that he wanted the ward for his medical students. Nightingale agreed, as she told Farr later.[12] However, her notes also make clear that the rules set up at the beginning for the ward were regularly flouted. Medical students were not to enter it "except in the regular course with their professor," but went in "perpetually, and straight from the post-mortems." Further, "the smell of the post-mortem theatre is *quite* perceptible in the ward," but the doctors would not believe it.

Jones had said that "no unmarried lying-in woman was to be admitted, *except* by an authority from her; they have admitted such, latterly five with disease upon them. And there had been pyemia in the ward." Jones thought that the ward would be closed only if she and Nightingale consented; the authorities would not otherwise "dare." Their consent depended, as Nightingale frankly put it, "upon whether we really think that we are killing women to teach midwives."[13] In fact, the doctors made the decision to close the ward.

Jones visited Nightingale early in December 1867 to discuss the order's "great affair" and "the poor midwifery ward." Nightingale considered it "quite settled that we leave K.C.H., and am rather glad that it is not left to *us* to say we *will* go." She noted Priestley's proposition "that *we* should build huts for them – everything else remaining as before." She did not want "to be under Dr Priestley at all – I was very glad to be under Dr Arthur Farre." She could not envision her Fund ever undertaking to provide "lying-in beds or wards or hospital again." Such would have to be provided in workhouse infirmaries, and she hoped that they could establish training there.[14]

Priestley's view was accepted by the hospital authorities, as Dr Lionel Beale (1828–1906), chair of the council of Jones's order, advised Henry Bonham Carter.[15] On the ward's closing in January 1868, an unsigned article in the *Medical Times and Gazette* reviewed the "dangerous experiment," but looked to a possible re-opening. Priestley was quoted as suggesting that "rooms could be built on the pavilion plan outside the hospital," or that rooms on "upper floors" in new houses near the hospital could be used." However, the anonymous author advised against any midwifery ward "in the immediate neighbourhood of a general hospital."[16]

Nightingale, much later, referred to Jones's "regret at ever having had lying-in women at K.C.H." at all. But, if there were fault, it was not Jones's but hers, Nightingale said, for she was "supposed to know more about hospital statistics ... and how bitterly I have repented it." Had she known earlier of statistics for Husson's general-hospital lying-in ward in Paris, she said, "I never would have done it." She also realized, however, that those data "were only brought out at our request." She hoped that "thousands of lives will be saved by the attention that has been aroused, and good sanitary legislation will proceed."[17]

Dr Semmelweis's Vienna Experience: Evidence Ignored

Nightingale did not know anything about the breakthrough made in 1847–48 by Hungarian Dr Ignaz Semmelweis (1818–1865) at the Vienna General Hospital. His name appears nowhere in her writing, and indeed his success in reducing mortality rates was not soon widely known. Nor was she aware of the work of Aberdeen obstetrician Alexander Gordon (1752–1799), whose 1795 book on puerperal fever dealt with his own experience of treating seventy-seven patients, of whom twenty-five died. Unlike Semmelweis's, his were private patients, not in hospital. He found that only women treated by a doctor or nurse who had previously attended other patients had died.[18]

The Vienna General, when Semmelweis was there, had the largest midwifery program in the world, divided into two clinics. In Clinic 1, under Semmelweis, births were attended by medical doctors and students; in Clinic 2, led by Dr Franz Hektor Arneth (1818–1907), by (women) midwives. Clinic 1 had a far higher death rate, despite the doctors and medical students' greater professional expertise.

Entry was effectively random: women were assigned to one or the other clinic depending on the day they entered. Semmelweis turned to the historical statistics to figure out the discrepancy. He used the same method Nightingale would apply, after Crimea, to mortality data: comparing outcomes with different conditions, without being able to identify the precise cause. He discovered that death rates were lower before autopsies became routine in 1822, instituted to instruct medical students. Before that date, mortality was 125 per 1,000 births, to rise to 530 afterwards. The two-clinic system was instituted in 1839. Mortality rose to 388 in Clinic 2 (midwives) and to a staggering 984 in Clinic 1. Students routinely did eight autopsies a day, the midwives none. Further, midwives were trained on "phantoms," or dummies, while medical students worked on deceased women and infants, increasing their exposure to the yet-unknown bacilli. Semmelweis acknowledged that he himself had caused deaths by assisting in deliveries after conducting post mortems, thus transmitting the pathogen to the next birthing mother.

In May 1847, Semmelweis began his experiment of requiring medical students to wash their hands in a solution of chloride of lime before entering the labour room. He reported deaths declining from 11 per cent to 2 per cent as a result. He erroneously thought that only "cadaveric" matter caused puerperal fever, and thus did not require handwashing between patients. A spike in deaths occurred when, in October 1847, a diseased woman, who was placed in the first bed and so was examined first, survived, but eleven of the next twelve patients died.[19] The practice was changed to require handwashing after every examination of a patient, but Semmelweis's only early publication, in 1848, did not include this crucial refinement.[20] He did not publish a full account of the lessons he learned until 1858, in Hungarian, and made up from his lectures. In 1861 he brought out a 543-page German edition.[21]

The tragic story of Semmelweis is well known, that he was not reappointed in Vienna in 1848 (he was offered an inferior appointment, which he did not take). He then returned to Hungary, although it was not until 1855 that he obtained a good appointment there, at the University of Pest, when he again reduced death rates.

It is hard to understand why it took so long for his discovery to be taken up. True, his first publication reflects a faulty understanding of the data, and his full book was late in appearing, but his colleagues spread the word, giving papers and publishing articles in German, English, and French. Herewith three examples:

Dr Arneth, who headed Semmelweis's Clinic 2 and who had a Scottish mother, wrote Dr James Simpson as early as 1848 with news of his colleague's discovery, only to receive a prompt and surly reply.[22] Arneth gave a paper in Edinburgh in April 1851, which appeared in a British medical journal; he also published accounts in French and German.[23]

C.H.F. Routh, a German-speaking British doctor, wrote an article for a British medical journal in 1849. He observed that a doctor's hands, after touching dead matter, "however well washed, still retain a *peculiarly fetid cadaveric odour,* which does not disappear for several hours, and sometimes not till the next day." Since midwives were taught on a wood "phantom," rather than corpses, they "did not get their hands infected with cadaveric matter." With the handwashing precautions, "the *number of deaths at once fell to seven per month,* or the usual average of the second division," the midwives.[24] Doctors attending childbirths should not "attend any woman in labour in clothes which might have been infected by 'cadaveric matters or other poisonous secretions from living persons.'" They should not just wash their hands carefully "but also make use of a solution of chlorine, to disinfect the hand from any poisonous matters with which it may have become contaminated, before they presume to enter the lying-in bedchamber."[25]

Public-health expert Dr John Simon, in his annual report to the General Board of Health in 1858, included highlights from Routh's account. This should have helped to push the message out to a broader medical–public health readership. His account was brief, but included the essentials: avoiding contact with cadaveric matter and, if one couldn't, not examining a vagina until the following day; "that, besides very thoroughly cleansing their hands they should systematically *disinfect them with a solution of chlorine.*"[26]

Semmelweis's findings came to be recognized around the world as a major step in reducing maternal deaths (and some infant deaths) after childbirth. An early comment likened it to Jenner's discovery of the cowpox vaccination.[27] He was not suitably honoured until more than a century after his death, when the medical faculty at Budapest was named the Semmelweis University Medical School.

Nightingale never saw Semmelweis's book or any of the shorter accounts, any of which could have reshaped the midwifery ward at King's College Hospital in 1861. She learned of his good results only through the meta-analysis done by Dr Léon Le Fort, a French Army doctor, who also published on the Crimean War. He had been commissioned by the director of the French public-hospital system, Armand Husson, to compare maternity hospitals. However, when Le Fort sent in his manuscript, Husson refused to publish it – it showed how high the Paris death rates were. Undaunted, Le Fort did some further research, including another trip to England. His 546-page *Des maternités,* with material from many countries, appeared privately, in a small press run, in 1866. In the preface, he reported Husson's commissioning of the book and subsequent refusal to publish it.[28] Nightingale saw a copy only thanks to Farr's tracking one down for her.

Husson himself proceeded to London and asked Nightingale's assistance with hospital introductions, as if he were embarking on his own study. She did not know any of this background and innocently told Dr Farr that Husson was going to publish mortality data from maternity hospitals for all of Europe.[29] She went to some trouble to gain him access to various hospitals.

Le Fort's study was impressive, but his treatment of Semmelweis was garbled, and he omitted some crucial points. None the less, when Nightingale finally saw a copy in 1869, she could not restrain her "ardour." It was "a most important work, though not however exhaustive" and "in some places disappointing." For example, while it showed how high the death rates were at the Paris Maternité, it did not give a plan of the building, while it did give that for other hospitals. She remarked that "M. Husson's tables" showed that the death rate at the Paris Maternité was 202 per 1,000 in 1864, much higher than the worst year at the King's College midwifery ward. She agreed, sardonically, with Le Fort "that, as women *will* have children (though they had much better not), there *must* be midwives – and as practical midwifery can only be taught *in hospitals*, what we have to do is to find out the form of hospital which is *not* destructive to lying-in women."[30] She quoted none of Le Fort's (faulty) coverage of Semmelweis, but concentrated on comparative death rates by country, and the comparison of home births with those in institutions.

Doctors gradually came to realize that they were responsible for many deaths by transmitting disease. Dr Farr reported to Nightingale on a paper by Dr Evory Kennedy (1806–1886), master of the Dublin Rotunda Hospital, at the Social Science Congress in Bristol. He said that Kennedy "came as a high priest to burn the idol to which he had offered holocausts."[31]

Introductory Notes on Lying-in Institutions

After the closing of the midwifery ward and program at King's College Hospital in January 1868, Nightingale began to investigate what went wrong. She received much help from Dr John Sutherland, and numerous physicians contributed data from their own practices and responded to her questions. Nurses were not involved. The research was interrupted in 1870 by the Franco–Prussian War, so that the book was not published until 1871. The "Introductory" of the title was to signify further work to follow for a more definitive edition. Nightingale hoped that Dr Sutherland would write it. No second edition ever appeared.

For one thing, definitive answers never emerged during Nightingale's working life, which continued into the 1890s. She was frequently asked to open a midwifery ward, or to advise on a new maternity institution, but she never saw her way to doing this. She could not find a way to train midwives in a maternity institution without causing maternal deaths, that is, more deaths than would have happened with home births, even in the worst of home circumstances. She had protracted correspondence on alternative sizes and designs of maternity wards, including suggestions about iron buildings and one-woman huts, pursued with James Y. Simpson.

Simpson was a prime person for Nightingale to consult on the failure at King's. He wrote her at length about the general issue of such wards, and that at King's in particular, which he had visited. From seeing it, he told her, he could not help looking on "the magnificent staircase there as a great magazine of deteriorated and malefic air collected from the wards and ready to be sent back into the wards."[32] It should be rebuilt to be "a magazine of fresh air to feed the wards." His conclusion, in other words, was the same as Jones's.

In the same letter, Simpson gave as the three causes of puerperal fever: "deteriorated air" from wards, crowding, and doctors and nurses. He advised isolated buildings and isolating birthing women in wards of one or two patients only, the nurse sleeping there. Iron would be good as a construction material, as the building could be easily taken down and put up again. He referred to examples (Melbourne and Copenhagen) of separate small rooms. He asked Nightingale if she had seen Le Fort's "large work" on the subject. Semmelweis received not a mention, nor did Arneth, Routh, Simon, or the much earlier fellow Scot, Gordon.[33]

The following year, Nightingale was anxious to "hunt up anything for you from Sir James Simpson," she told Dr C.J.B. Williams (1805–1889), who specialized in diseases of the chest. She wanted to know if Simpson had approved of "*any* form of lying-in hospital."[34] Simpson had stated the dangers of including a maternity ward in a general hospital, advocating instead temporary iron buildings. But he died in 1870, so the matter could not be pursued. His advice on iron buildings was ignored.

The data Nightingale gathered showed unequivocally that deaths were lower at workhouse infirmaries than in regular hospitals, in spite of the poorer general health of the inmates. Mortality from puerperal fever was the exception to the general rule in society of death rates falling as people's social class and income rise.

· Dr J.H. Barnes (1833–1880), of the Liverpool Workhouse Infirmary, was a major informant for Nightingale on maternal deaths, especially welcome because his institution had an "enviable notoriety from its absence of puerperal fever."[35] She obtained extensive data on home births from Dr George Rigden of Canterbury, Dr Farr acting as intermediary. Farr reported back to her that he believed in Rigden's "accuracy" and regretted that he had received "little recognition" for his work. Farr joked that, on her next pilgrimage to Canterbury, she should go not to the cathedral crypt, but to the local waterworks – the softening process was so "beautifully carried out."[36] Army doctors forwarded material from their "soldiers' wives hospitals."

Drs Farr and Sutherland both assisted in Nightingale's quest to ascertain the "normal death rate" of birthing mothers. Such a statistic would then enable comparison across different types of institution from maternity to general hospitals, versus home births. The sanitarian Edwin Chadwick proposed comparing "rich" and "poor" mothers, to which Sutherland commented that the range would have to include those "comfortably" off and working class, not just the extremes.

With the benefit of hindsight, we can readily see the reason for the reversal in death rates by class: better-off women received more specialist care, and hence were more likely to be infected by another mother's post-mortem examination. Post mortems were not conducted at workhouse infirmaries. That the Paris maternity hospitals had such high death rates was counterintuitive, for they had the best-trained midwives, with two full years of instruction. But Paris midwives conducted post mortems. Nightingale would frequently rail against acceptance of a mere month of training for British midwives. However, they did not do post mortems.

After *Introductory Notes on Lying-in Institutions* appeared in 1871, Nightingale sent a copy to Dr C.J.B. Williams: "You cannot do me a greater service than to criticize it, for the little book is put forth merely to collect opinions." She invited him to note in the margin what alterations or additions were needed for "a future and (it is to be hoped) better edition."[37] When she sent one to Dr Barnes at Liverpool, she combined her request for comments with great appreciation of his work: "to whom so remarkable a portion of this little book is due – with the earnest request and hope that he will begin – with the first word he reads – to note on the margins the omissions to be supplied – the additions to be made – and that, having contributed so much valuable information, he will afford still more with his great kindness – for a future and (it *is* to be hoped) better edition."[38]

The *British Medical Journal's* review of *Introductory Notes* was patronizing and sexist, that in the *Lancet* highly favourable.[39] There were also anonymous letters to the editor.[40] Nightingale was frustrated with the reviews. She sent on "three critiques" to Sutherland, complaining of the lack of "real criticism" from anyone who knew anything about the subject.[41]

Nightingale had sent a copy to J. Braxton Hicks (1823–1897), president of the London Obstetrical Society and lecturer on midwifery at Guy's Hospital.[42] In the accompanying, deferential letter, she acknowledged omissions and sought improvements. He wrote to the editor of the *Medical Times and Gazette* to counter one point, her proposal to educate women "physicians-accoucheuses to take charge of lying-in institutions." He would not take a position on whether or not women should be in medicine, but worried that their deficient education in midwifery made them unable to deal with medical complications, which he enumerated. He understood the "physician accoucheuse" to be at a lower level than a (male) doctor. Obstetricians, meaning medically trained men, were the desirable option. Women either had to be as fully educated as men, or not be in the profession at all. The only exception would be a woman directly supervised by a medical practitioner.[43]

Nightingale fumed to Dr Sutherland about Hicks's remarks, for she essentially agreed with him on the level of training required.[44] She drafted a letter to the editor in response, but did not send it.[45] Hicks also must have seen some merit in the book, for he asked her about the hoped-for "second edition" and offered more data. He also had more questions for her about the handling of the data.[46]

When the reviews of *Introductory Notes* appeared, Dr Sutherland thanked Nightingale for sending on the *Medical Times and Gazette*, whose "droll" notice would serve better than the *Lancet* in promoting the book "and help to sell it." However, he did not agree with her siding with Evory Kennedy: "He committed a capital mistake about the Rotunda and gave the enemy cause of great rejoicing." He thought that "none of them had any knowledge of the real sanitary principles involved in the question." They floundered about "amidst misunderstood facts." Sutherland did not think they would see any more "philanthropic hospital builders."[47]

Nightingale met with Kennedy in 1879, about "Dr [Æneas] Munro's lying-in cottage scheme," which the latter outlined in his *Deaths in Child-bed and Our Lying-in Institutions, together with … a Model Maternity Institution* (1879), dedicated to William Farr, MD. Nightingale told Henry Bonham Carter that Kennedy "deplores his having been responsible for many, many deaths" at the Rotunda.[48]

Later Developments in Midwifery

When a new district-nursing organization was opened in London in 1875, there were implications for midwifery cases. Nightingale was concerned with the high death rates reported by Liverpool district nurses on women delivered at home. However, as she observed, "the same nurse nurses fevers and childbirth." She remarked also on the (continuing) low death rate of birthing women in the workhouse infirmary.[49] She would soon advise that visiting nurses keep midwifery and sickness cases strictly separate: "One should never take the other's cases," and the organizations would ideally be separate.[50]

Physicians continued to write to Nightingale for advice on midwifery. Dr Heywood Smith (1838–1928), for example, in 1876 sent her "a long and valuable letter." She replied that he could do "so much to induce the medical profession to turn their attention in the right direction as regards the training of midwives." She thought his British Lying-in Hospital, in Holborn, London, was better than others. She called her own book "a sort of guidepost, based on melancholy experience – a sort of town crier inviting further consideration – begging and crying out for further statistics, especially from men of weight like yourself."[51]

How little understood puerperal fever was can be seen in a paper of 1887 by William S. Playfair (1835–1903), then professor of midwifery at King's College Hospital. Puerperal fever was "practically the same thing as surgical septicemia," he said, caused by poison being absorbed through the genital tract. The poison could either originate "*de novo* from the decomposition of some of the organic matters resulting from childbirth" or be conveyed from without, "by septic channels as foul sponges, infected hands of practitioners or nurses, or suspended in the atmosphere, as in rooms into which sewer gas finds its way." This shows no advance in aetiology since Nightingale's own research twenty years earlier. "De novo" generation actually heads his list of causes, followed by such better candidates (as it turned out) as infected hands and foul sponges.[52]

Improvements at the General Lying-in Hospital, in Lambeth, London, could be seen in the 1894 book by Robert Boxall (1858–1915), by which time "Listerian measures" had been adapted for obstetric practice. That had taken a closing of the hospital for massive renovations.[53]

Women in Medicine

Nightingale knew the women "firsts" in medicine: the first woman to qualify anywhere (in the United States), the first to qualify in England, and the first qualified Englishwoman to practise in India, among others.

The English-born Dr Elizabeth Blackwell (1821–1910) was the first woman to qualify as a physician, in 1849, which she did in the United States, where her family had moved when she was a child. It took her several years of work to save enough money to pay the medical tuition fees. She was then turned down by twenty-five schools but accepted finally by the small Geneva Medical School in upstate New York. The sympathetic dean there consulted the students, who rose to the occasion with a letter espousing the principle that "one of the radical principles of a republican government is the universal education of both sexes," that every branch of scientific education "should be open equally to all." They not only approved Blackwell's application "to become a member of our class," they pledged themselves "that no conduct of ours shall cause her to regret her attendance at this institution."[54] Moreover, they kept that pledge, as can be seen in her account of their respectful conduct in classes, where they treated her like an "older sister." The only hitch she experienced, apart from being lonely, occurred when she was told not to attend a particular class. She wrote to the professor, most politely, of her desire to attend all classes. He let her in and there were no further bans.[55] When she graduated at the top of the class, her classmates congratulated her. Early women students elsewhere were treated miserably by male students, and sometimes by the professors.

Blackwell subsequently studied midwifery at the Maternité in Paris, where she lost an eye from an infection and had to give up surgery as a career. Her younger sister, Emily Blackwell (1826–1910), became the third woman to qualify as a doctor in the United States, at Case Western Reserve, and became a surgeon.

Back in England in 1851, Elizabeth Blackwell met Nightingale, and they became friends. Blackwell described her first visit to Embley in her memoir:

> The laurels were in full bloom. Examined the handsome house and beautiful grounds. Walked much with Florence in the delicious air, amid a luxury of sights and sounds, conversing on the future. As we walked on the lawn in front of the noble drawing room, she said 'Do you know what I always think when I look at that row of windows? I think how I should turn it into a hospital ward and just how I should place the beds!' She said she should be perfectly happy working with me – she should want no other husband.[56]

With Nightingale family friend Selina Bracebridge, they went on a day-long expedition to the parish of a reform-minded priest, William Quekett, visiting his schools, savings' bank, gardens, and cottage garden boxes, all work for which Nightingale envied him. She joked in a letter to her sister, "But oh! there's another *Mrs Quekett* on the tapis [carpet] – how I hate her."[57]

Blackwell's memoir acknowledged Nightingale's influence on her own "awakening" to the importance of sanitation: it was "the supreme goal of medicine, its foundation and its crown." She described Nightingale as "one of my most valued acquaintances ... then a young lady at home, but chafing against the restrictions that crippled her active energies."[58]

When Blackwell decided to return to the United States later that year, the two had one last full day together. They went to a lecture on political economy, then visited Dr Charles Verral's spine hospital, and both women wrote comments. Nightingale was impressed with how diffidently her friend gave her views, critical of how the child patient was being treated.[59] Blackwell noted that they were "not favourably impressed by the judiciousness of the exercises." After dining with the Bracebridges, recalled Blackwell, she "parted from her with tears."[60] The two, however, had at least one other expedition together, in June 1851, visiting the German Hospital at Dalston.[61] That hospital would be something of a model for Blackwell for her small women's hospital in New York.

Nightingale wrote Blackwell in 1852 from Umberslade, Warwickshire, where she was doing a water cure. The letter discusses the state of Europe, the education of women, Auguste Comte, J.S. Mill, and a female priesthood. Blackwell published a book that year, and gave Nightingale a copy: *The Laws of Life, with Special Reference to the Physical Education of Girls.*

Early in 1854, Blackwell wrote from New York to introduce her sister and "fellow worker," Emily, who was about to travel in Europe to obtain wider experience. She also provided an update on the dispensary that she, her sister, and another woman doctor had opened, preliminary to founding a small hospital.[62] She was assisted in this by gynaecologist Dr James Marion Sims, who founded the Anglo-American Ambulance (recounted in chapter 4). He gave a "convincing address" on the need for a women's hospital.[63] The New York Infirmary for Women and Children opened on Nightingale's birthday in 1857, 12 May, with Harriet Beecher Stowe giving the address.

The letter Nightingale wrote Emily Blackwell (they had not met) was sombre. She warned about the need to be "an apostle of the cause," committed to not marrying or flirting.[64] Elizabeth asked Nightingale's help for obtaining British qualifications for herself.[65] Nightingale made inquiries, wrote her associate Sir James Clark and the eminent physician and medical writer Sir Benjamin Brodie (1783–1862) to introduce her and ask their assistance.[66] Blackwell in fact became the first woman listed on the Medical Register. The following year, she helped to form the London School of Medicine for Women, in Bloomsbury, where for many years she was professor of gynaecology.

When "Mrs Dr Blackwell," as Nightingale called her to Sidney Herbert, was back in England in 1857, she asked her to Malvern, in Worcestershire, where she was doing a water cure. She was considering Blackwell for the head of her new nursing school, but undertook to Herbert to make no firm proposal without consulting him.[67] In his reply, he referred to her schemes as being "without a corporeal entity ready to work them."[68] Blackwell rejected the proposal, reasonably enough, as the proposed focus was nursing and she wanted to establish a private medical practice and promote women in medicine.

While in London in 1859, Blackwell gave a series of public lectures at the Marylebone Literary Institute on health issues related to women. Nightingale gave tickets to Mrs Farr and a Farr daughter.[69] The lectures received good newspaper coverage[70] and helped to establish Blackwell's reputation as a woman doctor. The young Elizabeth Garrett attended the first, and was motivated to think of a medical career for herself.[71]

Also in 1859, Blackwell sought Nightingale's "counsels" on establishing a "sanitary professorship," for which funding was promised by the *comtesse* de Noailles, an Englishwoman. Nightingale responded that it should be attached to "an old established hospital," and that the professor should "*not*" be the director. A complication: Nightingale was still expecting / hoping that hospitals would be located in countryside, for reasons of air quality. She advised on possible trustees (Lord Brougham too old; Lord Ashburton or Lord Cranworth would be better).[72] However, the *comtesse* kept changing her mind, so that negotiations with Blackwell came to nothing.

Nightingale recalled that she and Blackwell "were on different roads (although to the same object)." Her friend wanted "to educate a few highly cultivated" women, and she, "to diffuse as much knowledge as possible." Nightingale wrote her again that she did not want to prevent her from making any use of her ideas – "There is no copyright in 'ideas'" – but thought her plan for her next lecture "dangerous," that is, that it would prevent her from carrying out her own ideas. It would set the medical staff of the great hospitals against her. She would go into the plan with Blackwell, "if you think that it would clear up anything to your mind to see me again." If she gave out her "ulterior object," she warned, she could not make a case "for establishing a special hospital of the kind you mention, as against the great general hospitals. The patients themselves would prefer going to the latter." Blackwell could end up in debt. It would "strengthen the male feeling against your M.D.ship."[73]

Blackwell was in the United States during the Civil War, but her early leadership in organizing aid there did not result in any official appointment. She started the Women's Central Relief Association and assisted in the Ladies Sanitary Aid Association, but Dorothea Dix (1802–1887) was chosen to superintend the army nurses.

Blackwell returned to England permanently in 1869, to die in 1910 only months before Nightingale. The friendship, however, was not resumed. Each tried to recruit the other to her causes, and neither succeeded. Their differences grew as Blackwell became more conservative in her social views, as we see below. While Nightingale's early letters to her were to "my dear friend," they later deteriorated to "dear Miss Blackwell."

Blackwell's correspondence shows that she held mixed views of her friend throughout. She certainly misjudged Nightingale's mission in the Crimean War, telling her sister that the episode would be "instructive" and "useful," a chance for her to "sow her wild oats in the shape of unsatisfied aspirations and activity," then to come home to "marry suitably to the immense comfort of her relations."[74] She also misjudged her friend's *Notes on Nursing*, a "capital little book in its way," useful, practical, and readable. But "Florence cannot write a book in the usual meaning of the word. She can only throw together a mass of hints and experiences ... but she is not able to digest them into a book which will remain as a classic." She was not disappointed with it, however, as she "expected nothing higher."[75]

Blackwell learned about Britain's nefarious Contagious Diseases Acts at the Social Science Congress in Bristol in 1869. The legislation targeted women for compulsory internal examination (nothing for the men), to be followed by a month or longer in a lock hospital for treatment. Nightingale had led the fight against the law since 1860, produced a statistical analysis showing regulation to be ineffective in reducing syphilis in the army, and probably held back passage of the law by two years.[76] Blackwell was late in joining the struggle, and needed coaching.

Nightingale urged her friend to consult Dr William Farr on the matter, and warned at length about mistaken opinions. It was a battle of "the frogs and mice," she wrote, an allusion to Homer's *Iliad*, of "mere talk and opinion." It would take straining "every nerve ... as a general does in a campaign, with professional ability and devotion" to win. She regretted that she was unable to take it on; in fact, she continued to give some assistance, though not leadership.

She looked up "old documents as well as new," and sent them to Blackwell. On the inspection of troops for syphilis, she noted that they were "as utterly useless as they were degrading to the men and to the officers, and that voluntary application and appeal to honour have greater success."[77] Her next letter urged her friend "to study out the case." Opinion was typically substituted for investigation. "Some men" have the "opinion" that legislation was required, without any facts. There were also men on the other side, so who should decide? It was a practical question, for which the "opinion of physicians, however eminent," was not wanted. "What is wanted is *clear, connected, statistical detail* showing what is the amount of syphilis among a population 'unprotected'? What is the amount under 'protection,' and, lastly, what results when 'protection' is withdrawn?"[78]

In 1870, Blackwell put out a pamphlet containing (part of) her extreme position on sexually transmitted disease. She held that "all forms of chronic disease are so many disqualifications for marriage," naming "scrofulous or consumptive tendencies or any danger of insanity" as the worst. She would forbid marriage when both partners possessed "one of these diseased tendencies," forecasting that their "OFFspring would be 'certain to be either idiots, cripples or defective in organization.'"[79]

In 1871, Blackwell agreed to testify before a commission on the Contagious Diseases Acts and wrote to ask for advice. She sought no less than an inquiry into "the causes and remedy of prostitution," to go on to propose more draconian measures, even making "the voluntary communication of contagious disease a penal offense." Instead of the existing "lock hospitals," Blackwell wanted "lock-up houses, managed by women, under the superintendence of a lady who is a government officer and responsible for her subordinates." She ended, however, diffidently, asking if she should confine herself to the direct point of evidence, on compulsory examination of the women, and if her correspondent would add any suggestions.[80]

Nightingale, a liberal, and more realistic about human behaviour, was horrified, as was Dr Sutherland, who drafted some of her reply. "Be a woman ever so vicious, she has inalienable personal rights, which none but such idiots as social legislators would venture to interfere with." The act itself "should go." Government should cease to interfere "beyond its function." Further, while Blackwell wanted an inquiry on the causes of prostitution, Nightingale asserted that they were "perfectly well known," to be dealt with "by moral means," meaning "gentleness and considerate charity," for those who sought help voluntarily. All procuring should be felony.

"Voluntary infection" could not be made a crime, Nightingale wrote; it would have to extend to both sexes, "and the *animus* could never be proved." She was firm that "compulsory locking up under women is as bad as under men." She urged Blackwell to keep to "the only practical matter, namely the cruelty of forced examinations."[81]

In 1872, Blackwell established the "National Health Society," modelled somewhat on the Ladies' Sanitary Association, but for both men and women. She had spoken at meetings of the latter at the Bristol congress in 1869.[82] In 1871, she asked Nightingale if she approved of the new organization, then in planning, and if she would be on its board. The letter ends philosophically: "Dear friend, the never-ceasing effort to make God's laws the rule of life seems to me the only thing worth living for, and I do long to render good service to my dear native land."[83] Nightingale did not join.

She was not keen either on Blackwell's acceptance of medicine as it was, that "the ordinary male medical education should be given to women," as she saw it. "I have never known her enter in the least into any idea that there could be reform."[84] Both women saw midwifery as the obvious choice for women doctors, but they differed on how to educate them. Blackwell seemed to favour studies of one field, then the other, while Nightingale wanted them integrated.

In 1883, Blackwell, calling herself "your old friend," proposed "a thorough school of *midwifery for women*." She was not pleased with the London School of Medicine for Women, for neglecting the subject, and disliked the "moral tone" given it by leading medical women.[85] She recalled Nightingale's earlier work on the subject, which was for training midwifery nurses. But she was seeking a base for women doctors and added that Dr Mary Ann Scharlieb, after graduating with distinction, could not convince obstetricians in London to allow her to operate. They "told her emphatically that they wished to keep all operative midwifery to themselves." Scharlieb then went to Vienna.[86] Clearly women badly needed opportunities to obtain clinical experience and then to practise.

Dr Sutherland evidently saw more merit in Blackwell's proposal than Nightingale did, especially on connecting midwifery practice with "male aid" in cases of danger. French midwives were required to call in a physician in such a situation. Sutherland contended that medical training had been "making great strides among men," while women had been "kept simply to midwifery work," so that the gap in expertise between the sexes was growing.[87] In any event, Blackwell did not open a midwifery school, and the London School of Medicine for Women carried on as before.

Blackwell's views on social purity took her into positions unjustifiable even by the knowledge of her day. In an 1897 address, she again held that promiscuity was the cause of venereal disease. The bacillus that causes gonorrhea was identified in 1879, that for syphilis not until 1903. She lumped the two diseases together for purposes of causation: "Promiscuous intercourse inevitably tends to give rise to varying forms of venereal disease, no matter what precautions may be taken." In women, inflammation and irritation, from the "unnatural repetition of the sexual act," rendered the natural secretions "morbid." For men, similarly, the "natural secretions" became "morbid," developing into "blennorrhagia, or purulent gonorrhea." Further, she presented the "well-known fact," without producing a reference, of disease arising from "the congress of different races."[88] This material was given as an address to medical women in 1897.

Blackwell's *Essays in Medical Sociology* (2 vols, 1902) is misnamed, because it not only consists mainly of talks that give their author's opinions and moral values, but reports no research. Much in the book is neither medicine nor sociology – for example, the statement that "unchecked licentiousness or promiscuity contains in itself the faculty of *originating* venereal disease."[89] Blackwell reaffirmed her opposition to the compulsory inspection and treatment of women, also the right of society to make the transmission of disease a "legal offence." She now wanted the police to hire "superior women," a change from more ordinary women running lock hospitals.[90] Her essays also show concerted opposition to vaccination.[91] There are two chapters on "the abuses of sex," meaning masturbation and fornication, subjects Nightingale never discussed.

When the two women's years of meetings and correspondence are reviewed, we see that Nightingale was the leader, beginning with the centrality of sanitation and prevention, and moving on to such specifics as the Contagious Diseases Acts. Blackwell, however, could speak well in public, something Nightingale never did. She wrote and gave talks on human sexuality, including female enjoyment of sex, another non-starter for Nightingale. She published a number of books, but was not nearly as effective a writer. Both had a gift for friendship, maintained contact with numerous people, including leading scientists. Blackwell deserves celebration for leading the way for women to enter the medical profession, but her "social purity" leanings, not shared at all by Nightingale her colleague, mar some of what she wrote.

The First Woman to Qualify in England: Elizabeth Garrett

Dr Elizabeth Garrett (1836–1917), later Garrett Anderson, was the first woman to qualify as a doctor in England, by sitting the examinations of the Society of Apothecaries, which promptly changed its rules to prevent a recurrence. She in due course became professor of gynaecology and dean of the London School of Medicine for Women. She had shaky relations with Nightingale, who considered her position on nursing not only wrong but badly misguided. Her paper on "Hospital Nursing" to the Social Science Congress in Manchester in 1866 was not only published in its *Transactions*,[92] but covered by newspapers and the *Illustrated London News* and *Macmillan's Magazine*. The *Lancet* quoted her as saying that nursing by *ladies* was the "very best nursing England has seen." Nightingale huffed in a letter to Dr Farr that, because ladies happened "to produce nurses who are better than drunken old sots, therefore *all* 'ladies' are good nurses," likening it to the patient who recovered even if the doctor gave something he did not understand.[93]

Nightingale deprecated Garrett's focus on social class – the "lady superintendent" to be over the ordinary hospital nurses of the "lower middle classes." Her own criterion was training, which Garrett seemed to downgrade. She fully expected that "ladies" would usually be given the administrative posts, but they had to be trained for them and qualify on the basis of merit; working-class women could and did rise from the ranks. As well, while she wanted regular, paid positions for all nurses, including matrons, Garrett would perpetuate the "lady volunteer" in hospitals. Someone who did not need the salary, Nightingale explained, could give it away, but the very existence of unpaid personnel lowered salaries, making it hard for women who had to earn their living. "I think just the contrary from Miss Garrett – that we ought to *train* 'ladies' up to such a point that they will *command* high *pay*." She did not think there was "the least danger of 'ladies' crowding into hospitals as nurses," but rather the other way, "of 'volunteer' *untrained* ladies offering themselves for war and emergencies."[94]

Nightingale did not reply publicly to the coverage given the issue, but did comment to Drs Sutherland and Farr, Henry Bonham Carter and Sir Harry Verney.[95] Farr had presided over the section in which Garrett gave her paper. He advised Nightingale to submit a "correction," but not be controversial, and in time to do an additional paper.[96] She did neither.

Nightingale wanted midwifery practice to be chiefly in the hands of female physicians, but they could not "fancy they can '*pick up*' medical knowledge" in six months or so. She told Sir Harry Verney that she thought that Garrett could help in the reform: "It has been suggested to me that, if one of the lying-in hospitals could be reformed and placed under the supervision of Miss Garrett, with children added – Miss G.

being the resident medical officer – a real school for female physicians would thus best be established." Nightingale was pleased that the women doctors did not want to treat men.[97]

Dr Frances Hoggan (1843–1927) thought that Garrett did high-risk abdominal surgery and resigned from the New Hospital for Women on that account. She helped Blackwell found the National Health Society in 1871 (Hoggan was honorary secretary).

Whatever Nightingale's judgment of Garrett on nursing, she was willing to help her later when women doctors were ready to establish their own (small) hospital. There was an urgent need for one, for women doctors were kept out of the regular hospitals. Nightingale's help is related in chapter 5 as her advice largely concerned hospital design.

A footnote: Garrett Anderson's daughter, Dr Louisa Garrett Anderson (1873–1943), was Nightingale's last doctor and signed her death certificate in 1910.

Women Doctors for India

British-born Dr Mary Ann Scharlieb (1845–1930), CBE, later Dame, was a pioneering woman physician in India. She studied and then practised medicine in Madras, where her husband was a barrister. She studied later in London and obtained English qualifications. On her husband's death in 1891, she became the breadwinner for the family. She was that rare woman doctor for whom Nightingale's respect was unmixed. She also helped set up hospitals and medical training for women in India. The initiator, however, was no less than Queen Victoria, who had been influenced by a woman missionary, Elizabeth Bielby (1849–1929), who was not then medically qualified (she later was) but had successfully treated the maharani of Punna. The maharani gave Bielby a locket for the queen, with her message inserted in it. The queen's journal records her being moved by hearing of "the dreadful need" of women who were ill but who would not have a male doctor.[98]

When Lord Dufferin was appointed viceroy of India in 1884, the queen commissioned Lady Dufferin to organize medical care for women. She rose to the occasion, with much help from Nightingale. The National Association for Supplying Medical Aid to the Women of India was established, with the queen as patron, the viceroy as patron in India, the vicereine as president, and the various governors as vice-presidents.[99]

When Scharlieb left again for Madras in 1885, Nightingale wrote the governor, M.E. Grant-Duff, to introduce her and urge his active support for her work. Scharlieb needed a salary not only for herself as chief medical officer, but for an assistant, and money to buy drugs.[100] Nightingale described her to the governor as differing from the typical lady who would be content to "pick up" nursing and doctoring for India, believing instead that "nothing was good enough for India." With five years of medical training, "she goes out as the first fully qualified lady doctor." The letter ended with a typical Nightingale refrain on sanitation: "I long to hear about the Madras drainage and water supply."[101] Letters to Grant-Duff in 1885 went on to deal with the practicalities of establishing a "Caste and Gosha" women's hospital, that is, one that had separate quarters for Hindu, and Muslim women, and "Brahmin ladies."[102]

Scharlieb also assisted Nightingale by reading and criticizing her material in draft. Businesslike, on one manuscript she was reviewing, she suggested that the alterations could be made in proof. She was also a person of faith, dedicated to serving the poorest, least educated women. Yet she was careful not to let her faith interfere with good practice. When Nightingale described her to Lady Dufferin, she called her "a devoted Christian," who for that reason would not make "medicine a vehicle for proselytism."[103]

Dr Scharlieb proved a valuable source for Nightingale on child marriage and enforced widowhood, meaning the punitive treatment of child brides on the death of their husband, even if the marriage had never been consummated. The husband's death was proof of the wife's sinfulness, for which she had to atone by numerous privations. The British government had banned suttee, but not the "death in life" of enforced widowhood. Scharlieb's memoir records her describing the misery to Nightingale; a year after the husband's death the widow "is stripped very roughly of jewellery and rich clothes," for "a length of unbleached long cloth."

Her head is shaved … she is immersed in the sacred water, a mystical washing away of sin. She emerges dripping, shivering with cold, with sorrow and with fear. Her calico shroud must dry on her person, and from this time until the day of her death, she knows no comfort, no consolation … no nourishing and pleasant food, only cold rice and water – her touch, her very presence, is pollution …

Who can wonder at Florence Nightingale's generous sorrow for such sufferings, and who cannot understand her desire to help anyone who was able and willing to give such relief as might be possible to these patient sufferers?[104]

In 1887, Scharlieb had to return to England, her health broken. Nightingale was disappointed – her friend had gone into private practice to pay for her son's education: "No one can fill her place at Madras, hundreds could do so in England. Her work was immense, unique. She was 'facile princeps' [easily the first] and now it is all over."[105]

Nightingale assisted behind the scenes, but probably never met, one of the first Indian women to qualify as a doctor, Rukhmabai (1864–1955), who came to prominence for her refusal to consummate a childhood marriage. At age nineteen, she filed to have the marriage annulled. A favourable decision was reached, but her husband appealed, and in 1886 the decision was reversed. Rukhmabai was liable to six months in prison, which term could be renewed with her continued refusal. Men could marry a series of wives, but, as she pointed out, a woman could not marry again even if her husband died. Her husband appealed to public opinion with a pamphlet, citing his property rights. A compromise was reached in 1888, with Rukhmabai paying restitution to her husband. This decision led to the formation of a Rukhmabai Defence Committee to repeal prison sentences to enforce consummation. The case showed how British rule could make matters worse. Indian courts could not send a wife to prison for failure to consummate, but British courts could. British authorities, moreover, were reluctant to go against Indian customary or religious practices.[106]

Rukhmabai defended herself eloquently in the press, in both India and England, in letters by "A Hindoo Lady."[107] She explained her rebellion by reference to her "love for education and social reform," so that she wanted to continue her studies as much as she could. She wanted to do what was in her power to alleviate the sufferings of Hindu women. The bishop of Carlisle (Robert Goodwin) and numerous academics and journalists took up her cause, which was embarrassing to the British government.[108]

Nothing survives of Nightingale's writing on the case, but she is known to have prepared a brief for the Privy Council Office.[109] She received access to the relevant papers from Dadabhai Naoroji, founder of the East India Association, whom she assisted when he ran for Parliament. Lady Wedderburn, wife of a Liberal MP and India expert, provided Nightingale with correspondence from Rukhmabai and an extract on her "second trial" from the *Bombay Gazette*.[110] Her friend Benjamin Jowett later used his contact with Lord Lansdowne, then viceroy of India, on the matter.[111]

Rukhmabai was brought to England by the Liberal women who took up her cause. In 1889, she began studies at the London School of Medicine for Women, assisted by the Lady Dufferin Fund. She qualified in 1893 and returned to India, to practise for years, rising to be head of the Zenana State Hospital. She never (re-)married.

Nightingale's first acquaintance with a married woman medical student was with Mrs Kadambin Gangooly (Ganguly) (1861–1923), who trained at the Medical College at Calcutta. She had married after having made up her mind to do medicine, and had since had one or two children: "But she was only absent thirteen days for her lying-in!! And did not miss, I believe, a single lecture!!"[112]

Encouragement to the First Greek Woman Physician

It seems that Nightingale, late in life, gave encouragement to the first Greek woman to qualify as a medical doctor, Maria Kalapothake (1859–1941), who trained in Paris and travelled to London in 1894 to see British hospitals. The intermediary was a childhood friend of Nightingale's, Katharine M. Lyell, herself an expert botanist and sister-in-law of geologist Charles Lyell. Her father, Leonard Horner, FRS, took his daughters to meetings of the British Association for the Advancement of Science, as Nightingale's father had her. Katharine Lyell contacted Nightingale in 1894, to ask for a meeting for a Greek friend.[113] No meeting took place, but Nightingale wrote a letter of introduction for "Mlle Kalapothake" to the matron at St Thomas'.

In 1896, then Dr Kalapothake wrote Nightingale from Athens with what must have been a cheering letter on her work in Greece:

> Since then, I have been at home, practising in Athens, and have had occasion to feel the need of good nursing, a thing still in its infancy in Greece. When the war seemed imminent, the [*illegible*] of Greek women furnished the means to send out a completely equipped hospital to [*illegible*] and at the same time lectures were started for the ladies wishing to serve as nurses. I gave them lectures with the aid of several lady medical students as demonstrators. And,

notwithstanding the short time we had before us, managed to give the nurses the necessary rudiments of anatomy and physiology, with practical demonstrations in bandaging and practical operation to the use of antiseptics. The result was above all one could have hoped for, although undisciplined from an English standpoint. The Greek ladies made excellent nurses and were untiring in the performance of their duties.[114]

The letter went on to describe their goal of opening a training school for nurses and asked Nightingale to be an "honorary member" of the committee, a role she typically declined.

Last Work on Midwifery

Dr Priestley, the doctor who closed the Nightingale midwifery ward at King's College Hospital in 1868, gave a paper in 1892 to the Seventh International Congress of Hygiene, London, on the improvements made in maternity hospitals. For it, he had the president of the Actuarial Society, Benjamin Newbatt, compute an estimate, for six data sets, of lives saved by the introduction of antiseptics.[115] Newbatt compared actual deaths with an estimate based on Le Fort's pre-antiseptic data. Nightingale commented, in marginal notes: "Not anything else?" evidently believing that the use of antiseptics was not the only cause of the lower rates. She highlighted Priestley's remarks on the danger of disregarding "other sanitary conditions" and on the use of the pavilion model with careful aseptic and antiseptic practices. Where he stated that "a thoroughly antiseptic plan is greatly facilitated by other sanitary arrangements, such as ventilation and sufficient drainage," she added: "Voire [see] Maternité," the Paris hospital where these were lacking, and the death rates high. She continued to correspond with nurses and midwives, and track the medical literature on midwifery, until 1897.

PART THREE

Later Campaigns
(1880s and 1890s)

WRITING FOR DOCTORS, RURAL HEALTH VISITORS, STATE REGISTRATION OF NURSES, BACTERIOLOGY, AND GERM THEORY

Four distinct areas of Nightingale's late work with doctors are related in this chapter. This phase finds her updating previous material but also broaching entirely new subjects. The chapter looks first at what she wrote specifically for doctors, published in Quain's *Dictionary of Medicine*, on nurse training and hospital nursing, respectively. Both articles show the evolution of her ideas from her earliest books, reflecting substantial advances in medical science and practice. Second, a new project, on promoting rural health, follows, developed with the Buckinghamshire medical officer of health, hence a new initiative on an old concern.

The final two topics are matters on which copious misinformation about Nightingale is in circulation: third, her role in the state registration of nurses and, fourth, her role in germ theory. In both cases, primary sources tell us what she actually said and did, but they are typically ignored, even by eminent authors. How contentious the proposal for state registration was seems to have been little understood. That doctors and a financier–hospital administrator were the main forces against it, not Nightingale, will be shown. On germ theory, numerous writers have Nightingale proclaiming her opposition on her deathbed! Yet how she came to terms with bacteriology and the growing evidence for germ theory is of interest, as is her use of it to promote public health in India.

Nightingale's Articles in Quain's *Dictionary of Medicine*

The *Dictionary of Medicine* (1882), edited by Dr (later Sir) Richard Quain (1816–1898), gave Nightingale the opportunity both to update her material on nursing and to direct it to the *Dictionary's* readership, mainly doctors, who were also the main contributors. She produced two articles (one on nursing practice, the other on nurse training), as did Douglas Galton (on hospital construction and administration, respectively). Galton used her material in his articles, and she reviewed and commented on his drafts. He, her close associate, a royal engineer, and a leading hospital architect, acted as intermediary with Quain and helped format her material into dictionary style.

The resulting, compact articles are plodding in places (lists of antiseptics), but elegant in others, with those on health and healing among her very best writing. They generally show how far both nursing practice and training had evolved since 1860, when her school opened and her *Notes on Nursing* first appeared. She wrote the articles 1876–78, a few years before their publication. She revised them in 1889 for a new edition in 1890, which also appeared in the United States, and again in 1892 for an 1894 edition, 1895 in the United States. Colleague and cousin Henry Bonham Carter helped with those last revisions.

In Nightingale's article on nursing practice, various disinfectant solutions are specified for a number of uses, while in 1860 she advised only frequent washing of hands with soap. Soiled sheets, for example, are to be steeped in boiling water with carbolic acid 1 to 100, while a solution of 1 in 20 is given to coat the fingers for vaginal probes.[1] The heading, "Personal Cleanliness," is the same as in the original *Notes on Nursing*, but now there is much more detail. The essay is very similar to the Memorandum for Probationers on Beginning Ward Work issued in 1878 at St Thomas' Hospital.[2]

Nightingale gives no source for the quantities for carbolic solutions: perhaps it was the tutor at her school, Mary S. Crossland, as correspondence from her in 1878 reports on Dr Bernays's use of disinfectants: chlorine and carbolic were his top picks, although for scarlet fever he considered it cheaper to burn everything rather than disinfect. He had little faith in Condy's fluid, but believed in fresh air and cleanliness, she wrote.[3] A letter by Crossland in 1892 gave an update on antiseptic and aseptic use, with a copy of the St Thomas' "pharmacopoeia," which gave the strengths of the various solutions it used.[4]

Since doctors were the main readers of the *Dictionary*, Nightingale put in a word on benefits for hospital nurses, including regular breaks in the working day and a full month's holiday. Night nurses required adequate "undisturbed sleep."[5] Later editions called for a "second education" "every five or ten years" after training.[6]

Nightingale distinguished the nurse's and the doctor's roles more than ever: "The physician prescribes for supplying the vital force – but the nurse supplies it." She then cited a much-quoted definition: "Health is not only to be well, but to be able to use well every power we have to use."[7] The World Health Organization would echo it when it was founded in 1948: "Health is a state of complete physical, mental and social well-being and not merely the absence of disease or infirmity."

Nightingale defined sickness and healing with clarity and confidence:

Sickness or disease is Nature's way of getting rid of the effects of conditions which have interfered with health. It is Nature's attempt to cure – we have to help her. Partly, perhaps mainly, upon nursing must depend whether Nature succeeds or fails in her attempt to cure by sickness. Nursing is therefore to help the patient to live. *Training* is to teach the nurse to help the patient to live. Nursing is an art, and an art requiring an organized practical and scientific training. For nursing is the skilled servant of medicine, surgery and hygiene.[8]

The article on nursing practice shows how many tasks nurses had taken over from junior doctors or medical students. When the Nightingale School opened in 1860, nurses were not trusted with the taking and recording of patients' temperatures. This changed in a few years. By the time of Quain's *Dictionary*, their tasks included: dressing blisters, burns, and sores; administering stimulants (alcoholic drinks) and medicines as ordered, enemas, injections, and suppositories; managing trusses, and appliances in uterine complaints; passing the catheter (at least for women); making and applying poultices and minor dressings, wet, dry, and greasy; syringing wounds and the vagina; managing helpless patients (move, change, and keep clean, warm, or cool); cleaning the patient's teeth, gums, and tongue; washing or sponging the patient without exposure to chill in any part; preventing and dressing bedsores; making bandages of various kinds, line and pad splints; taking temperature and pulse, sometimes every fifteen minutes in acute cases; and testing urine. A nurse doing home visits had also to be able to pass the speculum and the catheter for men. Two further tasks were added in 1894: giving subcutaneous injections and using a galvanic battery.[9]

Specifics for observation had also become more detailed. The nurse was now "to observe correctly and to report correctly on the state or character of secretions, expectoration, pulse, skin, appetite, effect of diet, of stimulants, and of medicines, eruptions, the formation of matters," on the patient's mental condition, to note delirium or stupor, plus the nature of breathing (quick, slow, regular, or difficult) and quality of sleep.[10]

Nightingale's often-misunderstood stipulation of obedience to doctor's orders here is well stated. In the article on nurse training, she distinguished between intelligent obedience and servility. Training made the difference, teaching the nurse to act "for the best" in carrying out orders, "not as a machine but as a nurse ... like an intelligent and responsible being." She was not to be "servile, but loyal to medical orders and authorities."[11] Similarly, in the practice article, the nurse was "to obey intelligently, using discretion."[12]

"Health Missioners" and the Medical Officer of Health for Buckinghamshire

In the 1890s, when Nightingale spent extended stays with her stepnephew and his wife, Sir Edmund and Margaret Verney, and their family at Claydon House, Bucks, her late sister's home, she took up the promotion of health visitors, called "health missioners," with the county medical officer of health, Dr George Hanby De'Ath (c. 1862–1901). He put on a program of lectures for the "lady visitors," augmented by practical visits to villagers' cottages. The Verneys, especially Frederick, also her stepnephew, then a member of the Bucks Sanitary Committee, later MP for North Buckinghamshire, strongly promoted the project.

Nightingale was worried: "What is read in a book stays in the book." Mothers and girls who did not believe that sanitation affects health and prevents disease had to be convinced.[13] She went to some trouble to promote the training, especially the cottage visits.

When Dr De'Ath was planning the classes, Nightingale ordered books for him: four copies of Huxley's *Physiology*, which she thought "rather a dead book," but which she was sure he would put "life" into, and three each of Morris, *Hair and Skin*, and Treves, *The Influence of Clothing on Health*, with an offer to obtain more.[14] When De'Ath started the classes in 1892, Nightingale sent him "a few criticisms" on his "missioner's form." She gave him "joy with all my heart and soul at the success of your opening lady lectures," especially because there were so many invitations for them to visit the cottages – proof, for her, that the village women were not put off by the "ladies."[15]

Among other tasks, Nightingale was set to find diagrams or models to be used in the lectures. Her own physician, Dr Ord, recommended that the heart and lungs, "freshly taken from a sheep," would be "infinitely more useful" than a diagram or model.[16] Perhaps nothing came of this, for Nightingale continued to pursue ordinary models. She asked De'Ath if he had tried the National Health Society, founded by Drs Elizabeth Blackwell and Ernest Hart. She enclosed £10.10 for expenses.[17]

Nightingale approved of De'Ath starting his lectures by "touching on the difference between health and sickness. Quite the best."[18] She approved also when the class did a "raid" on a supplier of bad milk: "No greater work is being done in these times than redressing sanitary evils. And I hope you will awaken the sleeping sanitary authorities. I give you joy of your great work."[19] The project's success can be seen in the fact that people in other counties sought out the lecturers trained in Bucks.[20] Dr Ord recounted that he had given lectures on sanitation to poor women in Brixton, but they would not change their ways – he wished them better luck in Bucks.[21]

Nightingale was asked the next year (1893) to contribute a paper for the Conference of Women Workers on Rural Health in Leeds. This turned out to be "Rural Hygiene," read by Maude Verney (wife of Frederick, her sister's stepson), well-structured and much longer than the Bucks paper. It began with early examples in India, where lecturers went around to villages to show people how to dispose of their refuse and keep their water supply pure. It went on to what women could achieve with "health-at-home training" and what responsibilities local authorities had.[22]

The medical officer of health at this time was expected to attend to "infected rooms," after being hermetically sealed, and to direct the "baking" of clothes in the case of a serious illness. Evidently "great surgeons" were "proverbially careless about infection," hence the need for these special measures. In this example, the patient, at Claydon House, was Nightingale's stepgrandniece, Ellin Verney, Edmund and Margaret's daughter. Her illness is unspecified, but of months' duration. Nightingale gave detailed instructions on the use of disinfectants, including 20 per cent carbolic soap for cleansing the child's heel, for "infectious skin has been known to harbour *under* that hard skin." She advised successive courses of application of disinfectant solutions to the child's body, leaving days between the various stages.[23]

De'Ath's only publication was a pamphlet, *Cholera: What Can We Do?* (1892), in which he quoted Nightingale's advice on prevention and included two pages written by her. He quoted also doctors Sir Andrew Clark (1826–1893), Ernest Hart, and Waller Lewis, and the Local Government Board. As well as stating his own advice on cleanliness measures, De'Ath related a range of death rates for Asiatic cholera, from 45 to 64 per cent, stating also that the disease "defied drugs ... It was eminently a case in which prevention was far more efficacious than cure."[24]

By 1892, the cholera bacillus was known, also that it was not transmitted by air, unlike many other diseases. It had been found to favour an alkaline fluid, and did not live in acid media.[25] The draconian treatments of early–mid-nineteenth century – blistering, emetics, purging, and the use of toxic metals – do not appear now. No effective treatment was yet known, but De'Ath's advice was in the right direction – for liquids, against dehydration.[26] Dehydration destroyed electrolytes needed to keep the heart pumping. The effective treatment for cholera, found only in the 1960s, is oral rehydration.

Nightingale must have liked De'Ath's warning against "too much reliance" on disinfectants, for possibly giving "a false sense of security." Cholera was not stopped "by merely substituting one smell for another," for it was possible "to remove the odour and leave the danger."[27] She contributed the last pages of the pamphlet, with stirring words for vigorous preventive measures: "Is not health the most precious thing of all – the capital of men, women, and children, especially every working man and woman?" The battle would never be lost by taking stringent measures, "for, if cholera does not come, we are winning the day against fever, diarrhea, against poor health and following out the laws of God, who means us all to be healthy."[28]

When Nightingale was reviewing De'Ath's syllabus in 1895, she complimented him for the "thought" he gave "everything he planned or said," which might be hasty but also, to some degree, from experience. However, his remarks on "burns" filled her with fear, "because he does what Sir J[ohn] Herschel said we all do, viz., forms and enunciates opinions *a priori*, without the slightest inquiry: 'has this been tried? What was the result?'"[29] Nightingale had read Herschel when an adolescent, and saw him at Oxford at meetings of the British Association for the Advancement of Science in 1847.

Prevention of Infantile Blindness

In 1895, Nightingale took up the prevention of infantile blindness with Dr De'Ath. She had been alerted to the issue in 1889 by Dr Frederick Mant Sandwith (1853–1918), then physician at the new Women's Hospital in Cairo. He told her that Muslim children (Coptic Christian infants fared even worse) developed ophthalmia in their first week of life from flies settling on their eyes: "If they don't come in [for treatment] the first week they are generally stone blind for life with those terrible white eyes. But now we insist upon their [mothers and children] coming before it is too late and we pay the greatest attention to teaching them sanitary habits."[30]

The issue came up again in 1894, when a Charlotte Smith, who was neither a doctor nor a nurse, sent Nightingale a copy of a paper she had presented to the British Institution of Public Health.[31] Nightingale evidently wrote back, as Smith later thanked her for information sent. Smith sent her details about what various cities were doing on the matter. She called for "all midwives" to learn to look for the signs.[32] Smith also published an article on ophthalmia in the *Medical Magazine*, excerpted in the *Review of Reviews*.[33]

Nightingale sent Dr De'Ath "unsatisfactory printed leaflets" on the prevention of infantile blindness for his comments, but whether they were Smith's or someone else's is not clear.[34] A month later, Nightingale sent him the following instructions, and possibly sent the same to Smith, source not specified:

> Prevention of blindness. After a newly born child is washed, great care should then be taken to clean the inside of the eyelids of each eye, as any collection of matter within the eyelids is very dangerous and must be removed. The outside of the eyelids should be well cleaned, and the eyelids separated and the edges cleaned. Each lower eyelid should be pulled gently down on the cheek and some water dropped on the inner surface, the eyelid should then be allowed to close. The water will thus wash the eyes. This should be done twice a day for a month.[35]

Nightingale's advice differs from what Smith published by being proactive. The *Review of Reviews* excerpt called for the infant to be taken to a doctor without delay if his or her eyes became red or swollen, or ran. What use was made of this advice is not evident, but it is an interesting example of networking across professional lines.

Also at this time, Nightingale had occasion to worry about De'Ath's health. She urged him to take time off and hire an assistant, chiding him about not going to another doctor. He should see the oculist at Guy's: "Great doctors never treat themselves," she told him.[36]

In 1898, Nightingale was "aghast" at De'Ath's losing his appointment, where he was "so necessary." She was not a Bucks ratepayer, but thought she might write the Local Government Board about it.[37]

The State Registration of Nurses – Doctors on Both Sides

It is unfortunate that Nightingale's last big campaign concerned a vexatious issue that took time and depleted her energy from what might have been productive work. She felt compelled to take on state registration, or rather the version proposed by the British Nurses Association, as harmful to nursing by giving too much power to doctors and promoting academic over practical learning. Its register would exclude good nurses from a working-class background, because they could not pass the written examination, yet it would not protect the public against unqualified nurses. The issue has been analysed at length, both in general,[38] and on Nightingale's role in particular.[39] My object here is to relate the central and contentious role doctors played from the beginning. A complication: some pro-registration doctors were Nightingale's close friends and colleagues, notably Drs Sir Henry Acland and Sir James Paget.

Dr Acland is credited with the first suggestion of a state register of nurses, akin to that for the medical profession. In his preface to Florence Lees's *Handbook for Hospital Sisters* (1873), he noted that, while women could be registered as medical practitioners, they could not be as nurses, a situation he thought ought to be remedied. Nothing happened to this suggestion until 1887, when Dr Bedford Fenwick and Ethel Fenwick, shortly after their marriage and her resignation as matron at St Bartholomew's, set up the British Nurses' Association (BNA). The founding meeting, held at their home, followed a meeting of the Hospital Association, an earlier organization founded by Henry Burdett, a banker and hospital administrator. Rivalry, rudeness, and lawyers' letters date from these first meetings.

The BNA proposal included some good measures, notably a three-year training program (the Nightingale School was still only one year), a benevolent fund, and pensions for nurses, although Burdett's Hospital Association was ahead of it on that score. Both also had a register, neither large, to identify qualified nurses, thus giving them advantages from their training, while protecting the public from untrained nurses. However, even the doctors supportive of the BNA acknowledged that there was no effective way of removing nurses for misconduct or incompetence. The BNA acquired the "Royal" prefix in 1891 and a royal charter in 1892.

Nightingale was annoyed that Acland, an early supporter of the BNA, asked Sir Harry Verney to attend a meeting about it: "I ENTREAT [underlined three times] you *not* to attend" it, she wrote her brother-in-law: "I cannot think how Dr Acland can ask you. I *implore* you not to go." She could not write the letters "which I have been ordered to write for it."[40] The meeting was held at St George's Hall, London, with an overflow audience, presided over by William Savory, president of the Royal College of Surgeons. Princess Christian of Schleswig-Holstein (Queen Victoria and Prince Albert's daughter Helena), the BNA's royal and very active patron, gave a stirring speech.[41]

Nightingale met with Dr Norman Moore (1847–1922), senior physician at St Bartholomew's Hospital, who confirmed much of what she did not like in the registration scheme, especially its control by doctors, not nurses. He justified this on the grounds that the matron would play favourites in making recommendations, and gave an example of Ethel Fenwick adjusting her marks in rating candidates for a prize, to ensure that her favourite won.[42] The two hospitals that most strongly opposed state registration were the two at which Fenwick had nursed, the London and St Bart's. Isla Stewart, Fenwick's replacement as matron at St Bart's, became a major BNA supporter.

Ethel Fenwick, at the request of Princess Christian, approached Nightingale for her support. The letter was deferential, asking for her "invaluable advice and any suggestions" on the BNA draft bylaws, before they were confirmed. The association's first and great aim (registration), she said, would "crown the edifice of which you laid the foundation and cornerstone so strongly, the establishment of nursing as a legally constituted profession."[43] Nightingale, of course, had never bothered about the legal constitution of nursing. She was next sent a printed invitation to attend a meeting on state registration, to hear Dr Bedford Fenwick speak.[44]

Nightingale described the registration conflict in 1888 to Frederick or Maude Verney, with an allusion to the Battle of the Frogs and Mice, a parody of Homer's *Iliad*:

> There is a great split: a Batrachyomachia – Burdett and £20,000 on the one hand, the matrons and Princess Christian on the other. Both are going to set up nurses' registers. Both are bidding for popularity on all sides. Henry Bonham Carter has declined to be vice president to one side – and I to t'other. We will talk about it when we meet ...
> They are trying to make a nurses' republic with a princess at its head, without the smallest idea of governing themselves or of *knowing how to raise their own standards. Training will be destroyed by registering.* But nursing will survive.[45]

Nursing academics tend to be critical of Nightingale's stance, ignoring how deeply the issue divided both doctors and nurses. Burdett's Hospital Association, which antedated the BNA and had established the National Fund for nurses, thoroughly and consistently opposed the proposal. Royal family members were divided, with the Prince and Princess of Wales (later Edward VII and Queen Alexandra) supporting the Hospital Association and its Pension Fund, while his sister Princess Christian backed the BNA. Each side attacked the other. Nightingale thought Burdett's "abuse of the BNA ... not quite as bad as the BNA's of him."[46] She declined to meet Henry Burdett when he asked her, but acknowledged that he "*is* doing one useful thing – the BNA, nothing but harm."[47] The gifted and tenacious Burdett carried on the fight for years after Nightingale quit it.

That Burdett was an avid royalist no doubt also helped. In 1889, he published a highly deferential account of the charitable work and public life of the Waleses: *Prince, Princess and the People.* He established and raised money for the Prince of Wales' Hospital Fund, which became, in 1902, the King Edward's Hospital Fund. Burdett was honoured with a knighthood in 1897. After her husband ascended the throne, Queen Alexandra insisted on replacing Princess Christian as president of the Army Nursing Service.

Nightingale was mightily miffed that so many of her medical friends joined the BNA, and that some even became vice-presidents. It was "thrown at my head,' she recounted, that Sir Henry Acland, Sir Rutherford Alcock, and Sir James Paget were all on the BNA. "O God, stop them."[48] However, they also passed information back to her, and they, like others who joined, had reservations. She had a lengthy interview with Paget, at Acland's request, prior to the Mansion House meeting of 17 July 1889. He advised delaying it, but the gathering took place as scheduled. Acland should speak at it, Paget advised, but "say nothing." They should sit back and let the now "Royal" BNA fight with the Hospital Association. Acland perhaps took this advice; at least he is noted as speaking only to propose a vote of thanks to Princess Christian for her support of the BNA.[49]

Some doctors who joined the BNA gave timely advice to Nightingale. For example, on the wording of the royal charter, Sir Rutherford Alcock (1809–1897) obtained a promise from the Privy Council "to let him know when the R. Charter is lodged." This induced her query to Henry Bonham Carter, "Then why does he not take his name off the BNA manifesto?"[50] Alcock later signed her public letter against registration.[51]

Physicians dominated the BNA / RBNA's council from the beginning. No nurses were vice-presidents, and only seven were on the twenty-one-member executive.[52] Princess Christian, as president, dominated. This caused a serious grievance for Nightingale: a nursing association headed by someone who had never trained or practised as a nurse. The British Medical Association passed a resolution in favour of registration in 1895. Paget predicted the RBNA's breakup because members fought at their own meetings, as became increasingly evident in newspaper reports. Members attacked each other, wrote letters to the editor with their grievances, even took legal action. Princess Christian, when she presided, could not control the members, Paget pointed out. He advised letting both associations have a register: the Privy Council would not give both of them a charter: "The queen *cannot* grant a charter except after the most ample time given for counter-pleas and examination. You may use this time. No charter can be passed in a hurry."[53]

Paget confirmed that the register gave no powers of exclusion from practice and no means of removing a nurse for misconduct or incompetence. It could do no more than indicate that someone had at one time trained and once was respectable, damning words. He thought that forty or fifty years hence a register would make sense, when the profession was filled with more educated women, to protect them against uneducated women. It was advantageous to have royals "on both sides." Yet, ostensibly, as Sir William Savory explained, the register was "to give a better guarantee to the public in regard to their qualifications."[54]

Acland tried for some time to bring the two sides together. He told Ethel Fenwick in 1889 that she could not proceed without Nightingale's approval.[55] Fenwick tried, but Nightingale would not budge – their differences really were fundamental. So were they with Princess Christian. In 1891, Nightingale remarked that she could not understand "how men of the world, as, e.g., Sir H. Acland, should, without my leave or previous knowledge, have crammed me down the princess's throat *in a way* which has created animosity and greatly injured the cause."[56] Philanthropist and ally William Rathbone, MP, told Nightingale that Acland and Paget lacked the courage to tell the princess to "get out" of the RBNA.[57]

The tactic of the anti-registration group was to have the registration provisions watered down. They drew up a detailed petition to the Board of Trade and collected a large number of signatures, many of them by profession leaders. The treasurer of St Thomas' Hospital was the main organizer.[58] The RBNA responded with a public letter, co-signed by Ethel Fenwick and Drs Brudenell Carter (1828–1912) and James (later Sir James) Crichton-Browne (1840–1938), criticizing the petition and its signers. It regretted that "medical men of respectability and, in a few cases, even of eminence, should have been induced, in ignorance of the facts and by the misrepresentations of interested persons," to have attached their signatures to the document.[59] Nightingale privately called this letter "very foolish and vulgar."[60]

She otherwise kept to the background. The petition to the Board of Trade worked, and the RBNA "Register" was reduced to a mere list of names not at all comparable to the medical register, meaning "no professional privilege," but simply RBNA membership. Nightingale set this out in a public letter, co-signed by seven hospital matrons, many eminent doctors (though fewer with titles than the other side), and senior hospital administrators.[61] Some signers had helped promote nursing, such as the Duke of Westminster, as chair of the Metropolitan and National Nursing Association, and William Rathbone, MP, who had financed the first professional nursing in Liverpool. The difference between this list and those of the RBNA is striking. Nightingale's includes trained matrons, with their job titles.

Dr Acland tried again in 1893 to bring Nightingale and Princess Christian together. He wrote the princess that she had to have Nightingale's "name," without asking the latter, who would never have consented, if he had asked, as she told him. The princess did not answer Acland's letter, but a secretary acknowledged its receipt.[62] He next asked Nightingale to write a letter for the 1893 annual meeting, which was to be held at Oxford University. He pressed her to "see," or to "ask to see" the princess, which distressed her "beyond anything you can imagine."[63]

Acland presided over the Oxford conclave. Still trying to reconcile the two sides, he asked Nightingale for her advice on how to handle the session. She proposed that "you, in taking the chair, should not commit yourself to approval of the whole scheme of the association, and that you should point out the difficulties which will occur in working the 'list' (we will not call it 'Register'). You might positively say that you 'are desirous of giving the association the opportunity of making its objects known to the public,' to 'dilate upon the benevolent objects.'" He should make it clear that he had taken the chair "at the request of H.R.H."[64] Whether or not he took this advice is not clear. If he did, he would have caused offence – the chair of a meeting inviting debate on the very purpose of the organization. Yet worse would soon happen to the RBNA.

Nightingale was bothered by the "Princess Christian party" seeking out Balliol College for the venue, the college where her good friend Benjamin Jowett was master. He told her that the princess had asked for Balliol Hall and that he felt that "he could not refuse." He considered that he would "go away" in order not to be there, although that would be rude, as she related the situation to Henry Bonham Carter. He presumably did absent himself, for the *Times* report of the meeting does not note his name, while it does those of the princess, Acland, as presiding, his daughter, Miss Acland, and a number of prominent doctors. Dr Bedford Fenwick moved a motion of gratitude on the part of British nurses to the princess for her efforts to improve their profession.[65] Again, this meant a doctor speaking for nurses to thank a non-nurse on what she did on a core nursing matter. Nightingale and Acland evidently had some exchanges on the subject in 1894, but what is not clear, for he burnt a letter from her, "as you desire."[66]

Sir Joseph Lister joined the RBNA, although his hospital, King's College, was one of those opposed, and he, according to Nightingale, knew "nothing at all about nursing." She did not know him, and he was not someone she could "send for," as she told Henry Bonham Carter.[67]

In the account of the 1894 meeting, the only nurse's name mentioned was that of "Miss Thorold," matron of the Middlesex Hospital, for presenting a bouquet to Princess Christian. Not relating experience, nor advising on policy, but handing over a bouquet! Many doctors' names are listed, plus a few other notable persons, some with their wives: Sir Henry Acland, Professor Brudenell Carter, Sir James Crichton-Browne, Sir Dyce Duckworth, Sir Joseph Fayrer, Dr Bedford Fenwick, Sir Francis and Lady Jeune, Sir Joseph Lister, Sir James Paget, Sir Richard Quain, Sir William Roberts, Sir William Savory, Sir Sidney and Lady Waterlow, Sir Spencer Wells, and Sir John Williams.[68]

In 1895, the bylaws were changed to end founders' permanent seats on the council. Nightingale subsequently noted the names of four persons "struck off the council": Bedford Fenwick, (Louisa) Hogg, Isla Stewart, and (G.M.) Thorold.[69] The Pension Fund people were also on the move. The matron at Oxford's Radcliffe Infirmary, Flora Masson, a Nightingale protégée, reported to her that "a grand function was held at which the Princess of Wales received the Pension Fund people."[70]

The worst blow, no less than a "betrayal," came to the RBNA in 1896, when a "fundamental principle" for its founding was reversed. Dr Bedford Fenwick had succeeded in having the British Medical Association agree to seek an act of Parliament for the state registration of nurses. The doctors' association called a meeting to confer with the RBNA on it. That gathering adopted, by a majority of one, an extraordinary resolution: "That a legal system of Registration of Nurses is inexpedient in principle, injurious to the best interests of nurses and of doubtful public benefit."[71] Even the medical secretary of the RBNA voted for it. The resolution was never repealed, so that new organizations had to be formed to promote registration.

The RBNA continued to meet on other business, held lectures, and still attracted members. Nurses used their membership in it and being on its register as a job qualification. The register served a useful purpose for some nurses, even with its legal limitations, but neither the RBNA's nor the Hospital Association's register had large numbers of names, nor was either well maintained.[72]

Also in 1896, a nurse, Margaret Breay, brought a legal suit against Sir James Crichton-Browne for his refusal to entertain a resolution of hers at an RBNA meeting. She won and was awarded a farthing in damages, and he appealed.[73] Meetings became more acrimonious, duly reported in the newspapers. Nightingale had nothing to do with any of these events.

A report of the RBNA's annual meeting of 1897 included complaints about "the removal of several matrons from the general council" and the packing of the general council with nurses from the Middlesex Hospital and the Chelsea Workhouse Infirmary, so that "paid servants of a public institution were employed by the superior officers for the fulfillment of private ends."[74]

Also in 1897, or ten years after the BNA's founding, both Dr Bedford and Ethel Fenwick sided with a protest group, the Members' Rights Defence Committee, to denounce the RBNA for mismanagement, specifying overspending and bringing in new bylaws without discussion by the members. Ethel Fenwick's motion called for a select committee to hold a public inquiry, which was passed unanimously. A doctors' organization, supported largely by general practitioners, the Incorporated Medical Practitioners' Association, supported the protest group.[75]

All this perhaps helps to explain why the state registration of nurses was not achieved in Britain until 1919, after the creation of several intermediate organizations to press for it, five select committees studying the matter, and six unsuccessful private member's bills. Registration came in earlier in some jurisdictions, such as New Zealand, Scotland, and some American states. Doctors contested it in others, notably in Canada.

Was Nightingale right? With the benefit of hindsight, it is hard to fault her for opposing such a defective measure, with its heavy domination by doctors. However, her insistence on the centrality of good character for nursing, and the inability to judge it by examination, entailed an obvious double standard. Doctors were qualified without such a requirement, as were and are other professionals. Many doctors objected to her position, including her friends. She was never persuaded to change her mind on it, but declining numbers supported it.

Nursing advocate Monica Baly assessed the result of the "Thirty Years War" for registration as a "Pyrrhic victory." The standard required, "when the smoke of battle subsided, would have satisfied neither Nightingale nor Mrs Fenwick," nor the College of Nursing when it was eventually established: "It was all an expedient compromise." The profession, moreover, had handed over its control to government, to the people "who had the responsibility for keeping the hospitals staffed as cheaply as possible."[76]

Bacteriology and Germ Theory

Bacteriology as a discipline is a product of the second half of the nineteenth century, after Nightingale's major writing on nursing, hospitals, and health care. "Germ theory" is the popular term for the view that diseases are caused by specific pathogens: bacilli or bacteria, viruses, and so on, as opposed to "spontaneous generation" from miasms (the Greek plural is *miasmata*, which is not used here). Nightingale never mentioned "spontaneous generation" in her writing, but clearly subscribed to the view that diseases emerge from miasms and could change from one to another, as in diarrhea turning into dysentery or cholera.

Louis Pasteur's research on hops, grapes, and silkworms dates to the 1860s, but the application to human diseases, such as gangrene, with post-surgery death rates of 50 per cent, was not then obvious. It is perhaps no coincidence that the surgeon who made the breakthrough on antiseptic procedures, Joseph Lister, was the son of a wine merchant who was an amateur scientist, FRS, and maker of an improved microscope. Joseph Lister began experimenting with a carbolic spray at the Glasgow Royal Infirmary in 1865. He did not mention "germ theory" anywhere in his landmark paper of 1867 reporting his results.[77] Rather he explained that it was not the oxygen that caused "suppuration" in surgical wounds, but "minute organisms suspended" in the air. They were living entities, or had "vitality," as he put it. His carbolic spray, then the strongest antiseptic available, "destroyed the life of the floating particles." The spray, however, irritated the patient's skin, and Lister stopped using it. This won him Nightingale's respect: "After having upset the whole world by his 'spray,' he has condemned his 'spray' in the face of the whole world and the stars," she wrote Henry Bonham Carter.[78] Antiseptics would instead, in varying solutions, be used on the operating bed and equipment.

Nightingale's espousal of miasma theory led to good results, for sturdy measures to do away with "filth," the habitat in which germs breed, destroy the unseen germs themselves. Her measures for thorough washing of floors and walls, with attention to avoiding porous materials in construction, were effective. She was attentive as much to fluid-borne as to air-borne sources, with rules about the removal of soiled bandages and bedding. Strict cleanliness went a long way to killing germs and preventing their multiplying. Lister, by contrast, considered only air-borne transmission of the pathogens. The sequence is instructive:

In 1854, Dr John Snow reduced cholera cases in London by having the Broad Street pump broken off – the water source in an area with a high number of deaths. However, the sight of "white flocculent particles" in a water sample did not lead to any general acceptance of germ theory. The bacilli seen under a microscope could have been products of the disease, it was thought, not the cause.[79]

No effective treatment for cholera was found, and periodic outbreaks continued. Followers of "heroic medicine" tried ever more toxic substances as treatments, such as mercury, lead, arsenic, and camphor, as is evident in numerous articles in medical journals, textbooks, and compendia of "materia medica."

The bacilli causing many of the greatest killer diseases were not identified until the 1880s and later. Major examples are typhoid fever (discovered 1880), tuberculosis (1882), diphtheria (1883), cholera (1884), tetanus (1884), pneumonia (1886), meningitis (1887), plague (1894), dysentery (1898), syphilis (1903), and whooping cough (1906).

German bacteriologist Robert Koch identified the bacillus for anthrax (1877), the mycobacterium for tuberculosis (1882), and the bacterium for cholera (1884). His authoritative "four postulates" paper, "The Etiology of Traumatic Infectious Diseases," appeared in 1879. He won the Nobel Prize in Medicine or Physiology in 1905 for his research on tuberculosis. It would be Koch's work on cholera that changed Nightingale's mind about germ theory, with Dr John Sutherland acting as the intermediary.

The Cholera Bacillus Identified

The British invasion of Egypt in 1882, at least partly over control of the Suez Canal (opened 1869), forms the background for the breakthrough on cholera. Medical teams from Britain, France, and Germany all went to Egypt after an epidemic broke out there in 1882. The British group was sent by the India Medical Board (cholera originated in India and epidemics persisted there). As we saw above, the group was led by Dr William Guyer Hunter, who had made his career in India. No member was a microscopist, and, not surprisingly, no microbiological cause was found. The epidemic was blamed on the weather reactivating cholera poisons dormant in the soil from the outbreak of 1865. Hunter was knighted for his efforts in ending the epidemic. This he did by employing vigorous sanitary measures, while getting the theory wrong.

A doctor on the French team died of cholera, and his colleagues returned to France. By the time Koch arrived in Egypt, with a substantial retinue of researchers, equipment, and animals for testing, the epidemic was over. Corpses lacking, the team moved to Calcutta, where they were plentiful. There Koch made the great breakthrough. Dr Sutherland read his findings and was persuaded. He purchased a "beautiful Vienna microscope" to see for himself, as he told Nightingale. The two were then occupied in briefing a new viceroy for India, Lord Dufferin, but Sutherland thought that Koch's discovery would save more lives than anything they might persuade Dufferin to do. Nightingale protested: "I did not know the bacillus was of more consequence than a viceroy," but Sutherland would not budge.[80] He evidently persuaded her (no correspondence is available on the point), for she changed her tune. She continued to stress prevention, reasonably enough, for identification of the bacillus resulted in neither prevention nor cure. She came to realize that bacilli, on a slide, could be used in teaching prevention. In a publication for an Indian health journal, she urged that slides – "magic lantern shows" – be projected in villages to show the people "the obnoxious living organisms in foul air and water." These had "produced a strong impression" at a recent hygiene congress, she noted.[81] The following year, she gave a microscope to a nurse departing for Bangkok (her practice was to ask nurses what they wanted as a gift).[82] At least as early as 1864, Nightingale had understood the value of microscopes for examining polluted water, without drawing conclusions regarding germ theory.[83]

Nightingale's nursing school at St Thomas' Hospital began teaching a rudimentary form of germ theory as early as 1873. Medical instructor John Croft's published lectures to the nursing students include a chapter, "Disinfectants and Antiseptics," which gives specifics on the available antiseptics and their preferred uses. It ends with the admonition that antiseptics were not substitutes for ventilation, fresh air, and cleanliness, Nightingale's point precisely.[84]

Her insistence on preventive measures, far from impeding progress, meshed with best practice. Conceptually, however, she did not want germs to be thought of as "the cause," when filth was, and the filth had to be dealt with. In 1890, she distinguished between the germs themselves and their origins, which could be traced to bad water and filth. She acknowledged Koch's demonstration of germ theory, with a qualification: "I think it is passing away in its dangerous aspect (Koch's), viz., that of considering the 'germs' as the origin, not the product of the disease, of which uncleanliness, bad drainage, bad water supply, etc., are the origin."[85] She was not disputing the *existence* of bacteria, but stressing the role played by unsanitary conditions. In 1893, Nightingale praised the sanitary commissioner of Bombay for being "full of information." He did not "talk bacilli but real practical uncommon common sense."[86]

Identification of the bacillus that causes a disease is essential for the development of a vaccine against it. The great Russian–French bacteriologist Waldemar Mordecai Haffkine developed a cholera vaccine while working at the Pasteur Institute in Paris. He went to India in 1892 to test it and remained there for most of the next thirty years. On route to India, he visited the British Army hospital at Netley.

On a visit to England in 1896, Haffkine wanted to meet Nightingale. Dr Acland tried to arrange that, but it probably did not happen (there is no correspondence to indicate any did). Acland wrote Nightingale to make the request, explaining that Haffkine had been working in India on cholera prevention for the past three years. Haffkine sent her a copy of his book, *Anti-Cholera Inoculation: Report to the Government of India* (1895), with a handwritten dedication.[87]

When plague broke out in Bombay in 1896, Haffkine was appointed bacteriologist to the government and given space at the Grant Medical School. He quickly developed an effective vaccine. The British government sent English nurses to work in a plague hospital, and Nightingale briefed them. Nurse Georgina Franklin told her about his inoculation, and that they would meet him.[88]

Nightingale worried about the encounter with the "great inoculator," as she and they called him. Franklin reported back that they were indeed inoculated, albeit by another doctor, using his method. She assured Nightingale, "Statistics prove the treatment to be of use as, out of a school of thirty boys, the one who would not be injected had plague and died, the twenty nine inoculated escaping. This is one instance out of many."[89] Haffkine was named a Companion of the Order of the Indian Empire (CIE) by Queen Victoria in 1897.

Wherever she stood on the theory, Nightingale continued to convey the right message on prevention. In 1883, when a cholera epidemic was looming in the United States, she was asked by a journalist for the *New York Herald* to provide advice. After some delay, this was published as "Scavenge! Scavenge! Scavenge!" and reprinted also in British newspapers.[90] It appeared also in public-health journals, both British and American.[91] An irate writer of a letter to a newspaper in Tasmania sent it along with pointed reference to the "disgraceful … swamp" of Launceston.[92]

When a cholera epidemic broke out next in 1892, Dr Hart, speaking to the National Health Society, quoted Nightingale's 1884 letter.[93] "Scavenge! Scavenge! Scavenge!" was again picked up in newspapers across the country.[94]

Nightingale as "Lifelong Opponent" of Germ Theory

Despite the ample evidence of her coming to accept germ theory and see its usefulness, numerous authors call Nightingale a "lifelong" opponent of germ theory. Those making the mistake include eminent historians, doctors, and nurses. Australian medical historian F.B. Smith had Nightingale vehemently opposed to germ theory,[95] while a review of his book drew dire consequences from her supposed opposition: "No one did more to keep cholera alive and well than Nightingale."[96] Charles Rosenberg, a Harvard historian of medicine, faulted "her certainty" and "strident and uncompromising" views on germ theory in his introduction to an edition of her *Notes on Hospitals*. Her "explicit rejection" of the theory, he stated, took her further from the "consensus of medical opinion during the last third of the nineteenth century."[97] A director of Army Medical Services incorrectly had her "never" believing in germ theory.[98] A fellow of the Royal College of Physicians had her "totally opposed to the very idea that diseases were caused by germs," so that, in retrospect, she deserved "mockery."[99] A historian, later editor of the *Oxford Dictionary of National Biography*, also had Nightingale "never" accepting germ theory, among other failings.[100] A book on hospital infections is equally firm, though incorrect, that she "never accepted, even in later years, the germ theory or the value of antiseptics."[101]

A historian writing in an epidemiology journal has Nightingale, with Edwin Chadwick, maintaining "their allegiance to the 'miasmatic' explanation of disease causation despite Koch's discovery many years before their deaths."[102] That same author, in a book with much positive material on Nightingale, had her going to her grave in 1910, "believing that disease was caused by a bad smell."[103] A recent book on Crimean War history faulted her for "not believing in germs," although the war ended years before Pasteur and Lister even began their research.[104] Nursing historians and nursing academics have been as inaccurate.[105]

Clearly the misinterpreting-Nightingale crowd is numerous, diverse, and still growing. In the next, final chapter, the subject turns to the smaller number who have seen great merit in her ideas and example, again a diverse and growing number.

8

CONCLUSION

The Enduring Legacy

Nightingale continued to work into the 1890s, or for more than thirty years after her first publications and the opening of her school, but by the late 1890s she did not go beyond making inquiries, keeping up on developments such as on antiseptic procedures, and sending greetings to nurses. She continued to meet with senior nurses as late as 1898. She retired about 1900, judging by her answer to occupation on the 1901 census, "living on own means," when earlier she had specified management of Nightingale Fund nurse training.[1]

This final chapter makes connections with developments that continued well after Nightingale's lifespan. This begins with parallels between the foundation she gave to nursing and that William Osler gave to modern medicine. Next comes recent work on neuroplasticity and sunlight that draws on her early advocacy of sunlight. Then we consider how her methods could be used on current health-care challenges, especially vis-à-vis today's state of hospital-acquired infections. This entails a revisit to the hospitalism of her time. Finally, we examine how her approach might help set (general) health-care priorities for today and the coronavirus pandemic more specifically.

Nightingale and Modern Medicine: Dr William Osler

Canadian-born Dr William Osler (1849–1919), who was knighted in 1911, is recognized as the "father of modern medicine" and the great influence in moving medical training from the lecture hall to the bedside. Nightingale, of course, insisted on bedside training for nurses from the founding of her school in 1860. It must be augmented by lectures, but would be primarily hands-on, the experienced nurse training the pupil. Nightingale was influenced on this by army doctors she respected telling her that newly graduated doctors did not know one organ from another when actually confronted with a living patient.

Nightingale and Osler never met or corresponded, but there is enormous overlap in their views on health, healing, and the respective roles of doctors and nurses. He knew her work well, owned copies of her major books and sources on her (a medical colleague of his, Maude Abbott, wrote an early book on her). Osler praised Nightingale in an article of 1891, where he credited her with turning nursing, "unsettled and ill-defined" at the time of the Crimean War, into its "modern position": "ever blessed be her name."[2] He did not cite her in his most famous book, *The Principles and Practice of Medicine* (1892), but several sections of it show a common approach.

When Osler began his clinical studies at the Montreal General Hospital in 1870, it was a modest 150 beds in size, "ill-lighted and ill-ventilated," "old, coccus-and rat-ridden."[3] Built in 1729, beside the St Lawrence River, it was no healthier in 1875 when five Nightingale nurses arrived to introduce professional nursing to Canada. The group was led by Canadian-born matron Maria Machin (1843–1905), who was keen to return to Canada after gaining nursing experience in Germany and then training very successfully at the Nightingale School. She was the well-educated daughter of a clergyman, had been principal of a girls' school, and was an excellent tutor at the Nightingale School. Nightingale's advice on a proposed new Montreal General, designed by English architect Alexander Graham but never built, is outlined in chapter 5.

The nurses' time at Montreal was difficult almost from the start. In October 1875, Machin reported "your little colony here is doing very well, all are well, in good heart."[4] Then, in 1876, an epidemic took the life of Nurse Martha Rice and Machin's fiancé, a doctor. She requested replacements, and two more nurses were sent in 1877. However, the situation worsened, and Machin and all the nurses returned to England in 1878. Four of the nurses (not Machin) on route, they were shipwrecked on route home on barren Anticosti Island in the St Lawrence. However, they were rescued by a ship conveniently heading for Britain.

When Machin wrote to Nightingale with her plans to return home, she was sent a moving letter: "You have created much at Montreal. Now perhaps God will send you to create somewhere else. I have had heavier falls than this. But I scramble up ... Do you know it is twenty three years today since I was in the thick of receiving the sick and wounded from the Battle of Inkermann, and with scarcely anything to do it with. I should despair, if God were not there."[5] Machin next became the first trained matron at the prestigious St Bartholomew's Hospital, London, with another Montreal nurse in a senior position.

Jane Styring, another of the Montreal nurses, later was superintendent of a London workhouse infirmary, at Notting Hill. She reported to Nightingale that antiseptics gave them "a great deal of work, however they had learned them at St Thomas', which was useful as they had just come in when I went to Montreal," so that she was "quite an authority" there.[6]

Osler's Principles and Practice of Medicine

It is easy to see why Osler's *Principles and Practice* would become such a useful reference work for doctors. The original, 1892 edition is 1,079 pages long, divided into eleven sections by type of disease. Most sections have multiple chapters, again by type of disease. Section I, for example, "Specific Infectious Diseases," has thirty chapters, beginning with typhoid fever, given thirty-five pages. There are then subsections on definition, symptoms, a historical note, aetiology, discovery of the bacillus and points on how it fulfils Koch's law on bacillus identification, modes of conveyance, contagion, varieties, diagnosis, prognosis, prophylaxis, treatment, and comparison with typhus fever. *Principles and Practice* was translated into French, German, Spanish, Russian, and Chinese. Revisions were made by later doctors so that new editions continued to appear into the 1930s.

The book has no general introduction nor definitions of health or illness, or the roles of nurses or doctors in healing. Osler's views on these key points, however, spring up unannounced in various places in the text. The lengthy treatment of typhoid fever, still then a great killer, is a good source both on general points and similarity of approach with Nightingale, who never wrote on typhoid fever and seldom on specific diseases.

Osler gave great attention to environmental factors in aetiology: filth and bad sewers. He offered examples of mortality rates, citing a major medical source, Murchison, with 19 per cent of a large number of cases, adding the mortality rate for the Montreal General Hospital of 11.2 per cent over twenty years. He was firm on prevention, asserting occurrence to be in direct proportion "to inefficiency of drainage and water supply." Much could be done "to prevent the spread of the infection" by recourse to "the most rigorous methods of disinfection." He advised boiling drinking water and milk "when epidemics are prevalent."[7] A later paper noted the "great victory" over typhoid fever: "with a pure water supply and perfect drainage, typhoid fever almost disappears from a city."[8] All this is similar to Nightingale's earlier advice.

The section on treatment is especially revealing, for there was then no effective remedy for typhoid fever:

> The profession was long in learning that typhoid fever is not a disease to be treated by medicines. Careful nursing and a regulated diet are the essentials in a majority of the cases. The patient should be in a well-ventilated room (or in summer out-of-doors during the day), strictly confined to bed from the outset, and there remain until convalescence is well established. The bed should be single, not too high, and the mattress should not be too hard. The woven wire bed, with soft hair mattress, upon which are two folds of blanket, combines the two great qualities of a sick bed, smoothness and elasticity. A rubber cloth should be placed under the sheet. An intelligent nurse should be in charge. When this is impossible, the attending physician should write out specific instructions regarding diet, treatment of the discharges and the bed linen.[9]

Nightingale put it more forcefully, that medicine and nursing do not cure, but only nature, by God's laws. The nurse's function was to put the patient in the best condition for healing to take place. This is precisely what Osler advised for typhoid fever. His specifics on the type of bed, mattress, and ventilation are all standard Nightingale fare.

Details he next gave on diet again echo hers. Milk was "the most suitable food," with a substitute noted for those who do not like it. Beef tea, chicken broth, and consommé also feature, with barley, gruel, and something akin to Nightingale's "egg flips."

Osler reviewed the use of "antiseptic medication" to treat typhoid fever, that is, the attempt to destroy the bacilli or the toxic agents they produced. These endeavours had been "laudable," he said, but so far "without success." Good results had been claimed from carbolic and iodine treatment; he could testify to the inefficacy of corrosive sublimate.[10] He then went on to the relief of symptoms, the risk of heart failure, and avoidance of bedsores.

Finally, Osler gave specifics on convalescence that again remind one of Nightingale, a great advocate of separate, well-situated convalescent institutions. He considered that the management of convalescence was "often more difficult" than the disease in the acute stage, and he had firm rules for diet.[11]

The "intelligent nurse" clearly was key to the success of treatment for Osler. If there was no such person available, he resorted to the usual substitute, that the physician write out instructions for the patient's diet, observation of discharges, and changes of bed linen, all matters known to be done badly all too often by helpers without training.

Nightingale evidently knew Osler's *Principles and Practice*, for she gave a copy of it to a nurse leaving for a plague hospital in India.[12]

Osler was more optimistic than Nightingale about the possible good effects of pharmaceutical research:

> The growth of scientific pharmacology, by which we now have many active principles instead of crude drugs, and the discovery of the art of making medicine palatable, have been of enormous aid in rational practice. There is no limit to the possibility of help from the scientific investigation of the properties and action of drugs. At any day, the new chemistry may give to us remedies of extraordinary potency and of as much usefulness as cocaine. There is no reason why we should not, even in the vegetable world, find for certain diseases specifics of virtue fully equal to that of quinine in the malarial fever.[13]

Osler was writing decades after Nightingale, when pharmacology and bacteriology were both more advanced. She had come to accept germ theory, without realizing how much bacteriology would benefit medical science. Osler did: "Preventive medicine was a blundering incomplete science until bacteriology opened unheard-of possibilities for the prevention of disease."[14] The effects of antibiotics were then still decades off. The same holds for radiation treatment, stem cells, and microscopic surgery – all unthought of in their day.

A later Osler paper adds further points on the important role of the nurse and the limits to chemical / pharmaceutical interventions. Never as extreme as Nightingale in denigrating the uses of chemicals or drugs, Osler, however, comes across as conservative. There were only a "few great medicines," he said, naming six: digitalis, iodine of potassium, iron, mercury, opium, and quinine. It was better for the doctor to rely on them than "employ a multiplicity of remedies the action of which is extremely doubtful."[15] He regretted that the public had "not yet been fully educated to this point," so that doctors sometimes had to order medicines for the sake of their patients' friends. He battled "poly-pharmacy, or the use of a large number of drugs (of the action of which we know little, yet we put them into bodies of the action of which we know less)." This battle had not been "fought to a finish," he said.

Osler then applauded what he saw as a "return to what used to be called the natural methods – diet, exercise, bathing and massage." The value of diet in prevention and cure was more fully recognized than before: "One of the great lessons to be learned is that the preservation of health depends in great part upon food well cooked and carefully eaten," again, all very much in accord with Nightingale's views.

The same paper went on to praise the progress made by nursing care:

Nursing. Perhaps in no particular does nineteenth-century practice differ from that of the preceding centuries more than in the greater attention which is given to the personal comfort of the patient and to all the accessories comprised in the art of nursing. The physician has in the trained nurse an assistant who carries out his directions with a watchful care, is on the lookout for danger signals and, with accurate notes, enables him to estimate the progress of a critical case from hour to hour. The intelligent, devoted women who have adopted the profession of nursing are not only in their ministrations a public benefaction, but they lighten the anxieties which form so large a part of the load of the busy doctor.[16]

Osler, in another essay, ranked the nursing profession with that of medicine and the clergy: the trained nurse had become "one of the great blessings of humanity, taking a place beside the physician and the priest, and not inferior to either in her mission. Time out of mind she has made one of a trinity." He then made a point Nightingale had stressed throughout her working life, the great privilege of nursing the neediest: "There is no higher mission in this life than nursing God's poor."[17] Osler's father was an Anglican priest, and Osler himself had attended one year of theological college before taking up medicine.

Osler and Nightingale Nurses

Exceptionally for that period, Osler worked with Nightingale nurses from 1875 in Montreal to his last position at Oxford in 1905. His second contact with them took place at his next medical appointment, in 1884 at Philadelphia. The first trained matron, Alice Fisher (1839–1888), had studied at the Nightingale School in London and pioneered trained nursing in three British hospitals. Fisher died in Philadelphia after only four-and-a-half years as matron. Osler attended her on her deathbed and published a tribute to her in the *Medical News*.

He praised Fisher for the changes she had effected in Philadelphia: "The good work which she has accomplished has stimulated other hospitals of the city, and training schools have been established at the Pennsylvania, Episcopal and University Hospitals. By no means the least important lesson Miss Fisher's too brief life in this community has been the demonstration of the fact that the profession of nursing affords a most suitable field for women of the highest culture and intelligence."[18] Fisher herself was the daughter of a noted astronomer-priest. She had published two novels before entering the Nightingale School. She subsequently wrote a book with another Nightingale matron, Rachel Williams, *Hints for Hospital Nurses* (1877).

Osler moved in 1889 to Baltimore, where he became physician-in-chief at the new Johns Hopkins University Hospital, and when its medical school opened, in 1893, one of its first four professors of medicine. The founding superintendent of nursing and principal of the nursing school at Johns Hopkins was Canadian-born Isabel Hampton (1859–1910). The two can be seen to have worked together amicably, for there is surviving correspondence from the period.[19] Osler was on the selection committee that interviewed the leading applicants for the position. Also on it, with the president of the university, was Dr John Shaw Billings, the army doctor who designed the hospital, with advice from Nightingale.[20]

In 1894, Hampton married Dr Hunter Robb (1863–1940), who was then on the staff of the hospital and a colleague and friend of Osler's. The wedding took place in England – Nightingale sent the bridal bouquet. She and Hampton had corresponded earlier on a nursing paper for the world congress in Chicago in 1893, "Sick-Nursing and Health-Nursing," which Hampton read on her behalf. Hampton Robb duly resigned her position to move with her husband to his new appointment at Case

Western Reserve University in Cleveland, Ohio. As a wife and mother, she could not hold a nursing position, but found a new realm of influence writing three nursing books, forming nursing organizations, and helping to found other nursing schools.

The title of her major book, *Nursing: Its Principles and Practice for Hospital and Private Use* (1893), echoes Osler's title of the previous year. Her volume is remarkable for uniting the best from Nightingale – the stress on biophysical conditions such as cleanliness, light, nutrition, and ventilation – with copious examples of recent practice. The first edition was 484 pages, expanded to 565 pages in 1907, compared with a mere 79 pages for the first edition of Nightingale's *Notes on Nursing* (1860), then 222 pages on revision. Neither Nightingale nor Osler appears in Hampton Robb's index, but the connections are obvious. As well as containing material on Nightingale's core ideas on environmental conditions, her work has much on the nurse's role in observation and reporting to the doctor.

In preparing her volume, Hampton Robb drew on the notes she had used in teaching. She is said to have been an excellent and innovative instructor, at the bedside as well as in the classroom. She was keen on teaching aids, using a skeleton, a mannequin for visceral organs, specimens, charts, and pictures.[21] In contrast with the Nightingale School, nursing students at Johns Hopkins heard lectures, from her as well as from medical doctors.

Hampton Robb sent Nightingale a copy of *Nursing* and hoped that she would "approve of it, in part at any rate." She asked for her "criticism upon it and any suggestions," which would meet with her "careful consideration."[22] Her mentor undertook to send a critique, but evidently lost the author's new address in Cleveland. Hampton Robb made one further attempt to obtain her views, probably in 1896, when she was revising the book for use in a three-year program. That program, incidentally, would limit nurses' workday to eight hours, the longest period she thought possible in the United States to keep them strong and healthy. She had given a paper on the subject the previous year at their superintendents' convention (Hampton was a founder of the organization).[23]

Nightingale did a very rough draft on the differences between English and American society that would affect nursing, but it is not at all clear if she ever sent it. It would not have helped in a book revision.[24]

Hampton Robb's *Nursing* was intensely practical, heavy on what nurses were to do in what situations. However, she also increased the academic content of training, expanding the two-year program to three years, with the first six months devoted to theory. She had earlier organized the first graded course in nurse training in the United States, at the Illinois Training School in Chicago. Hampton Robb was an advocate generally of high standards of training for nurses.

Especially in its expanded, later editions, her *Nursing: Its Principles and Practice* represents professional practice as it was in the 1900s and 1910s. It also marks a change in style of titles: Nightingale favoured the modest "Notes on," and for her midwifery book the more diffident "Introductory Notes on." Williams and Fisher's book is more humble still, "Hints on." Hampton Robb confidently promised more – and delivered.

Both Hampton Robb and Osler, however, differed from Nightingale in including private nursing in their writing. "Private Use" appears in Hampton Robb's subtitle. Correspondence shows Osler's concern for better care for private patients at the hospital, not a matter Nightingale would have countenanced. Her own *Notes on Nursing*, in another major difference, was written for mothers and girls in the family giving health care and informal nursing, not for professional nurses or students. Both Hampton Robb and Osler wrote for professionals and for students preparing for professional work.

Osler also knew Hampton's assistant matron at Johns Hopkins, Devon-born Nightingale nurse Louisa Parsons, RRC (1855–1916), who became the first superintendent of the nursing school at the University of Maryland Hospital, also in Baltimore. In 1882, Parsons had served as a British military nurse in the first Egyptian campaign. In 1885, she received the very prestigious Royal Red Cross (Nightingale received the award at its inception, in 1883, for her work at Scutari in the Crimean War). Parsons also won a medal from the Egyptian khedive (ruler). She later headed nursing for the Red Cross at Fort McPherson, in Atlanta, during the Spanish–American War (1898), and served the British Army again nursing in the (Second) Boer War. Parsons never met Nightingale personally (not all pupils did), but she identified strongly as a Nightingale nurse. While in Baltimore she wore her old "Nightingale cap."

Parsons became terminally ill while visiting Oxford many years later, when Osler was there. Alerted to her condition, he visited her regularly in hospital and kept in touch with the nurses looking after her. On her death, he attended her funeral and sent a wreath, on behalf of the "Medical and Nursing Staff of the Johns Hopkins Hospital." Parsons, as a member of the Reserve Nursing Staff, was given a military funeral. Lady Osler wrote to a mutual friend with details of the ceremony, from her husband's description: "The coffin was carried to the church on a gun carriage – a company of soldiers, buglers, and a firing party – rifles fired over the grave and the 'Last Post' called by the buglers. Sir William said it was immensely impressive – a gorgeous autumn afternoon, with wonderful lights and shades – the roadside lined with people from far and near. Isn't it nice it could be so done?"[25]

The fact of Parsons being buried with military honours – though probably not the pomp, – represents a step Nightingale had long wanted for army nurses: officer status. By the end of the Crimean War, she had begun to call for it, arguing for non-commissioned status for untrained assistant nurses, when the British Army had never had any nurses above the rank of private. Again, as we saw in chapter 1, the census then grouped nurses in with domestic employees, not health professionals.

Neuroplasticity, Healing, and Sunlight

Canadian psychiatrist Norman Doidge, a leading author on "neuroplasticity," or the brain's ability to reprogram itself, credits Nightingale with advocacy of a key related process: the effect of sunlight on healing. He praised her promotion of the pavilion style of hospital design, for its maximizing patients' exposure to sunlight, in structures "designed to expose patients to as much sun as possible," but unfortunately that "brief, sunlight-friendly period in the nineteenth century ended with the invention of the artificial light bulb." The bulb was believed to contain the same full spectrum of light as direct sun, but it did not. The next stage of hospital design "no longer favored natural light, because science could not explain Nightingale's insight that sunlight actually heals."[26]

Nightingale did not know the causal mechanism, but had read the available medical literature. She drew on an 1858 speech on sunlight as a hygienic agent by the president of the New York State Medical Society.[27] She quoted from a British journal article reviewing many recent publications, notably one by Sir James Wylie, a British doctor who was physician to three Russian tsars, with his observations of St Petersburg hospitals. He had found that hospital rooms without windows, but otherwise adequately heated and ventilated, had only one-quarter the recoveries of well-lit hospital rooms. The article flagged the "exquisite sensibility" of the eyes to light, which rendered them "peculiarly adapted *to transmit the influence of this agent throughout the system.*" The retina transmitted not only through visual rays, but healing and chemical rays, although only the "visual nerves" were required for vision. Both Nightingale and Wylie also made references to observations by Arctic explorers.[28]

Nightingale devoted a full chapter in her *Notes on Nursing* (1860) to light, as "essential to both health and recovery." The points are repeated in all the editions of the book, slightly abbreviated for *Notes on Nursing for the Labouring Classes*, perhaps a concession to the reality of poor light in workers' homes.

Not coincidentally, Nightingale's Crimean War colleagues shared her views on the value of sunlight. Robert Rawlinson, the civil engineer on the Sanitary Commission, used language similar to hers in an article in a major architectural journal: "Sunlight is of the utmost importance; any plan which renders sunlight impossible is defective. Architectural grandeur cannot compensate for such defect."[29]

Sidney Herbert was onto the issue of light early in the days of his Royal Commission on the Crimean War. He wrote that he agreed with Dr R.G. Whitfield at St Thomas' (whose letter is not extant), that we do not "yet know the laws or the powers by which it is effected. But there is little doubt that the sun's rays have a direct effect upon atmosphere and upon human health, and no one but an engineer would ever have dreamed of constructing a hospital as to disbar the wards from being visited by the sun's rays."[30]

Nightingale was neither prescient nor lucky in her belief in sunlight's role in healing. While she knew nothing of neurotransmitters, she could compare outcomes between places with varying amounts of sunlight. From Quetelet she found out the harmful effects of "dark, unaired sides of deep valleys" on development that he described in his influential *Physique sociale.*[31]

Nightingale had learned something of sunlight's influence as early as her 1849–50 travels in Egypt. There she deprecated "the northern sunlight" for being "like lamplight": "I shall never forget my first sight of the sun behind the masts of Alexandria, taking possession of his own land of the East." She praised the Moorish architecture of Egypt for its latticed windows, so that one could look "up to the blue sky and golden sunlight." In bazaars, the sunlight poured in "through the square holes left in the roof."[32] She noted that Apollo, the Greek sun god, was considered to be a god of healing.

In her chapter on light in *Notes on Nursing*, she said that the "best rule" was to give patients "direct sunlight from the moment he [the sun] rises till the moment he sets."[33] She added further examples in later editions and other writing, for example, in Quain's *Dictionary of Medicine*: "*Light*. Second only to air is light as an essential for growth, health, and recovery from sickness – not only daylight, but sunlight – and indeed *fresh* air *must* be sun-warmed, sun-penetrated air ... People say the effect is on the mind. So it is, but the enlightened physician tells us it is on the body, too. The sun is a sculptor as well as a painter. The Greeks were right as to their Apollo."[34] Doidge particularly appreciated her "sculptor" metaphor, suggesting no skin-deep effect, but that light and colour could "sculpt the circuitry of the brain." Her "sculptor" expression appears in three editions of her *Notes on Nursing* as well as the Quain's article.

An early, 1858 paper she wrote on hospitals proposed that sunlight, second only to fresh air, was essential for "speedy recovery," except perhaps for certain ophthalmic and a few other cases. She noted medical research by Dr Milne-Edwards, Mr Ward, and Sir Andrew Wylie: "Dark barrack rooms, and barrack rooms with northern aspects, will furnish a larger amount of sickness than light and sunny rooms." Further, "window space should be one third of the wall space," and the windows "from two or three feet of the floor to one foot of the ceiling." Warmth was easier to control, but "we cannot generate daylight, or the purifying and curative effect of the sun's rays."[35]

The time of day was also relevant. As she wrote architect William Beckett Dennison: "The morning sun is always advantageous, the south sun not so much so." North–south wards were preferable because they ensured that the "whole wall surface" would be exposed to sunlight. North walls (when east–west), were "always more or less damp and cold." Wards should have "sweeping light," so waste "no ray of sun."[36]

Sunlight, naturally, was just as important for army hospitals. Her (unsigned) article in the *Builder* in 1858 asserted: "In the teeth of all these popular fallacies, we assert that every sick ward should be capable of being flooded by sunlight; and, consequently, that the windows should bear a large proportion to the wall space in all hospitals. Experience appears to prove that window space should not be in a much less proportion to wall space of a hospital than one to two.[37]

Sunlight was also essential for learning. A letter of 1874 advises:

That it is quite out of the question to build an *infant school* with so little sunlight or indeed window space at all. An infant school ought to have its *two long* sides and one of its short ones quite *open* to the *sun and air,* so that the children may have the sun from the moment they come into school till the moment they leave; *S.E., S.W., N.W.* (closing it to the *N.E.).* It is well known that both health and power of learning depend on this – in infants especially. This school has only *one S.E.* and one N.W. window.[38]

In 1885, when advising architect Alfred Waterhouse on plans for the Liverpool Royal Infirmary, Nightingale stated firmly: "The pavilions appear far enough apart and not high enough to shut out sun from one another – a point of great importance. (In the most recent and largest pavilion hospital, Edinburgh, the pavilions are too near, 88 ft. apart, and the walls too high, 63 ft., and they shut out sunlight.)."[39]

Hospital-Acquired Infections Today: Revisiting "Hospitalism"

Modern hospitals continue to produce hospital-acquired infections, now often called healthcare-associated infections (HAIS). American data indicate that one in twenty-five hospital patients on any day acquires such an infection. An estimated 722,000 HAIS occurred in acute-care hospitals in 2011, while about 75,000 hospital patients with HAIS died.[40] National Health Service data show that about 300,000 patients develop an infection each year in England while being treated.[41]

Canadian data are no better. The Canadian Nosocomial Infection Surveillance Program, while admitting the poor collection of data, estimates that roughly 10.5 per cent of hospital admissions result in an HAI, or 330,000 patients each year, with an estimated 12,000–18,000 deaths. HAIS are thus the third leading cause of death, after cancer and heart disease.[42] Should we be surprised that rates are higher with crowding and cutbacks in cleaning?

Another Canadian study shows lower estimates, with the conclusion that half the infections could be prevented by proper hand hygiene.[43] A detailed report on hand-hygiene practices in Canada and internationally notes that Canadian hospitals seeking accreditation since 2009 have been required to audit compliance by doctors and nurses, and to correct practice if inadequate.[44]

Pathogens resistant to antibiotics are on the rise and threaten to become worse. Nightingale, from the period before the discovery of antibiotics, has been a positive source for administrators and medical specialists on preventive measures. As an antibiotic-resistant era threatens, prevention becomes even more essential.

Nightingale was a pioneer in advising frequent handwashing for nurses. It features in her *Notes on Nursing* (1860): "Every nurse ought to be careful to wash her hands very frequently during the day."[45] How to do so received several paragraphs. Further details as to antiseptic solutions and particular procedures appear in later advice, notably in her Quain's *Dictionary* article,[46] but the basics were there as early as 1860. An American surgeon, Atul Gawande, as we saw in chapter 2, gave her too much credit for bringing down the death rates in the Crimean War hospitals, but he was fully justified in citing her on handwashing. Reviewing deaths in his own unit, Gawande concluded: "Proper hand hygiene is the primary method for reducing infections."[47]

Nightingale also understood the challenge of convincing medical doctors, notably surgeons, to use washable clothing, instead of the conventional business suits of professional men. She advised further that hospitals should assume the responsibility of washing surgical garments for both doctors and nurses.

Her enormous contribution to reducing hospital death rates would continue to be cited after her own active career. During the Spanish–American War of 1898, US soldiers died in large numbers from the unsanitary conditions of camps and hospitals, reminiscent of Crimea. They died also in large numbers at Chickamauga, a staging ground in Tennessee for troops before invading Cuba, and then later in Montauk, Long Island, where the sick and wounded were sent to recover: "Forty years after Florence Nightingale's achievement in the Crimean War, we ought to feel ashamed of the conditions at Chickamauga and Montauk. A typhoid epidemic should disgrace any civilized community."[48]

Nightingale Principles on Funding and Avoiding Waste

Misused and wasted resources pose another vexatious challenge in health care today. Nightingale wanted careful spending on health care. Hospitals should be adequately funded, but managers had a duty to ensure value for money. Hospitals should be large enough to benefit from economies of scale in ordering supplies, but not so large as to risk errors from administrative complications.

A national health service was well beyond her view, although her principles and years of effort led in that direction. Now that many countries have national systems for medical care, hospitals, and pharmaceuticals, the potential for waste is enormous. Wastage in private systems, of course, tends to be higher, as the profit motive is well known to encourage unnecessary tests and surgery. While, in Britain, 10–15 per cent of medical and surgical treatments offer little or no benefit, or do more harm than good, in the very privatized United States, the figure goes up to an estimated 40 per cent.[49]

A study conducted by the Academy of Medical Royal Colleges found enormous over-prescribing and over-use of X-rays and drug "cocktails" – practices that result in longer hospital stays, waste resources, and increase risk to patients' health. An estimated 6 per cent of all English hospital admissions and 4 per cent of all hospital beds were required to deal with over-drugging.[50]

Might Nightingale's core principles help us now to address the great health-care problems of our day? How would she select the subject of her next campaign? Presumably she would consult the numbers, as she did after Crimea. We should then ask what are the major causes of preventable mortality, and determine for which ones we can make a difference.

The World Health Organization publishes estimates of the top ten mortality "risk factors," for the whole world, and separately for low-, middle-, and high-income countries. The order of risks varies greatly by income level. For low-income countries (US$825 or less per year), childhood underweight tops the list, and for high-income (US$10,066 or more), tobacco use. The categories "unsafe water, sanitation, and hygiene" and "indoor air smoke from solid fuels" (cooking with wood or dung) were significant for low-income countries, but off the list for the wealthiest.[51] The above estimates were for 2004.

The health consequences of global warming are now on the agenda, with documentation of sickness and death caused by climate change (floods and fires) and air pollution from burning fossil fuels. Health practitioners are urged to be "at the centre of climate change strategies," giving leadership, as they did in the past.[52]

According to the chair of the Intergovernmental Panel on Climate Change (IPCC), Dr R.K. Pachauri, "Climate change appears to be more rapid, more serious and more dangerous than was thought even several years ago. It looks increasingly likely that the worst-case scenarios projected by the [IPCC's] Fourth Report in 2007 will be realized. Even worse, as is suggested by the rapid melting of ice at the poles, there is increasing risk that many of the trends will accelerate, leading to abrupt or irreversible climatic shifts."[53]

The World Health Organization has begun to re-examine its data to take into account air pollution, mainly from burning of fossil fuels. In 2014, it published estimates of 7 million premature deaths a year worldwide from this cause,[54] a figure rivalling tobacco smoke as a cause of preventable mortality.

Nightingale took on the major challenges of her day: care for the poorest and famine relief and prevention. She worked with the leading progressive doctors, and they made great strides, even on the toughest issues. From the disastrous Crimean War she learned that good can come out of evil, not in any simplistic way, and with no guarantee that the best expertise and concerted effort will work – but the potential for change for the better was there. It is a good philosophy still now for the great health challenges from global warming and the injustices of our world. Her method, policy savvy, and activism are needed at least as much today for the challenges our world faces.

The Effect of the Coronavirus Pandemic

The usefulness of Nightingale's principles for disease prevention, such as frequent handwashing and ventilation, was noted in the Introduction. So also was her pioneering work (with William Farr) on presenting data effectively. With the COVID-19 pandemic, people have become accustomed to seeing charts, with upward or downward curves showing infections, hospitalizations, and deaths, and then vaccination rates for first, second, and subsequent doses.

As I conclude this work, another notable contribution of Nightingale's merits mention: the establishment of a public-health infrastructure. She, with doctors, promoted the adoption of and amendments to Britain's laws on public health in favour of increased powers for inspection of houses and stronger requirements on sewers and drains, for clean water.[55]

She also promoted public-health measures in India. One of the first acts of Sir John Lawrence, on his installation as viceroy in 1864, was to appoint sanitary committees for Bombay, Calcutta, and Madras. He reported this in his first letter to Nightingale after his arrival. He noted that the committees were composed of five members, a civilian at the head, and the medical officer of health as secretary.[56] Nightingale would be in frequent touch with these medical officers of health.

In the COVID-19 pandemic of 2020+, countries with an established public-health infrastructure have done better in combatting infections and minimizing death rates. In them, access to vaccination has been based largely on need, not ability to pay, so that residents of long-term care facilities, health-care and other essential workers, and the elderly preceded even the wealthy and powerful. Housing plays a role here, of course, so that those in more crowded areas, with greater density per dwelling, had higher death rates than those with more space, another issue Nightingale raised as early as 1860.

The distribution of vaccines among countries remains on the basis of what-you-can-pay-for rather than need. The World Health Organization, and numerous public-health experts, warn that no one will be safe while large numbers of people (billions as this is written) remain unvaccinated. Nightingale was a pioneer in making those links between environmental and social conditions and outcomes. The viruses will change, but the broad principles of how to meet new challenges remain.

A final note on recognition – or not – of Nightingale's closest "medical men": Drs John Sutherland and William Farr. Neither was ever given a knighthood or other honour such as a C.B., while Drs Andrew Smith, director-general of the Army Medical Department, and John Hall, principal medical officer in the Crimea, were both knighted. Yet Nightingale and her medical men pursued their goals of saving lives and improving health care by analyzing data, and ignored the views of their seniors. Perhaps there is a lesson here, that it is essential to know what not to do and whose advice not to follow when embarking on reform. Nightingale indeed may have had this in mind when she gave as the title to her best-known book: *Notes on Nursing: What It Is and What It Is Not.*

NOTES

Letters in the notes not otherwise indicated are by Nightingale. For letters, the date and archive are given, plus the volume in the *Collected Works*. Estimated dates are indicated in square brackets, as are translations, brief editorial explanations, and biblical citations.

Abbreviations of Primary Sources

Add. Mss.	British Library Additional Manuscripts
BL, Asia	British Library Asia, Pacific and Africa Collections, London
Bodleian	Bodleian Library, University of Oxford
Boston	Boston University Archives
Cambridge	Cambridge University Archives
Claydon House	Claydon House, Middle Claydon, Buckinghamshire
Clendening	Clendening History of Medicine Library, Kansas University Medical Center, Kansas City
Columbia	Columbia University Presbyterian Hospital School of Nursing, New York
Edinburgh, LHB	Lothian Health Board, Edinburgh Edinburgh University Archives
LMA	London Metropolitan Archives, London
Osler Library	Osler Library of the History of Medicine, McGill University, Montreal
Radcliffe	Radcliffe College, Schlesinger Library, Boston
Toronto	Thomas Fisher Rare Books, University of Toronto
Wellcome	Wellcome Collection, London
Wellcome, RAMC	Wellcome Library, London, Royal Army Medical Corps Archives
Wiltshire	Wiltshire County Record Office, Trowbridge, Pembroke Collection
Woodward	Woodward Library, University of British Columbia

The Life and Times of Florence Nightingale

1 D.A.B. Young, "Florence Nightingale's Fever," *British Medical Journal* 311 (23–30 Dec. 1995): 697–700.
2 Farr letter, 16 Nov. 1858, Add. Mss. 43398 f92.
3 Nightingale, "Essay in Memoriam," Add. Mss. 45942 ff142–99, in 5:60.
4 "Is God in Our Social Life?" in *Suggestions for Thought*, vol. 2, in 11:510.
5 "What Would a Perfect God Create?" Vol. 1, in 11:217.
6 Letter, 8 Jan. [1852]. in Cook, *Life of Florence Nightingale*, 1:117.
7 Letter, 21 July 1870, Add. Mss. 45802 f149, in 8:230.
8 Letter, 30 July 1892, Hampshire Record Office, F/582/21, in 13:56.
9 Mackowiak, *Post-Mortem*.
10 *Times*, 22 Aug. 1860, 4A.
11 *Times*, 22 April 1872, 5B.
12 "Military and Naval Intelligence," *Times*, 6 April 1857, 5D.
13 "Neapolitan Exiles," *Times*, 20 April 1859, 6E.
14 "The Indian Famine Relief Fund," *Times*, 1 April 1861, 5F.
15 "Florence Nightingale Fund for the Relief of the Sick and Wounded and the Destitute Families of Polish Patriots," *Times*, 23 March 1863, 8A.
16 "The Wreck Register and Chart for 1864," *Times*, 26 Sept. 1865, 10.
17 "Advertisement for a ragged school," *Times*, 25 Jan. 1867, 8F.
18 "The British and Colonial Emigration Society," *Times*, 13 Jan. 1870, 7.
19 "The Distress in Paris," *Times*, 8 Feb. 1871, 11B.
20 "The Livingstone Expedition," *Times*, 31 Jan. 1872, 8B.
21 "Bosnia and Herzegovina," *Times*, 16 Nov. 1875, 7F.
22 Stopford Brooke letter, 20 Jan. 1878, Woodward, B38.
23 "*The Goliath*," *Times*, 12 Jan. 1876, 5E.
24 "The Atrocities in Bulgaria," *Times*, 18 Sept. 1876, 6.
25 "The Famine in India," *Times*, 17 Aug. 1877, 6E.
26 "Volunteer Ambulance," *Times*, 18 March 1878, 4F.
27 "The Prevailing Distress," *Times*, 30 Dec. 1878, 8D.
28 "Childhood without Toys," *Times*, 1 Jan. 1878, 9D.
29 "The Coffee Publichouse Association," *Times*, 27 March 1878, 11D.
30 "The Loss of the Princess Alice," *Times*, 19 Sept. 1878, 8C.
31 "London and Ascot Convalescent Hospital," *Times*, 30 June 1882, 13B.
32 "Building Fund for the New Hospital," *Times*, 6 March 1889, 1B.
33 "The Hurricane in the West Indies," *Times*, 20 Oct. 1898, 6C.
34 "The Proposed Memorial to Sidney Herbert," *Times*, 22 Oct. 1861, 12A.
35 "Frere Memorial Fund," *Times*, 7 July 1884, 8D.
36 Letter, 23 Jan. 1862, Add. Mss. 45790 f245, in 16:608.
37 Letter to Louisa Ashburton, 11 March 1861, National Library of Scotland, Acc. 11388/90, in 8:719.

38 "Building Fund for the New Hospital," *Times*, 6 March 1889, 1B.

39 "Hundred Thousand the Goal," *New York Times*, 21 April 1893, 9.

Chapter One

1 Hoyos, "How Would Florence Nightingale Have Tackled COVID-19?"

2 Allitt, "What Would Florence Nightingale Prescribe?"

3 Harford, "Florence Nightingale."

4 McDonald, "Nightingale and the Coronavirus Pandemic."

5 Letter, early 1880s, Add. Mss. 45824 f13.

6 Young, "Florence Nightingale's Fever."

7 Gill and Gill, "Nightingale in Scutari."

8 Letter, 13 June 1876, Wellcome, Ms. 9007/36.

9 Rothstein, *American Medical Schools*; Arikha, *Passions and Tempers*.

10 Thomas, "The Demise of Bloodletting."

11 List, 17 May 1855, Add. Mss. 43401 f61.

12 Letter, 24 Feb. 1879, Wellcome, Ms. 9007/182, in 15:855.

13 Letter to Mrs. Cox, 14 Sept. 1882, LMA, H1/ST/NC82/5/26.

14 Incomplete letter, c. 1888, Add. Mss. 68885 f72.

15 Fraser, *A History of English Public Health*; Hamlin, *Public Health and Social Justice*.

16 Hamlin and Sheard, "Revolutions in Public Health," 497.

17 Notes for Sidney Herbert, Wiltshire, 2057/F4/65, in 14:496.

18 Letter, 12 Dec. 1858, Wellcome, Ms. 5482/30.

19 Letter to Elizabeth Herbert, 11 Feb. 1858, Add. Mss. 43396 f57.

20 Goldman, *Science, Reform and Politics*, 189.

21 Chadwick letters, 19 and 29 Aug. 1871, Add. Mss. 45771 ff125 and 127, respectively.

22 Wyatt letter, 25 Nov. 1871, LMA, H1/ST/NC2/V29/71.

23 Wyatt letter, 13 March 1872, Add. Mss. 45786 f186.

24 Letter, 16 Dec. 1871, Wellcome Ms. 9005/110, in 6:549.

25 Letter, 16 Dec. 1871, Wellcome Ms. 9005/110, in :550.

26 Michael, "The Public Health Act, 1872"; (untitled), *Lancet* (28 Feb. 1874): 306; "Mr Stansfeld's Sanitary System." *Lancet* (23 Jan. 1875): 112–13.

27 Stansfeld letter, 4 April 1872, Woodward, c.5.

28 Letter, 15 March 1872, Wellcome, Ms. 9005/119.

29 Letter, 18 June 1874, Add. Mss. 45757 f246.

30 Skretkowicz, Introduction, in *Florence Nightingale's Notes on Nursing*, xxxiii–xxxviii.

31 Richards, *Samuel Gridley Howe*, 145.

32 Letter, 20 Aug. 1844, Claydon House, bundle 322.

33 Richards, *Julia Ward Howe*, 1:112–13.

34   Letter, 23 July 1845, in Richards, "Letters of Florence Nightingale," in 8:792–3.

35   Letter, 26 Dec. 1845, in ibid., in 8:794–8.

36   Letter, 7 June 1877, Add. Mss. 45804 f205, in 8:799.

37   Bowman letter, 3 March 1868, Add. Mss. 45800 f261.

38   Bowman letter, 15 June 1868, Add. Mss. 45801 f68.

39   Letter, 12 Oct. [1847], Columbia, C2.

40   Clark, "Introduction by the Editor," in Clark, ed., *The Management of Infancy*, xi.

41   Ibid., 206.

42   Letter, 20 Dec. 1856, National Library of Scotland, Ms. 7356.

43   Combe letter, 23 Dec. 1856, Add. Mss. 45796 f114.

44   Clark letter, 30 June [1861], Add. Mss. 45772 f164.

45   Letter, 25 Dec. 1858, Wellcome, Ms. 8997/83.

46   Letter, 23 Aug. 1856, Add. Mss. 45792 f40.

47   Letter, 5 Oct. 1858, Wellcome, RAMC, 1139/s4/5.

48   Letter, 16 July 1860, Wellcome, RAMC, 1139/s4/11.

49   Letter, 29 July 1863, Wellcome, RAMC, 1139/s4/22, in 9:232.

50   Letter, 25 July 1860, Wellcome, RAMC, 1139/s4/16, in 15:380.

51   "The Employment of Dr Sutherland," *Lancet* (24 June 1865): 683–5.

52   Cook, *Life of Florence Nightingale*, 2:344.

53   Sutherland letter, 16 July 1858, Add. Mss. 45793 f163, in 11:210–11.

54   McDonald, ed., *Florence Nightingale's Suggestions for Thought*, in 11:698–781.

55   S. Sutherland, letter, 30 Oct. 1887, Add. Mss. 52417 f101.

56   Woodham-Smith, *Florence Nightingale*, 584.

57   Letter, 25 Aug. 1856, Add. Mss. 45751 f1.

58   Letter, 22 July 1891, Times Newspaper Limited Archive.

59   Letter to J.J. Frederick, 22 July 1891, LMA, H1/ST/NC5/91/15, in 14:1037.

60   Herbert letter, 25 Nov. 1856, Add. Mss. 43393 f252.

61   Farr letter [23 July 1857], Add. Mss. 43398 f22.

62   Farr letter, 22 April 1858, Add. Mss. 43398 f53.

63   Farr letter, 10 Aug. 1858, Add. Mss. 43398 f72.

64   Nightingale, "Sanitary Statistics of Native Colonial Schools and Hospitals."

65   Farr letter, 1 Aug. 1857, Add. Mss. 43398 f24.

66   Farr letter, 11 Nov. 1857, Add. Mss. 43398 f37.

67   Farr letter, 21 May 1857, Add. Mss. 43398 f12.

68   Undated letter, Add. Mss. 43398 f13.

69   Farr letter, 17 June 1862, Add. Mss. 43399 f65.

70   Clode letter, 13 Jan. 1865, Add. Mss. 45799 f78.

71   Farr letter, 9 Jan. 1862, private collection, copy, Wellcome, Ms. 8033/3.

72   Farr letter, 17 July 1857, Add. Mss. 43398 f14.

73   Farr Letter, 25 Dec. 1857, Add. Mss. 43398 f40.

74 Farr letter, 23 Feb. 1858, Add. Mss. 43398 f44.
75 Farr letter, 25 Dec. 1857, Add. Mss. 43398 f40.
76 Letter, 29 April 1861, Add. Mss. 43399 f20.
77 Farr letter, 21 June 1861, Add. Mss. 43399 f29.
78 Farr letter, 19 Dec. 1864, Add. Mss. 43399 f235.
79 Letter, 16 Jan. 1871, private collection, copy, Add. Mss. 434000 f247, in
    8:231.
80 Letter, 14 May 1879, private collection, copy, Wellcome, Ms. 8033/17.
81 Letter, 23 March 1875, Wellcome, Ms. 5474/126.
82 Letter, 17 Oct. 1878, LMA, H1/ST/NC18/21/60.
83 Letter, 14 May 1879, private collection, copy, Wellcome, Ms. 8033/19.
84 Letter, 27 Oct. 1879, private collection, copy, Wellcome, Ms. 8033/17.
85 Letter, 30 Dec. 1879, Add. Mss. 50210 f134.
86 Letter, 3 May 1883, private collection, copy, Add. Mss. 43400 f281.
87 Letter, 25 June 1883, Farr Collection, British Library of Political and
    Economic Science, 1/78.
88 Eyler, *Victorian Social Medicine*.
89 Humphreys, *Vital Statistics*.
90 Graves, *A System of Clinical Medicine*, 60–4.
91 *British Medical Journal* (24 June 1865): 644.
92 Allen letter, 23 July 1867, Add. Mss. 45800 f127.
93 Dedication on *Notes on Hospitals*, School of Medicine, Mount Sinai, New York.
94 Letter, 26 May 1859, Wiltshire, 2057/F4/68.
95 Letter, 13 June 1874, Add. Mss. 47719 f40, in 13:726.
96 Letter, 17 March 1879, Add. Mss. 45805 f159, in 13:476.
97 Letter, 8 July 1880, Add. Mss. 47720 f100, in 13:166.
98 "On Different Systems of Hospital Nursing," in *Notes on Hospitals*, in 16:223.
99 Notes from a meeting with Dr. Toner, 8 Aug. 1881, Add. Mss. 47761 f22,
    in 13:513.
100 Letter, 17 March 1879, Add. Mss. 45805 f160, in 13:476.
101 Letter, 17 March 1879, Add. Mss. 45805 f159, in 13:476.
102 Nightingale, "Hospitals," in *Chambers's Encyclopaedia*, in 16:915.
103 Nightingale, "Sick Nursing and Health Nursing," 186, in 6:208.
104 Forbes, *Of Nature and Art*, advertisement.
105 Ibid., 11.
106 Ibid., 31.
107 Ibid., 244.
108 Ibid., 261.
109 Alfred Collinson letter, *Lancet* 69, no. 1754 (11 April 1857): 389–90.
110 Letter, 14 Feb. 1860, Add. Mss. 45751 f149, in 16:541.

111   Letter, 23 Feb. 1860, in Agnew, "Sir John Forbes and Miss Florence Nightingale," 41.

112   Baly and Mathew, "Nightingale, Florence," 910.

113   Armstrong, *The Gospel According to Woman*, 147.

114   Vicinus, *Independent Women*, 72.

115   Letter to Mme Mohl, 13 Dec. [1861], in Cook, *Life of Florence Nightingale*, 2:13–16.

116   Davies, "Making Sense of the Census," 595–6.

117   Kuhn and Wolpe, *Feminism and Materialism*, 114.

118   Iveson-Iveson, "A Legend in the Breaking."

119   Letter, 9 Oct. 1868, State Library of New South Wales, Sydney, in 13:420–1.

120   Letter, 27 March 1872, Staatsarchiv, Darmstadt, box 27, no. 14, in 13:455.

121   Nightingale Address 1, Florence Nightingale Museum, St Thomas' Hospital, Lambeth, London, 1.0725, in 12:766.

122   Nightingale Address 5, Florence Nightingale Museum, 1/0475.2, in 12:827.

123   Nightingale, "Sick Nursing and Health Nursing," 187, in 6:208.

124   Steven, "A Lecture on the Duties and Training," 332.

125   Singh and Ernst, *Trick or Treatment*, 133, and Speck, "Cholera."

126   Nightingale, "Trained Nurses for the Sick Poor," *Times*, 14 April 1876, 6CD.

127   Gairdner, *Public Health in Relation to Air and Water*, 92.

128   Review. "Notes on Hospitals," *Medical Times and Gazette* (30 Jan. 1864): 129–30.

129   Farr letter, 12 Feb. 1864, Add. Mss. 43399 f190.

130   W. Farr, "Miss Nightingale's 'Notes on Hospitals,'" *Medical Times and Gazette* (13 Feb. 1864): 186–7.

131   Farr, "Hospital Mortality," *Medical Times and Gazette* (27 Feb. 1864): 242.

132   "General Correspondence," *Medical Times and Gazette* (13 Feb. 1864): 188.

133   Murchison, "On the Isolation," *Medical Times and Gazette* (20 Feb. 1864): 210–11.

134   J. Bristowe, "Miss Nightingale on Hospitals." *Medical Times and Gazette* (20 Feb. 1864): 211.

135   *Medical Times and Gazette* (20 Feb. 1864): 211.

136   "Relative Mortality in Town and Country Hospitals." *Lancet* (27 Feb. 1864): 248 and 250.

137   Ibid., 250.

138   T. Holmes, "Mortality in Hospitals," *Lancet* (16 April 1864): 451.

139   W. Farr, "Mortality in Hospitals," *Lancet* (9 April 1864): 420–2.

140   Galton, *An Address on the General Principles*.

141   Nutting and Dock, *A History of Nursing*, 1:208.

142   Martin, "On Hospitals," in Holmes, *System of Surgery*, 3:962.

Chapter Two

1   Kirby, *Sir Andrew Smith*, 307.

2   Ibid., 311.

3   Copy of a letter, 1 Nov. 1856, Wellcome, Ms. 8997/10.

4   United Kingdom, *Second Report from the Select Committee on the Army before Sebastopol*, para. 14625.

5   Andrew Smith, *Medical and Surgical History*, 1:116.

6   Fred Smith, *Short History*, 11–14.

7   Nightingale, "Note on the Proportion of Attendants to Sick in Different Classes of Hospitals," in *Notes on Hospitals*, in 16:123.

8   Cyrus Hamlin, *My Life and Times*, 330.

9   Nightingale, *Notes on Matters Affecting* ... , 259, in 14:733.

10   Fenwick, ed., *Voice from the Ranks*, 57.

11   Ibid., 65.

12   Letter, 21 Feb. 1855, Add. Mss. 61991 f69, in 14:147.

13   Letter, 29 Dec. 1854, Leicestershire County Record Office, Raglan Collection, in 14:100–1.

14   "The Sick and Wounded Fund," *Times*, 8 Feb. 1855, 7E.

15   Soyer, *Soyer's Culinary Campaign*, 142.

16   Tyson, ed., *Letters from the Crimea*, letter 1.

17   Cook, *Life of Florence Nightingale*, 1:210.

18   Nightingale, *Notes on Matters Affecting* ... , 93, in 14:707.

19   United Kingdom, *Second Report*, evidence 19 March 1855, 1:362, para. 7523.

20   Letter, 12 Feb. 1856, in Hall letterbook, Wellcome.

21   Mitra, *Life and Letters of Sir John Hall*, 315.

22   "The Crimean Expedition," *Times*, 20 Sept. 1854, 7C.

23   "Professor Syme on Chloroform in Operations," *Times*, 12 Oct. 1854, 9A.

24   Myrtle Simpson, *Simpson the Obstetrician: A Biography*, 215.

25   *General Orders Issued to the Army of the East*, 77–8.

26   Nightingale, "Answers to Written Questions," No. 24.

27   Farr letter, July 1857, Add. Mss. 43398 f16.

28   Nightingale, *Notes on Matters Affecting* ... , 53, in 14:642–3.

29   United Kingdom, *Report of the Proceedings of the Sanitary Commissioners dispatched to the Seat of War in the East*.

30   Hall, *Observations on the Report of the Sanitary Commissioners*, 51.

31   Hinton, "Reporting the Crimean War."

32   Letter, 12 June 1857, LMA, H1/ST/NC3/SU85, in 14:513.

33   [Wheeler], "The Military Hospitals at Scutari," *Times*, 8 Dec. 1854, 8D.

34   "Miss Elizabeth Wheeler, one of the Nurses of the Scutari Hospital under Miss Nightingale," in United Kingdom, *Report upon the State of the Hospitals*

of the British Army in the Crimea and Scutari, 329–30; and "Miss Florence Nightingale," in ibid., 330–1, in 14:88–90.
35 Robert G. Richardson, *Nurse Sarah Anne: With Florence Nightingale at Scutari,* 176, endnote 27.
36 List, Wellcome, Ms. 8995/79.
37 Cumming letter, 22 Dec. 1854, Add. Mss. 43401 f23.
38 Frederick Robinson, *Diary of the Crimean War,* 314.
39 Reid, *Memories of the Crimean War,* 41.
40 Shepherd, *The Crimean Doctors,* 2:376–8.
41 Letter, 19 Jan. 1857, Wiltshire, 2057/F4/66, in 14:476.
42 Copy of letter, 1 Nov. 1856, Wellcome, Ms. 8997/10.
43 Sutherland letter, 12 Nov. 1856, Add. Mss. 45751 f3.
44 Letter to Herbert, 8 Sept. 1857, Wiltshire, 2057/F4/66, in 14:535.
45 Letter, 25 April 1857, Wiltshire 2057/F4/66, in 14:505.
46 Letter, 1 May 1857, Wiltshire 2057/F4/66, in 14:506.
47 Letter [April 1857], Add. Mss. 50134 f2, in 15:263.
48 Letter, 22 June 1857, Columbia, C33.
49 Letter, 15 July 1857, LMA, H1/ST/NC3/SU90, in 14:527.
50 United Kingdom, *Report upon … the Hospitals … in the Crimea and Scutari,* 99.
51 Longmore, *Sanitary Contrasts of the British and French Armies.*
52 Letter, 21 March 1863, Add. Mss. 43546 f29, in 15:387.
53 "M. Lévy on Hospitals," *Medical Times and Gazette* (19 April 1862): 407–9.
54 McDonald, "Biographical Sketches," on Sutherland in 6:674–6, on Rawlinson in 16:950–1.
55 Spriggs, "Hector Gavin."
56 Battiscombe, *Shaftesbury: A Biography,* 247.
57 Palmerston letter, 22 Feb. 1855, in Ashley, *Life and Correspondence,* 2:208–9.
58 United Kingdom, *Report of the Commission of Inquiry into the Supplies of the British Army,* hereafter *Supply Commission,* 1:9–10 and 2:39.
59 Letter to Sidney Herbert [5 Nov. 1855], Florence Nightingale Museum, 0858, in 14:257.
60 United Kingdom, *Supply Commission,* 2:23.
61 Ibid., 1:13.
62 Ibid., 2:37.
63 Tulloch, *The Crimean Commission and the Chelsea Board.*
64 Nightingale letter before 19 Jan. 1857, Add. Mss. 43394 f9, in 14:475–6.
65 United Kingdom, *Report of the Pathology of the Diseases of the Army in the East.*
66 Lyons letter, 11 Aug. 1861, Add. Mss. 45797 f252.
67 Lyons, *A Treatise on Fever;* Lyons letter, 16 Jan. 1861, Add. Mss. 45797 f160.

68 Koch, "The Etiology of Traumatic Infectious Diseases."

69 Small, *Florence Nightingale: Avenging Angel*, 126.

70 Royle, *Crimea*, 540, and Ponting, *Crimean War*, 199; for detailed refutations of his claims, see McDonald, "Florence Nightingale, Statistics and the Crimean War," "Statistics to Save Lives," and "Secondary Sources on Nightingale and the Crimean War," all in 14:32–40.

71 Small, *Florence Nightingale*, 185.

72 Letter, 3 Nov. 1858, Add. Mss. 50134 f54, in 14:568.

73 Soyer, *Soyer's Culinary Campaign*, 150.

74 www.uoguelph.ca/~cwfn/archival/index.htm <10 Oct. 2021>.

75 Robert G. Richardson, *Nurse Sarah Anne*, 176, endnote 29.

76 William N. Boog Watson, "An Edinburgh Surgeon – Patrick Heron Watson," 168.

77 Ibid., 169.

78 Ibid., 170.

79 Ibid., 171.

80 Letter, 30 March 1855, in United Kingdom, *Report upon … the Hospitals … in the Crimea and Scutari*, 449.

81 Luddy, *The Crimean Journals of the Sisters of Mercy*.

82 Chenu, *De la mortalité dans l'armée*, 131.

83 Letter [5 Nov. 1855], Florence Nightingale Museum, 0858, in 14:257.

84 Letter, 5 March 1856, Add. Mss. 43397 f96, in 14:349.

85 Letter, 10 Dec. 1860, Add. Mss. 45770 f211, in 14:1011–12.

86 Cyrus Hamlin, *My Life and Times*, 335.

87 Widmer, "Grandfather and Florence Nightingale," 571.

88 Nightingale, "Answers," Question 14.

89 Preface, *Notes on Matters Affecting …* , 7, in 14:584.

90 Nightingale, *Army Sanitary Administration*, in 15:348.

91 McDonald, "Florence Nightingale, Statistics and the Crimean War."

92 Kopf, "Florence Nightingale as Statistician," 389.

93 Cohen, *The Triumph of Numbers,* chap. 9.

94 Cohen, "Florence Nightingale," 132.

95 Richards, *Florence Nightingale*, 68.

96 Marshall, *Our Island Story*, 482.

97 Chung, "Florence Nightingale," 19.

98 Nightingale, *Notes on Matters Affecting …* , in 14:584, 857 and 859; regiments named at 315.

99 Woodham-Smith, *Florence Nightingale*, 258.

100 Winslow, "Florence Nightingale and Public Health Nursing," 330.

101 Ibid., 331.

102 Winkelstein, "Florence Nightingale," 311.

103 Dolan, *History of Nursing*, 216; first nine editions as Goodnow, *Outlines of Nursing History*.

104 Jacob, "The Evolution of Professional Nursing," in Cherry and Jacob, *Contemporary Nursing*, 8.

105 Hegge, "Nightingale's Environmental Theory"; Munro, "The 'Lady with the Lamp,'" 315; Shelly and Miller, *Values in Conflict*, 42–3; Maurer and Smith, *Community / Public Health Nursing Practice*, 162; Grypma, "Florence Nightingale's Changing Image?"

106 Lundy and Bender, "And Then There Was Nightingale," 80.

107 Hoffman, *Women Who Changed the World*, 64; Chung, "Florence Nightingale"; Purvis, *Women's History*, 2.

108 De Marco, *Performance-Based Medicine*, 74.

109 Gawande, "Notes of a Surgeon," 1285.

110 Goldie, ed., *"I Have Done My Duty."*

111 Letter, 10 Nov. 1855, LMA, HI/ST/NC1/55/6, in 14:265.

112 Robert Robinson, Narrative, Add. Mss. 45797 ff94–5.

113 Letter, 8 Oct. 1861, Wellcome, Ms. 8999/39, in 15:326.

114 Letter to family, 14 July 1856, Wellcome, Ms. 8996/74, in 1:143.

115 Letter, 8 April 1856, Convent of Mercy, Bermondsey, in 14:377.

116 Letter, 10 May 1856, Wellcome, Ms. 8996/55l, in 14:401–2.

117 Lind, *An Essay*.

118 Letter, 4 Jan. 1855, Add. Mss. 43393 f60, in 14:105.

119 Nightingale, *Notes on Matters Affecting* ... , Preface to Section I, in 14:594.

120 Ibid., in 14:596.

121 Ibid., in 14:597–8.

122 Porter, *Life in the Trenches*, 175.

123 United Kingdom, *Supply*, 1:15.

124 Pollock, "Florence Nightingale," 388.

125 Letter, March 1879, Add. Mss. 45750 f162, in 13:461–2.

126 Letter, 10 Feb. 1856, BL, RP 8997, in 14:331.

127 Letter, 10 Dec. 1854, BL, RP 8897, in 14:75.

128 Nightingale letter, 26 Feb. 1855, Wellcome, Ms. 8995/5, in 14:151.

129 Robert Robinson, Narrative, Add. Mss. 45797 f99.

130 Letter, 5 March 1856, Add. Mss. 43397 f96, in 14:349.

131 Letter, 7 June 1856, Add. Mss. 43397 f122, in 14:419.

132 Chenu, *Rapport au Conseil*, 647 and 695.

133 Letter, 7 June 1856, Add. Mss. 43397 f122, in 14:419.

134 Scrive, *Relation médico-chirurgicale*, 1:367–8.

135 Le Fort, "Guerres de Crimée et d'Amérique," in *Oeuvres*, 3:57.

136 Baudens, *On Military and Camp Hospitals*, 74.

137 R.H. Bakewell, "Notes on the Diseases," *Medical Times and Gazette* (3 Nov. 1855): 441–2.

138 Andrew Smith, *Medical and Surgical History*, 2:63–4.

139 Nightingale, "Notes on the Sufferings and Privations of the Army," in *Notes on Matters Affecting* … , 3, in 14:610.

140 Letter, 8 June 1861, Wiltshire, 2057/F4/69.

141 Reid, *Memories of the Crimean War*, 41.

142 Andrew Smith, *Medical and Surgical History*, 2:209.

143 United Kingdom, *Report of the Commissioners Appointed to Inquire into the Regulations Affecting the Sanitary Condition of the Army, the Organisation of Military Hospitals and the Treatment of the Sick and Wounded.*

144 Herbert letter, 20 Nov. 1856, Add. Mss. 43393 f258.

145 Herbert letter, 8 July 1857, Add. Mss. 43394 f100.

146 Letter, 7 July 1857, LMA, H1/ST/NC3/SU87, in 14:526.

147 Letter, 7 July 1857, Add. Mss. 43394 f95, in 14:524.

148 Letter, 7 July 1857, Add. Mss. 43397 f97, in 14:525.

149 Copy of a note, July 1857, Add. Mss. 43394 ff116–17.

150 Woodward, B64.

Chapter Three

1   Whitfield letter, 20 Feb. 1858, Add. Mss. 47742 f61.

2   South, *Facts Relating to Hospital Nurses*, 7.

3   Ibid., 24.

4   Peacock letter, 20 Aug. 1871, Add. Mss. 45802 f238.

5   Whitfield letters, 20 Feb. 1868 and 21 Sept. 1878, Add. Mss. 47742 ff209 and 220, respectively.

6   Letter, 21 May 1872, LMA, H1/ST/NC1/72/13, in 12:206.

7   Whitfield letter, 27 Oct. 1872, Add. Mss. 47742 f237.

8   Four British Library volumes, Add. Mss. 47738–41.

9   Reverby, *Ordered to Care*, 89.

10 Letter, 24 March 1873, Add. Mss. 47742 f245.

11 Croft, *Notes of Lectures at St. Thomas' Hospital.*

12 Letter, 24 March 1873, Add. Mss. 47742 f245, in 12:261.

13 Letter, 24 March 1873, Add. Mss. 47742 f245, in 12:259–60.

14 Letter, 17 March 1878, Add. Mss. 47742 f282, in 12:338.

15 Letter, c. May 1887, Add. Mss. 47738 f365, in 12:383.

16 Note, 3 Feb. 1890, Add. Mss. 45772 f09, in 12:431.

17 Letter, 26 Nov. 1892; Add. Mss. 47742 f16, in 12:450.

18 "Florence Nightingale's Last Will and Codicils," in 1:853.

19 Letter, 1 May 1873, Add. Mss. 47718 f173, in 13:504.

20 Note, 21 Feb. 1892, Add. Mss. 47761 f78.

21 Note, 21 April 1892, Add. Mss. 47764 f15.

22 Letter, 26 Dec. 1892, LMA, H1/ST/NC18/28/8.

23 Note, 21 Feb. 1892, Add. Mss. 47761 f76.

24 Crossland letter, 12 May 1893, Add. Mss. 47741 f22.

25 Haig Brown letter to Bonham Carter, 26 Aug. 1896, Add. Mss. 47727 f172.

26 Letter, 30 July 1892, Hampshire Record Office, F582/21.

27 Letter, 6 Dec. 1893, Wellcome, Ms. 9014/133.

28 Note, 29 Sept. 1892, Add. Mss. 47724 f146.

29 Simon, *Public Health Reports*, 2: 256.

30 Lowe letter, 6 Feb. 1864, Add. Mss. 45798 ff230–3.

31 Simon letter, 13 Nov. 1897, Add. Mss. 45815 f37.

32 Bristowe, *A Treatise on the Theory and Practice of Medicine*, 107–8.

33 Bristowe, "How Far Should Our Hospitals Be Training Schools for Nurses?"

34 Letter, 24 Sept. 1859, Add. Mss. 45797 f61, in 5:76–7.

35 Letter, 24 Sept. 1859, Add. Mss. 45797 f61.

36 Letter, late 1861–early 1862, Clendening, in 16:572.

37 Letter, 1 May 1861, Add. Mss. 45797 f200, in 5:90–1.

38 Letter, 23 April 1861, St Bartholomew's Hospital Archives, x102/2–3, in 13:62.

39 Letter, 10 May 1862, Clendening, in 10:574.

40 Letter, 21 Feb. 1863, Add. Mss. 45798 f93, in 16:577.

41 Letter, 18 Sept. 1869, Wellcome, Ms. 9003/118.

42 Letter, 26 June 1862, Wellcome, Ms. 9005/150, in 1:271.

43 Letter, 27 April 1874, Clendening, in 1:276.

44 Jowett letter, Dec. 1873, in Quinn and Prest, *"Dear Miss Nightingale"*, #320.

45 Letter, 13 June 1876, Wellcome, Ms. 9007/36.

46 Letter, 6 Aug. 1876, Wellcome, Ms. 9007/50.

47 J. Paget, *St. Bartholomew's Hospital and School*, 26–7.

48 J. Paget letter, 9 Jan. 1887, Add. Mss. 45808 f14.

49 S. Paget, *Memoirs and Letters*, 406.

50 Letter, 2 Dec. 1881, Clendening.

51 Bence Jones letter, 10 Aug. 1855, Add. Mss. 45808 f190.

52 Letter, 1 March 1856, Cambridge Add. 8456/I/161, in 6:233–4.

53 Bence Jones, "Report on the Accommodation in St. Pancras Workhouse," 465.

54 Letter, 29 Nov. 1871, Cambridge, Add. 8546/I/172.

55 Letter, 27 May 1872, Cambridge, Add. 8546/I/173, in 1:810.

56 Sieveking, *Training Institutions for Nurses and the Workhouses*.

57 Sieveking, "On the Importance of Supplying the Labouring Classes," 392, *Lancet* (1854): 391–2.

58 Sieveking letter, 31 Dec. 1864, Add. Mss. 45799 f67.

59 Twining, *Recollections of Workhouse Visiting*, 17–18.

60 F.B. Smith, *Florence Nightingale: Reputation and Power*, 169–70.

61 Sieveking letter, 31 Dec. 1864, Add. Mss. 45799 f169.

62 Rogers, *Joseph Rogers, M.D.*

63 Ruth Richardson, "Middlesex Hospital Outpatients Wing / Strand Union Workhouse."

64 Rogers, *Joseph Rogers, M.D.*, xv.

65 Barnes letter, 21 March 1866, Add. Mss. 45799 f252.

66 Gee letter to the chairman of the Workhouse Committee, Liverpool Workhouse Infirmary, 10 May 1866, Add. Mss. 45799 f250, in 6:273–3.

67 Ayers, *England's First State Hospitals*, 7.

68 Hart, *An Account of the Condition*.

69 Note [after 1 July 1865], Add. Mss. 45787 f61, in 6:337–8.

70 Letter, 16 Sept. 1874, Wellcome, 9006/234. in 6:557–8.

71 Letter c. 1867, Wellcome, Ms. 9002/167, in 6:433.

72 Letter, 18 Jan. 1867, Add. Mss. 45764 f10, in 16:730.

73 Anstie letter, 8 Oct. [1867], Add. Mss. 45790 f356.

74 Anstie letter, 8 Oct. [1867], Add. Mss. 45800 f152.

75 Letter, 14 Dec. 1867, Wellcome, Ms. 9002/194.

76 Letter, 30 Oct. 1866, Add. Mss. 45763 f234, in 6:358.

77 Nightingale, "Suggestions on the Subject of Providing," in 6:367–90.

78 Letter, 14 Nov. 1874, Royal Free Hospital Archives.

79 "The Hampstead Hospital," *Times*, 2 Nov. 1871, 11B.

80 Letter, 8 Nov. 1858, LMA, H1/ST/NC1/58/6.

81 Letter, 21 Oct. 1872, LMA, H1/ST/NC1/72/26, in 13:312.

82 Turner, *Story of a Great Hospital*.

83 Letter, 9 May 1873, LMA, H1/ST/NC1/73/2a, in 13:320.

84 Letter, 13 Jan. 1873, Add. Mss. 47717 f176.

85 Fasson letters in Add. Mss. 45803, Bonham Carter letters, in Add. Mss. 47718.

86 McDonald, "Alcohol and Opiates," in 13:318–38.

87 Bell, *Notes on Surgery for Nurses*.

88 Letter, 31 Aug. 1881, Add. Mss. 47734 f144.

89 Letter, 15 June 1882, Wellcome, 9009/50.

90 Undated draft, Add. Mss. 45806 f268.

91 Letter extract, 21 Aug. 1886, Edinburgh University, 104.

92 Letter extract, 7 Nov. 1886, Edinburgh University, 105.

93 Letter extract, 20 Dec. 1886, Edinburgh University, LHB1/111/8, in 13:366.

94 Ibid.

95 Letter, 28 Sept. 1859, St. Mary's Hospital, Paddington, Board of Governors Minute Book, in 16:523.

96 Farr letter, 19 Dec. 1864, Add. Mss. 43399 f235.

97 Note [beginning June 1875], Add. Mss. 47747 f32.

98   Letter, 14 June 1876, LMA, HI/ST/NC3/SUI80/29, in 13:109–10.

99   Letter, 17 June 1876, LMA, HI/ST/NC3/SUI80/76/32, in 13:111.

100 Letter, 19 Jan. 1877, LMA, HI/ST/NC3/SUI80/77/44, in 13:116.

101 Williams letter, 20 Oct. 1876, Add. Mss. 47747 f38.

102 Lorentzon and Brown, "Florence Nightingale as 'Mentor of Matrons,'" 279.

103 Sieveking letter, 19 May 1877, LMA, I/ST/NCI8/12/22.

104 Letter, 1 Jan. 1882, LMA, HI/ST/NCI/SUI80/82/94, in 13:131.

105 Letter, 20 July 1884, LMA, HI/ST/NC3/SUI80/107.

106 Letter, 21 Oct. 1884, Wellcome, Ms. 5483/39, in 13:133.

107 Letter, 21 Oct. 1884, LMA, HI/ST/NC3/SUI80, in 13:133–4.

108 Letter, 25 Oct. 1884, LMA, HI/ST/NCI/SUI80/84/117, in 13:135.

109 Letter, 25 Oct. 1884, Wellcome, Ms. 9010/37.

110 Letter, 1 Nov. 1884, Wellcome, Ms, 9010/41.

111 Letter, 1 Nov. 1884, LMA, HI/ST/NC3/SUI80/119, in 13:135.

112 Letter 6 November 1884, LMA, HI/ST/NC3/SUI80/121, in 13:135–7.

113 Williams letter, 10 Jan. 1885, Add. Mss. 47747 f114.

114 Williams letter, 17 Jan. 1885, Add. Mss. 47747 f117.

115 Williams letter, 24 Jan. 1885, Add. Mss. 47747 f119.

116 Letter, 25 Jan. 1885, with "Conversion of St. Paul" noted.

117 Letter, 19 Feb. 1885, Edinburgh University, f97, in 15:967.

118 Letter, 18 March 1885, Wellcome, Ms. 9010/66, in 16:476.

119 Minute book, LMA, A/NFC-2/1.

120 Note, Add. Mss. 47747 f136.

121 Williams letter [5 Nov, 1885], Add. Mss. 47747 f138.

122 Note 1885, LMA, HI/ST/NCI5/27.

123 "The Princess of Wales Branch of the National Aid Society," *Times*, 6 May 1885, 10D.

124 *Times*, 1 Sept. 1885, 5B.

125 Acland, *Memoir on the Cholera at Oxford in the Year 1854*.

126 Letter, 3 Dec. 1895, Bodleian, Acland d70 f183, in 13:222.

127 Letter, 26 June 1901, Add. Mss. 68889 f115.

128 Letter, 7 Nov. 1882, Bodleian, Acland d70 f106.

129 "The New Hospital for Women," *Times*, 9 July 1888, 4E.

130 "The General Medical Council," *Times*, 16 Feb. 1887, 4D.

131 Letter, 19 April 1876, 6:30 a.m., LMA, HI/ST/NCI/76/a, in 8:365.

132 Letter, 17 Dec. 1885, Bodleian, Acland d70 f16, in 10:739.

133 Letter, 30 Oct. 1866, Add. Mss. 45763 f234, in 6:357.

134 Letter, 31 March 1876, Bodleian, Acland d70 f51.

135 Letter, 3 Dec. 1895, Bodleian, Acland d70 f183, in 13:222.

136 Letter, 4 Dec. 1896, Add. Mss. 45814 f25, in 12:492.

137 Letter, 24 Jan. 1900, Bodleian, Acland d70 f189.

138 Letter, 2 Jan. 1865, Royal College of Physicians of London, 2415/1, in 16:707.
139 Letter, 29 May 1865, Royal College of Physicians of London, 2415/2.
140 McDonald, "Derby Infirmary," in 16:705–21.
141 Announcement, *Derby Mercury*, 19 Nov. 1869.
142 "The Nightingale Wing of the Derbyshire General Infirmary," *Derby Mercury*, 24 Nov. 1869.
143 Davico, ed., *Autobiography of Edward Jarvis*, 140.
144 Letter, 18 Sept. 1872, Yale University, Manuscripts, in 13:500–4.
145 Letter, 1 July 1873, Add. Mss. 47718 f121, in 13:505.
146 Letter, 1 May 1873, Add. Mss. 47718 f73, in 13:504.
147 Letter, 26 Feb. 1873, Add. Mss. 45803 f42.
148 Wylie, *Hospitals: Their History*, 45.
149 Letter, 6 Aug. 1881, Library of Congress, in 16:864, and notes 8 Aug. 1881, Add. Mss. 47761 ff21–2.
150 Notes from a meeting with Dr. Toner, 8 Aug. 1881, Add. Mss. 47761 f22.
151 "On the Occasion of the Opening for the Season of the Washington Training School for Nurses," *Toronto Globe*, 7 Nov. 1881, 9.
152 Letter, Oct. 1893, Add. Mss. 45812 ff27–50, in 13:525; Bonham Carter letters, 2 and 16 Sept. 1893, Add. Mss. 47725 f115 and f117, respectively.
153 Letter, Oct. 1893, Add. Mss. 45812 f37, in 13:526.
154 Worcester, *A New Way of Training*, 29.
155 Letter, 5 May 1895, Waltham Training School for Nurses Collection, Pkg #1 2/v/A; notes on a meeting, 9 May 1895, Add. Mss. 47761 ff82–3, in 13:517–18.
156 Notes, 9 May 1895, Add. Mss. 47761 f82.
157 Macleod letter, 10 Dec. 1897, Add. Mss. 45815 f48.
158 Lady Aberdeen letter, 13 Dec. 1897, Add. Mss. 45815 f51.
159 Pringle letter, 6 Aug. 1905, Add. Mss. 47736 f244.
160 Godden and Forsyth, "Defining Relationships and Limiting Power."
161 Roberts letter, 24 Jan. 1867, Add. Mss. 47757 f176.
162 Copy of Wardroper letter, 18 Oct. 1866, Add. Mss. 47729 f193.
163 Roberts letter, 23 May 1867, Add. Mss. 47757 f185.
164 Roberts letter [c. April 1868], Add. Mss. 47757 f229.
165 Letter, 14 July 1868, Add. Mss. 47757 f76.
166 Osburn letter, 14 July 1868, Add. Mss. 47757 f76.
167 McDonald, "Australian Hospitals," in 13:404–39; Godden, *Lucy Osburn: A Lady Displaced*.
168 Jenner letter, 4 July 1876, cited in Cook, *Life of Florence Nightingale*, 2:192.
169 "Legislative Assembly," *Australian Town and Country Journal*, 17 Sept. 1870.
170 Bonham Carter letter, 26 Oct. 1872, LMA, H1/ST/NC2/V50/72.
171 New South Wales, *Second Report of the Commission*.

172 Osburn letter, 11 July 1873, in MacDonnell, *Miss Nightingale's Young Ladies*, 84; "Public Charities Commission," *Sydney Morning Herald*, 19 Sept. 1873.

173 Windeyer letter, 4 July 1873, Add. Mss. 47757 f275.

174 Letter, 28 March 1874, Sydney University Archives, in 13:433–7.

175 "Near and Far," *Sydney Morning Herald*, 16 Oct. 1922.

176 "Public Charities Commission: First Report of the Commissioners." *Sydney Morning Herald*, 19 Sept. 1873.

177 Roberts letter, 8 Aug. 1873, Add. Mss. 47757 f279.

178 Osburn letter, 5 Sept. 1873, Add. Mss. 47757 f146.

179 Letter, 18 Sept. 1880, Add. Mss. 47757 f284.

180 Roberts letter, 24 July 1889, LMA, H1/ST/NC2/V45/89.

181 Letter, 29 July 1889, Wellcome, Ms. 9012/224.

182 Journal, Wellcome Ms. 9025.

183 Letter, 23 Jan. 1871, Wellcome, Ms. 9005/6.

184 Note from a meeting with Dr. Sutherland, 2 Dec. 1868, Add. Mss. 45753 f11, in 5:542.

185 Letter, 11 Oct. 1871, Wellcome, Ms. 9005/97.

186 Letter, 9 Oct. 1884, Johns Hopkins University Archives, in 9:922.

187 Note, April 1881, Add. Mss. 47763 f51, in 13:463.

188 Osburn letter, 24 Dec. 1885, Add. Mss. 47757 f148.

189 Husson, *Étude sur les hôpitaux*; Nightingale letter, 5 June 1864, Add. Mss. 45771 f42, in 16:616.

190 Letter, 15 Nov. 1865, Add. Mss. 45763 f196, in 16:444. Galton, *Report ... Descriptive of the Herbert Hospital at Woolwich.*

191 Letter, 23 July 1865, Boston, 2/20/13.

192 Letter, 23 June 1866, Add. Mss. 45763 f198.

193 "National Association of Social Science," *Times*, 15 and 16 Oct. 1858, 6EF and 7F, respectively.

194 Nightingale, *Army Sanitary Administration and Its Reform*, in 15:342–51.

195 "Sanitary Statistics of Native Colonial Schools and Hospitals," 556–8.

196 "Social Science Congress," *Times*, 13 Oct. 1863, 4BC.

197 "Aboriginal Races," *Adelaide Observer*, 21 Nov. 1863, 5.

198 Letter, 8 June 1881, Add. Mss. 45806 f157, in 13:664.

199 Letter of Emily Aston, 11 April 1890, Add. Mss. 45809 f318.

200 Dictated draft note, 3 Jan. 1890, Add. Mss. 47758 f198, in 13:176.

201 Bonham Carter letter, 29 Dec. [1893], Add. Mss. 47725 f164.

202 Letter, 27 Dec. 1893, Add. Mss. 47725 f154, in 13:182–3.

203 Letter, 29 Dec. 1893, Add. Mss. 45767 f10, in 13:184.

204 Letter, 31 Dec. 1893, Add. Mss. 47725 f166.

205 Letter, 30 Dec. 1893, Add. Mss. 47735 f171, in 16:930–1.

206 Letter, 3 Jan. [1894], Add. Mss. 47725 f175.

207 Goodall, "Nova et Vetera: Florence Nightingale and Nursing in Fever Hospitals," *British Medical Journal* (27 Oct,1928): 763.

208 Note, 7 March 1895, Add. Mss. 45813 f27, in 12:464.

209 McDonald, "Books on Nursing," in 12:27; Bradshaw, *The Nurse Apprentice*.

210 Cullingworth, *The Nurse's Companion*, 4.

211 Letter, 11 June 1892, LMA, HI/ST/NC1/92/8, in 8:403.

212 Note from a meeting with a nurse, 17 May 1892, Add. Mss. 47764 f27, in 12:444.

213 Crossland letter, 7 June 1892, Add. Mss. 47740 f219.

214 Masson letter, 2 Jan. 1890, Add. Mss. 47750 f5.

215 Letter, 7 Oct. 1886, Florence Nightingale International Foundation, Geneva, f98, in 10:758–9.

216 Letter extract, 20 Dec. 1886, Edinburgh University, LHB1/111/106, in 13:366.

217 Steven, "A Lecture on the Duties and Training," 337.

Chapter Four

1 Letter to Sir James Clark, 20 Feb. 1860, Wellcome, RAMC, 1139/54/7, in 15:374.

2 "The Late Thomas Alexander, C.B." *Lancet*, 27 Sept. 1862, 336.

3 Letter, 7 Oct. 1863, Wellcome, RAMC, 1139 S4/23.

4 Letter, 28 March 1857, LMA, HI/ST/NC3/SU76, in 14:501.

5 Letter, 16 Jan. 1857, Wiltshire, 2057/F4/66, in 16:245.

6 "Military and Naval Intelligence," *Times*, 27 March 1857, 10C.

7 Pincoffs letter, 22 Jan. 1857, Add. Mss. 45796 f130.

8 Letter, 2 Feb. 1857, Add. Mss. 45796 f134, in 14:478–81.

9 Letter, 24 Sept. 1861, Add. Mss. 45788 f127, in 15:597.

10 Letter, 22 Oct. 1862, Add. Mss. 45771 f14.

11 Nightingale, "Obituary: Dr. Sutherland." *Times*, 24 July 1891, 8D.

12 Letter, 21 July 1864, LMA, HI/ST/NC3/SU154, in 15:403–4.

13 Letter, 31 Aug. 1864, Wellcome, RAMC, 1139 LP/54, in 15:404.

14 Letter, 4 Oct. 1865, Wellcome, RAMC, 1139 LP54/10, in 15:412.

15 Wardroper letter, 26 Aug. 1880, Add. Mss. 45733 f104.

16 Note, 27 Aug. 1880, Wellcome, Ms. 9008/86.

17 Note, 20 Aug. 1880, Add. Mss. 47761 f23.

18 Notes from a meeting with Dr. Dugald Blair Brown, 23 May 1882, Add. Mss. 45827 f231, in 15:537–8.

19 Undated note to Dr. Sutherland, Add. Mss. 45753 f179.

20 Parkes letter, 4 Aug. 1860, Add. Mss. 45773 f9.

21 Farr letter, 9 Aug. 1860, LMA, HI/ST/NC3/SU197.

22 Parkes letters, 22 Dec. 1860 and 3 Jan. 1861, Add. Mss. 45773 ff15 and 20, respectively.

23 Parkes letter, 1 Dec. 1861, Add. Mss. 45773 f37.

24 Aitken letter, 9 April 1857, Add. Mss. 45773 f68.

25 Aitken letter, 30 Jan. 1861, Add. Mss. 45773 f144.

26 Add. Mss. 45773 ff1–63.

27 Letter, 17 March 1876, Add. Mss. 45786 f45.

28 Letter, 13 March 1876, Wellcome, RAMC, 1139 LP53/11.

29 Letters, 28 April, 12 and 20 July 1876, Bodleian, Acland d70 f93, in 15:513–16.

30 De Chaumont, *Lectures on State Medicine*.

31 Letter, 29 Jan. 1881, Bodleian, Acland d70 f97, in 15:530.

32 Letter, 1 March 1857, LMA, H1/ST/NC3/SU74, in 14:500.

33 Letter to Lord de Grey [Nov. 1869], Add. Mss. 43546 f134–6, in 15:484.

34 Farr letter, 16 May 1857, Add. Mss. 43398 f10.

35 Farr letter, 21 June 1857, Add. Mss. 43398 f13.

36 Letter, 28 July 1864, Add. Mss. 45762 f158.

37 Letter, 22 Aug. 1864, Add. Mss. 45762 f184.

38 Nightingale, *Notes on Matters Affecting ...* , 328.

39 Letter, 24 Dec. 1858, Add. Mss. 50134 f65, in 16:333.

40 Letter, 10 Sept. 1872, Add. Mss. 50134 f142.

41 Letter, 27 June 1873, Add. Mss. 50134 f47, in 16:462.

42 Letter, 5 May 1858, Columbia, C39, in 14:558.

43 Letter, 23 April 1858, Columbia, C38, in 16:263.

44 Sutherland letter, 22–23 March 1858, Add. Mss. 45751 f55.

45 Ibid.

46 McDonald, "The American Civil War," in 15:592–603; Wylie, *Hospitals: Their History*, 50.

47 Moten, *The Delafield Commission and the American Military Profession*.

48 Calkins, "Florence Nightingale: On Feeding an Army"; Hertzler, "Florence Nightingale's Influence on Civil War Nutrition."

49 Letter to Harriet Martineau, 24 Sept. 1861, Add. Mss. 45788 f127, in 15:597–8; Martineau was, as an abolitionist, a strong Union supporter.

50 Letter, 28 Sept. 1864, Wellcome, Ms. 5474/74, in 15:600.

51 Stillé, *History of the United States Sanitary Commission*, 27.

52 "Nightingale Association," *New York Times*, 14 April 1861, 1.

53 "Heroine of the War," *New York Times*, 1 Jan. 1883, 1.

54 Sutherland undated note, Add. Mss. 45751 f252.

55 Chappell and Pollard, *Letters of Mrs. Gaskell*, in 15:593.

56 De Grey letter, 17 Dec. 1861, Add. Mss. 45778 f8.

57 Exchange with Lord de Grey, Add. Mss. 45778 f7, in 15:531.

58 Letters, 18 and 19 Dec. 1861, Add. Mss. 45760 ff38 and 41, in 15:331–2.

59 Letter, 10 Jan. 1862, Add. Mss. 43546 f7, in 15:332–3.

60 Letter, 5 Feb. 1864, Add. Mss. 45777 f31.

61 Cuningham, *Cholera: What Can the State Do to Prevent It?*

62 Hathaway letter, 5 May [1864], Add. Mss. 45782 f148.

63 Letter, 15 Oct. 1889, Add. Mss. 45766 f273.

64 Letter, 26 Aug. 1887, Add. Mss. 45766 f31.

65 Letter, 3 Jan. 1888, Add. Mss. 45766 f59.

66 Letter, 5 May 1888, Add. Mss. 45766 f63.

67 Letter, 8 Feb. 1881, International Museum of Surgical Science, Chicago, M1957.395, in 10:173.

68 Letter, 23 Feb. 1885, Florence Nightingale Museum, 0543, in 15:970.

69 "The General Election," *Times*, 28 June 1886, 6A.

70 Letter, 24 June 1886, Boston, 1/8/109A.

71 Nightingale, letter to the editor, *Lancet* 96, no. 2464 (19 Nov. 1870): 725.

72 Private diary, Dollar, Scotland.

73 Boissier, "The Early Years of the Red Cross," 126.

74 Sutherland undated note, Add. Mss. 45751 f252.

75 Letter, 1 Nov. 1870, Wellcome, Ms. 9004/132, in 15:730.

76 Hutchinson, *Champions of Charity*, 350.

77 Undated Sutherland note, Add. Mss. 45751 f253.

78 Letter, late July–early August 1870, Reynolds Library, University of Alabama, Birmingham, 115, in 15:630.

79 Letter, 2 Aug. 1870, Wellcome, Ms. 9004/46, in 15:632.

80 Letter, 9 Sept. 1870, Woodward, A24, in 8:579.

81 Lister, "A Method of Antiseptic Treatment Applicable to Wounded Soldiers in the Present War," *British Medical Journal* 2 (3 Sept. 1870): 243–4.

82 McCallum, *Military Medicine*, 127.

83 Letter to Sir Harry Verney, 22 Sept. 1870, Wellcome, Ms. 9004/114, in 15:712–14.

84 Letter to Sir Harry Verney, 19 Sept. 1870, Wellcome, Ms. 9004/110, in 15:709.

85 Letter to Sir Harry Verney, 21 Oct. 1870, Wellcome, Ms. 9004/128, in 15:728.

86 Lees, "In a Fever Hospital before Metz" and "The Crown Princess's Lazareth for the Wounded."

87 Letter, 21 Oct. 1870, Wellcome, Ms. 9004/128, in 15:728–9.

88 Lees letter, 9 Oct. [1870], Add. Mss. 47756 f68.

89 Letter, 28 Nov. 1870, International Museum of Surgical Science, Chicago, M1957.346, in 15:749.

90 Letter, 24 Nov. 1870, Wellcome, Ms. 9004/152.

91 Verney letter, 24 Nov. 1870, Wellcome, Ms. 9004/154.

92 Notes c. May 1871, Add. Mss. 45825 f165, in 15:797.

93 "Florence Nightingale and Sir William MacCormac," *St. Thomas's Hospital Gazette* 45 (1947): 134.

94 Scotland and Heys, *Wars, Pestilence and the Surgeon's Blade*, 303.

95   Letter, 21 Oct. 1870, Wellcome, Ms. 9004/28, in 15:728.

96   Letter, 1 Nov. 1870, Wellcome, Ms. 9004/132, in 15:731.

97   Letter, 22 Sept. 1870, Wellcome, Ms. 9004/114, in 15:712.

98   Letter to Dr Hahn, 19 Nov. 1870, Wellcome, Ms. 9004/146, in 15:741.

99   Undated note, Add. Mss. 45836 f211.

100 "Miss Florence Nightingale on British Soldiers," *Times*, 25 Oct. 1895, 6B.

101 Letter, 12 Feb. 1881, Wellcome, Ms. 9008/122, in 15:860.

102 Letter, 6 June 1881, Add. Mss. 45765 f15, in 15:873.

103 Hawthorn letter, 6 Feb. 1882, Add. Mss. 45776 f31.

104 Letter, 25 Feb. 1882, Wellcome, 9009/15, in 15:875.

105 Letter, 23 Feb. 1882, Wellcome, Ms. 9009/15, in 15:876–7.

106 Letter, 14 Oct. 1882, LMA, H1/ST/NC1/82/34, in 15:938.

107 Letter, 13 Nov. [1882], quoted in Cook, *Life of Florence Nightingale*, 2:335–6.

108 Note c. Nov. 1882, Add. Mss. 45826 f125, in 15:942.

109 Letter, 23 Nov. 1882, Add. Mss. 45758 f162, in 15:945.

110 List of questions, 14 Dec. 1882, Add. Mss. 45826 f78, in 15:948.

111 Notes, Dec. 1882, Add. Mss. 45826 f86, in 15:950.

112 Note, 30 Oct. 1882, Add. Mss. 45827 f63.

113 Notes, 9 Oct. 1882, Add. Mss. 47763 f110, in 15:937.

114 Airy letter, 30 Oct. 1883, Add. Mss. 45775 f140.

115 Dedication, Aug. 1883, Add. Mss. 45807 f98.

116 Airy letter, 4 Aug. 1883, Add. Mss. 45775 f133.

117 Airy letter, 19 Aug. 1883, Add. Mss. 45775 f138.

118 Acland, "The Public Health in Egypt," *Times*, 11 May 1886, 5F.

119 Letter, 18 March 1885, Wellcome, Ms. 9010/66, in 16:476.

120 Letter, 26 Feb. 1885, LMA, H1/ST/NC3/SU180/146, in 15:972.

121 Williams letter, 18 May 1885, Add. Mss. 47747 f146.

122 Letter, 29 May 1885, LMA, H1/ST/NC3/SU180/162, in 15:992.

123 Letter, 16 June 1885, Wantage Papers, British Red Cross Archives, D/WAN/8/3/8, in 15:995.

124 Letter of Charlotte Munro, 4 June 1888, Add. Mss. 45808 f92.

125 Letter, 5 June 1888, Add. Mss. 45808 f98.

126 Letter, 13 Nov. 1893, Add. Mss. 45812 f55.

127 Letter, 13 Nov. 1893, Add. Mss. 45767 f100–1.

128 Hansard, *Parliamentary Debates*, 20 Nov. 1893, cols. 1281–2.

129 Letter, late July [1896], Add. Mss. 45767 f173, in 15:575.

130 Letter, 29 July 1896, Add. Mss. 45767 f172, in 15:575.

131 Letter, 1 Aug. 1896, Add. Mss. 45767 f175.

132 Note from a meeting, 27 Oct. 1896, Add. Mss. 47764 f152, in 15:576–7.

Chapter Five

1 "Paris 8th District Elysée–Saint Honoré," in *Paris Ouest, Sotheby's International Realty*, https://www.parisouest-sothebysrealty.com/en/estimating-area-paris-8th-elysee-saint-honore/ <16 Nov. 2021>.
2 Tenon, *Memoirs on Paris Hospitals*. Pringle, *Observations on the Diseases of the Army in Camp and Garrison*.
3 Letter, 23 June 1866, Add. Mss. 45763 f198.
4 Roberton, "On the Defects," 138–40.
5 Editorial, *Builder* 14, no. 711 (20 Sept. 1856): 509–11.
6 "Notes on the Sanitary Condition of Hospitals," in 16:63.
7 "An Unpublished Letter," in 16:517.
8 Roberton, "On the Need of Additional as Well as Improved Hospital Accommodation."
9 Letter, 7 Oct. 1861, Wellcome, Ms. 8999/37, in 16:627.
10 Dr. Combe, "Plan Proposed for the Hospital of a Regiment," *Builder* 18, no. 920 (22 Sept. 1860): 666–8, in 16:374.
11 Duns, *Memoir of Sir James Y. Simpson*, 145.
12 James Y. Simpson, "Effects of Hospitalism upon the Mortality of Limb-Amputations," *British Medical Journal* 1, no. 422 (30 Jan. 1869): 93–4.
13 "Sir James Simpson and the New Hospital, Edinburgh," *British Medical Journal* (16 Jan. 1869): 53–4.
14 James Y. Simpson, "On the Relative Danger to Life from Limb-Amputations," 393.
15 Letter, 7 Oct. 1869, Add. Mss. 45754 f11, in 16:703.
16 "The Rational Construction of Hospitals."
17 McDonald, "Workhouse Infirmaries, 1865–68," in 16:721–35; "St Marylebone Workhouse Infirmary," in 16:840–51; "Metropolitan Fever Hospitals," in 16:927–33.
18 Letter, 29 April 1860, Add. Mss. 45797 f198, in 16:589.
19 Letter, 7 Nov. 1864, LMA, H1/ST/NC5/3/22, in 16:675–8.
20 British Association, *Official Guide and Hand-book*, 74.
21 B.W. Richardson [B.W.R.], "Commentary on Hospital Mortality," *Medical Times and Gazette* (5 March 1864): 262–3.
22 Letter to Williams in acknowledgment, 21 May 1864, LMA, H1/ST/NC1/64/6, in 16:658.
23 Letter, 21 May 1864, LMA, H1/ST/NC1/64/6, in 16:658–9.
24 Taylor, *The Rebirth of the Norfolk and Norwich Hospital*, 10.
25 Letter, 20 April 1867, LMA, H1/ST/NC2/V16/67. Re Forbes and Barber and connection: "(365) Barber of Lamb Close House, baronets" (21 February 2019), in *Landed Families of Britain and Ireland*, https://landedfamilies.

blogspot.com/2019/02/365-barber-of-lamb-close-house-baronets.html
<15 Nov. 2021>.

26 Greenway, "Improved Hospital Construction," *Medical Times and Gazette*
    (24 Sept. 1870): 32.

27 Sutherland letter, 18 Oct. 1870, Add. Mss. 45755 f175.

28 Greenway, "On a New Mode of Hospital Construction," *British Medical
    Journal* (11 May 1872: 495–7.

29 Extracts from Greenway, 1872, Add. Mss. 45803 f13, in 16:749–50.

30 Greenway, "On a New Mode of Hospital Construction"; Nightingale's
    comments in Add. Mss. 45803 ff13–14.

31 Letter, 28 Nov. 1871, West Glamorgan Record Office, D/D xe 25, in 16:768.

32 Letter, 16 May 1874, Add. Mss. 45757 f240, in 16:772–3.

33 "Obituary, Charles Chadwick," *British Medical Journal* (11 Sept. 1886): 537.

34 "The Leeds New Infirmary," *Leeds Mercury*, 11 May 1869.

35 "British Medical Association," *Leeds Mercury*, 27 July 1869.

36 "British Medical Association," *Leeds Mercury*, 31 July 1869.

37 Parsons, *The General Infirmary at Leeds*, 12–13.

38 Letter, 2 Jan. 1865, Royal College of Physicians of London, 2415 1, in 16:709.

39 Letter, 13 June 1865, Royal College of Physicians of London, 2415 4,
    in 16:710.

40 Letter, 10 Nov. 1865, Royal College of Physicians of London, 2415/6,
    in 16:711–12.

41 Letter, 18 May 1866, Royal College of Physicians of London, 2415/7,
    in 16:714.

42 Leveaux, "The Correspondence between Dr. Ogle and Florence Nightingale," 67.

43 "Anniversary of the Derbyshire General Infirmary," *Derby Mercury*,
    17 Nov. 1869.

44 "Derby and Derbyshire Nursing and Sanitary Association," *Derby Mercury*,
    23 April 1870.

45 Osburn letter, 20 May 1868, Add. Mss. 47757 f73.

46 Osburn letter, 14 July 1868, Add. Mss. 47757 f76.

47 Roberts letter, 23 June 1867, Add. Mss. 47757 f199.

48 Notes [April 1867], Add. Mss. 47757 f184.

49 "Sydney Infirmary and Dispensary," *Empire*, 2 March 1868, 3.

50 "Summary," *Sydney Mail*, 22 Aug. 1868, 4.

51 Roberts letter, 4 Aug. 1879, Add. Mss. 47757 f281.

52 "New Sydney Infirmary and Dispensary," *Sydney Morning Herald*, 1 Aug. 1881.

53 Gregory letter, 21 Aug. 1874, Add. Mss. 45804 f14.

54 Machin letter, 25 Aug. 1874, Add. Mss. 47745 f33.

55 Letter, 4 Jan. 1875, Add. Mss. 45757 f261, in 16:804–5.

56 McDonald, note, in 16:805.

57 Cope, "John Shaw Billings, Florence Nightingale and the Johns Hopkins Hospital."

58 Billings letter, 23 Oct. 1876, Add. Mss. 45804 f169.

59 Billings letter, 4 Dec. 1876, Add. Mss. 45804 f173, in 16:819–22.

60 Letter to Henry Bonham Carter, 1895, in LMA, HI/ST/NC18/11/95.

61 Wagenaar, ed., *The Architecture of Hospitals*, 30.

62 Notes by Nightingale and Sutherland, c. Dec. 1868, Add. Mss. 45753 f150, in 16:750–2.

63 Note, Add. Mss. 45753 f153.

64 Letter to Emily Verney, 11 Oct. 1871, Wellcome, Ms. 9005/97.

65 Lees letter, 26 Jan. [1879], Add. Mss. 47756 f323.

66 "Construction of Hospitals: Wards," *Builder* 16, no. 816 (25 Sept. 1858): 641–3.

67 Letter, 4 Jan. 1875, Add. Mss. 45757 f261, in 16:804.

68 Letter, 26 Aug. 1874, Toronto, in 16:810.

69 Letter, 8 May 1875, University of Toronto Archives.

70 Letter, 5 April 1876, University of Toronto Archives, in 13:536.

71 Bensley, "The Hospital That Never Was."

72 Letter, 20 June 1888, Add. Mss. 45766 f98, in 16:885–6.

73 Letter, 8 July 1888, Add. Mss. 45777 f102, in 16:886–7.

74 Letter, c. 1888, Add. Mss. 45808 f140, in 16:890.

75 "The New Hospital for Women," *Times*, 9 July 1888, 4E.

76 BBC *Online News*, "Nurses Ditch Florence Nightingale Image," 27 April 1999.

Chapter Six

1 McDonald, "Establishment of the Training School for Midwifery Nurses," in 8:153–247.

2 Nuland, *The Doctors' Plague: Germs, Childbed Fever, and the Strange Story of Ignác Semmelweis*, 81.

3 Rigby, *A System of Midwifery*, 458.

4 Holmes, *Puerperal Fever as a Private Pestilence*.

5 Jones letter, 17 May 1861, Add. Mss. 47743 f105; Bowman letter, 3 Jan. 1861, Add. Mss. 45797 f152.

6 Letter, 14 Oct. 1867, LMA, HI/ST/NC1/67/7, in 8:178.

7 Jones letter, 10 June 1863, Add. Mss. 47743 f194.

8 Jones letter, 11 Jan. 1867, Add. Mss. 47744 f99.

9 Jones letter, 18 June 1867, Add. Mss. 47744 f123.

10 Jones letter, 23 June 1867, Add. Mss. 47744 f125, in 8:194.

11 Letter, 1 Aug. 1867, Add. Mss. 47744 f132.

12 Letter, 3 March 1868, Wellcome, Ms. 5474/116, in 8:202.

13 Note [17 June 1867], Add. Mss. 45752 f184, in 8:194.

14 Letter, 2 Dec. 1867, Add. Mss. 47715 f128, in 8:197.

15 Letter, 16 Jan. 1868, Add. Mss. 47715 f153.

16 "The Nightingale Memorial and Lying-in Hospitals," *Medical Times and Gazette* (1 Feb. 1868): 121.

17 Letter, 9 Feb. 1872, LMA, H1/ST/NC1/72/2, in 8:344–5.

18 Gordon, *A Treatise on the Epidemic Puerperal Fever of Aberdeen*. See also Ian M. Gould, "Alexander Gordon, Puerperal Sepsis and Modern Theories of Infection Control – Semmelweis in Perspective." *Lancet: Infectious Diseases* 10, no. 4 (April 2010): 275–8.

19 McCrae, *Simpson*, 197–9.

20 Semmelweis, "Höchst wichtige Erfahrungen," with English translation.

21 Semmelweis, *Die Aetiologie*.

22 McCrae, *Simpsone*, 196.

23 Arneth, "Evidence of Puerperal Fever"; "Note sur le moyen proposé … par M Semmelweis"; and *Über geburtshilfliche Praxis*.

24 Routh, "On the Causes of the Endemic Puerperal Fever of Vienna," 35–6.

25 Ibid., 39.

26 Simon, "An Introductory Report," xxxix.

27 Editorial Board, "Continuation of the Findings."

28 Le Fort, *Des maternités*, v and vi.

29 Letter, 19 June 1866, Wellcome, Ms. 5474/101, in 8:171.

30 Letter, 7 Aug. 1869, Welcome, Ms. 5474/118, in 8:221–2.

31 Letter, 9 Aug. 1869, Add. Mss. 43400 f236.

32 James Y. Simpson letter, c. 20 June 1869, Add. Mss. 45802 f152, in 8:219.

33 Ibid., in 8:220.

34 Letter, 21 July 1870, Add. Mss. 45802 f149, in 8:230.

35 Letter, 25 March 1869, Add. Mss. 45801 f210, in 8:213.

36 Farr letters, 3 Feb. and 16 Oct. 1871, Add. Mss. 43400 ff252 and 261, respectively.

37 Inscribed book, Boston.

38 Dedication, 10 Oct. 1871, Add. Mss. 45802 f253.

39 *British Medical Journal* (11 Nov. 1871): 559; *Lancet* (4 Nov. 1871): 640–1.

40 McDonald, "Response to Introductory Notes on Lying-in Institutions," in 8:332.

41 Letter, 11 Dec. 1871, Add. Mss. 43400 f270, in 8:340.

42 Letter, 28 Nov. 1871, Boston, 1/5/61, in 8:331.

43 Braxton Hicks, "The Education of Women in Midwifery," *Medical Times and Gazette* (25 Nov. 1871): 659.

44 Letter, 23 Jan. 1872, LMA, H1/ST/NC1/72/1, in 8:343.

45 Draft letter, 6 Dec. 1871, Add. Mss. 45802 f259, in 8:339.

46 Hicks letter, 30 Jan. 1872, LMA, H1/ST/NC2/V2/72.

47 Sutherland note, c. 18 Nov. 1871, Add. Mss. 45756 ff62–3.

48 Letter, 13 July 1879, Add. Mss. 47720 f42, in 6:474. Æneas Munro, *Deaths in Childbed and Our Lying-in Institutions, together with a Proposal for Establishing a Model Maternity Institution for Affording Clinical Instruction and for Training Nurses* (London: Smith, Elder, and Co, 1879).

49 Letter, 13 March 1875, Add. Mss. 45757 f382, in 8:371.

50 Letter, 24 June 1876, LMA, H1/ST/NC1/28, in 8:374.

51 Letter, 10 May 1876, Royal College of Obstetrics and Gynecology, in 8:372–3.

52 Playfair, "Introduction to a Discussion on the Prevention of Puerperal Fever," *British Medical Journal* (1887): 1034–56.

53 Boxall, *The Uses of Antiseptics in Midwifery*.

54 Blackwell, *Pioneer Work in Opening the Medical Profession to Women*, 65–6.

55 On Blackwell, see Boyd, *The Excellent Doctor Blackwell*; Fancourt, *They Dared to be Doctors*; and McDonald, "(Dr) Elizabeth Blackwell," in 8:1035–7.

56 Blackwell, *Pioneer Work*, 184–5.

57 Letter c. 1851, Wellcome, Ms. 8993/55, in 1:311.

58 Blackwell, *Pioneer Work*, 176.

59 Letter 8 May [1851], Wellcome, Ms. 8993/42.

60 Blackwell, *Pioneer Work*, 186.

61 Visitors book, St Bartholomew's Hospital Archives, London.

62 Blackwell letter, 27 March [1854], Claydon House, bundle 370, in 8:22–3.

63 "Necrology," *Journal of the American Medical Association* (Dec. 1883): 659.

64 Letter, 12 May 1856, Radcliffe, Blackwell Family Collection, box 5:70, in 8:24.

65 Note [c. 1858], Add. Mss. 45797 f53, in 8:25.

66 Letters 10 and 13 Feb. 1859, Library of Congress, in 8:27–8.

67 Letter, 9 Jan. 1858, Wiltshire, 2057/F4/67.

68 Letter, 10 Jan. 1859, Add. Mss. 43395 f122.

69 Letter, 25 Feb. 1859, Wellcome, Ms. 5474/5.

70 "A Lady Physician," *Times*, 16 March 1859, 9E, reprinted in *Sydney Morning Herald*, 10 Aug. 1859.

71 Boyd, *The Excellent Doctor Blackwell*, 177.

72 Letter, 10 Feb. 1859, Library of Congress, in 8:25–7.

73 Letter, 7 March 1859, Library of Congress, in 8:28–9.

74 Letter, 13 Nov. 1854, cited in Boyd, *The Excellent Doctor Blackwell*, 159.

75 Letter, 25 April 1860, cited in ibid., 185.

76 McDonald, "The Regulation of Prostitution by the Contagious Diseases Acts," in 8:411–509.

77 Letter, 1 Feb. 1870, Library of Congress, in 8:472–3.

78 Letter, 7 Feb. 1870, Library of Congress, in 8:473–4.

79 Blackwell, "How to Keep a Household in Health," cited in Boyd, *The Excellent Doctor Blackwell*, 237.

80 Blackwell letter, 3 May [1871], Add. Mss. 45802 f222, in 8:478–9.

81 Sutherland draft, after 3 May 1871, Add. Mss. 45755 f235l, Nightingale letter to Blackwell, 6 May 1871, Radcliffe, Blackwell Family Collection, box 5:70, in 8:480.

82 "The Social Science Congress," *Times*, 1 Oct. 1869, 7A.

83 Letter, 25 July [1871], Add. Mss. 45802 f237, in 8:30.

84 Notes, 27 June 1872, LMA, HI/ST/NCI/72/18.

85 Blackwell letter, 16 Feb. 1883, Add. Mss. 45807 f36.

86 Letter, 16 Feb. 1883, Add. Mss. 45807 f137, in 10:905.

87 Sutherland letter, 6 Jan. 1872, Add. Mss. 45756 f132, in 8:342–3.

88 Blackwell, "Medical Responsibility in Relation to the Contagious Diseases Act," in Blackwell, *Essays in Medical Sociology*, 1: 94–5.

89 Blackwell, "Rescue Work," in Blackwell, *Essays in Medical Sociology*, 1:123.

90 Ibid., 1:131.

91 Ibid., 2:48–54.

92 Garrett, "Hospital Nursing."

93 Letter, 20 May 1867, Wellcome, Ms. 5474/114, in 8:39.

94 Note, Add. Mss. 45818 f33.

95 Letter, 13 Oct. 1866, private collection, typed copy, Add. Mss. 43400 f111, in 8:31.

96 Farr letter, 19 Oct. 1866, Add. Mss. 43400 f125.

97 Letter, 13 April 1867, Wellcome, Ms. 9002/138, in 8:33–4.

98 Entry, 13 July 1881, Queen Victoria's Journal, Royal Archives, Windsor Castle, in 10:719.

99 Balfour and Young, *The Work of Medical Women in India*, chap. 3.

100 Letter, 23 Jan. 1885, BL, Asia, Pacific and Africa Collections, Mss. Eur F234/32/6, in 10:728–9.

101 Letter, 20 July 1883, BL, Asia, Pacific and Africa Collections, Mss. Eur F234/32/2, in 10:727.

102 Letters, 23 Jan. and 15 May 1885, BL, Asia, Pacific and Africa Collections, Mss. Eur F234/32/4 and /8, respectively, in 10:728–9.

103 Letter, 3 Dec. 1885, Florence Nightingale International Foundation, Geneva, f19, in 10:734.

104 Scharlieb, *Reminiscences*, 47–8, in 10:723.

105 Letter, 12 May 1887, Wellcome, Ms. 9001/63, in 1:380–1.

106 McDonald, "Child Marriage: The Rukhmabai Case," in 10:774–5.

107 Burton, "From Child Bride to 'Hindoo Lady.'"

108 Rukhmabai, "A Jubilee for the Women of India," *Times*, 9 April 1887, 8AB.

109 Letter, 8 May 1886, Wellcome, Ms. 9011/19.

110 Letter to Lady Wedderburn, 18 May 1886, Bodleian, Ms. Eng.C.3336.

111 Letter, 20 Feb. 1888, Add. Mss. 45808 f41.

112 Note, 20 Feb. 1888, Add. Mss. 45808 f41.
113 Jowett letter, 20 Feb. 1888, in Abbott, ed., *The Letters of Benjamin Jowett*, 119.
114 Kalapothake letter, 6 Aug. [1896], Add. Mss. 45812 f230).
115 Priestley, "On the Improved Hygienic Condition of Maternity Hospitals," *Lancet* 138, no. 3547 (22 Aug. 1891): 441–7. Lyell letter, 11 Nov. 1894, Add. Mss. 45812 f217.

Chapter Seven

1 Nightingale, "Nursing the Sick," 1046, in 12:745.
2 Memorandum, July 1878, LMA, HI/ST/NC18/1/8/1, in 12:753.
3 Crossland letter, 12 March 1878, Add. Mss. 47738 f99.
4 Crossland letter, 7 June 1892, Add. Mss. 47740 f219.
5 Nightingale, "Nursing the Sick," 1048, in 12:750.
6 Nightingale, "Nurses, Training of," 236, in 12:734.
7 Nightingale, "Nursing the Sick," 1043, in 12:735–6.
8 Nightingale, "Nursing the Sick," 1043, in 12:736.
9 Nightingale, "Nursing the Sick" (1894), 243, in 12:748.
10 Nightingale, "Nursing the Sick," 1048, in 12:748–9.
11 Nightingale, "Nurses, Training of," in 12:735.
12 Nightingale, "Nursing the Sick," in 12:751.
13 Public letter, 17 Oct. 1891, Add. Mss. 68887 f22, in 6:587.
14 Letter, 27 Dec. 1891, Chiddingstone Castle, letter 18.
15 Letter, 13 Oct. 1892, Clendening, in 6:592–3.
16 Letter, 31 Dec. 1891, Wellcome, Ms. 5473/9.
17 Letter, 27 Jan. 1892, Chiddingstone Castle, letter 19.
18 Letter, 2 Jan. 1892, Wellcome, Ms. 5473/2.
19 Letter, 16 April 1892, Boston, 2/2/9, in 13:882.
20 Letter, 25 June 1892, Wellcome, 5473/6, in 6:592.
21 Nightingale letter, 31 Dec. 1892, Wellcome, Ms. 5473/9.
22 Nightingale, "Rural Hygiene," in 6:607–21.
23 Letter, 10 Dec. 1890, Wellcome, Ms. 9013/124, in 12:438.
24 De'Ath, *Cholera*, 4.
25 Ibid., 3–5.
26 Ibid., 6.
27 Nightingale, in ibid., 17.
28 Nightingale, in ibid., 19.
29 Letter, 10 March 1895, Wellcome, Ms. 9015/32.
30 Sandwith letter, c. 1889, Add. Mss. 45809 f210.
31 C. Smith letter, 31 Dec. 1894, Add. Mss. 45812 f232.
32 C. Smith letter, 15 Jan. 1895, Add. Mss. 45812 f247.

33 "How to Prevent Blindness among Children: Suggestions for our Municipalities," *Review of Reviews* 10 (1894): 563.

34 Letter, 26 Feb. 1895, Wellcome, Ms. 5473/15, in 13:857.

35 Nightingale note, to Dr. De'Ath, Add. Mss. 45813 f29in 16:575.

36 Copy of a letter, 9 March 1895, Chiddingstone Castle, letter 22, in 13:58.

37 Letter, 9 March 1898, Wellcome, Ms. 9015/114.

38 Abel-Smith, *A History of the Nursing Profession*, chap. 5; Baly, *Nursing and Social Change*, chap. 12; Rafferty, *The Politics of Nursing Knowledge*; White, "Some Political Influences Surrounding the Nurses Registration Act."

39 McDonald, "State Registration of Nurses," in 12:515–74; Helmstadter, "Florence Nightingale's Opposition to State Registration."

40 Letter, 13 Feb. [1888], Wellcome, Ms. 9011/84.

41 "The British Nurses' Association," *Times*, 14 Feb. 1888, 10B.

42 Note, 24 Feb. 1888, Add. Mss. 47761 f30, in 12:523.

43 Fenwick letter, 11 Feb. 1888, Add. Mss. 45808 f33.

44 Invitation, 10 May [1888], Add. Mss. 45808 f74.

45 Letter [16 Feb. 1888], Add. Mss. 68885 f176–7, and Notes, Add. Mss. 47766 f184.

46 Note, 12 July 1889, Add. Mss. 47722 f18.

47 Note for Henry Bonham Carter, 12 July 1889, Add. Mss. 47722 f19.

48 Note on a meeting, 13 July 1889, Add. Mss. 47761 f73, in 12:532.

49 "British Nurses' Association," *Times*, 18 July 1889, 5D.

50 Letter, 20 April 1889, Add. Mss. 47721 f184.

51 Nightingale, "Royal British Nurses' Association," *Times*, 3 July 1893, 7C.

52 Rafferty, *The Politics of Nursing Knowledge*, 62.

53 Letter, 14 July 1889, Bodleian, Acland d70 f127, in 12:533.

54 "British Nurses' Association," *Times*, 18 July 1889, 5D.

55 Letter, 11 July 1889, LMA, H1/ST/NC2/V31/89.

56 Letter. 5 June 1891, LMA, H1/ST/NC8/91/7, in 12:545.

57 Letter, 30 April 1891, Add. Mss. 47755 f219.

58 Wainwright, "To the Editor of Times," *Times*, 22 May 1891, 12E.

59 Letter, *Times*, 27 May 1891, 13C.

60 Letter, 25 June 1891, LMA, H1/ST/NC1/91/8.

61 Nightingale, "Royal British Nurses' Association," *Times*, 3 July 1893, 7C.

62 Letter, 17 July 1893, Add. Mss. 47725 f56, in 12:564.

63 Letter, 22 July 1893, Add. Mss. 45786 f138.

64 Letter, 22 July 1893, LMA, H1/ST/NC1/93/6 93/6.

65 "British Nurses' Association," *Times*, 26 July 1893, 2F.

66 Acland letter, 15 April 1894, Add. Mss. 45786 f161.

67 Letter, 18 July 1893, Add. Mss. 47725 f68, in 12:565.

68 "Royal British Nurses' Association," *Times*, 8 Dec. 1894, 9F.

69 Note, 18 June 1895, Add. Mss. 47726 f179.
70 Letter, 24 July 1895, Wellcome, Ms. 5476/55.
71 Nutting and Dock, *A History of Nursing*, 3:48.
72 Abel-Smith, *A History of the Nursing Profession*, 76.
73 "Nurses and Doctors," *Berrow's Worcester Journal*, 10 Oct. 1896, 2.
74 "The Royal British Nurses' Association," *Times*, 23 July 1897, 8D.
75 "Charges against the Royal British Nurses' Association," *Daily News*, 14 Oct. 1897.
76 Baly, *Nursing and Social Change*, 154.
77 Lister, "On the Antiseptic Principle in the Practice of Surgery," *Lancet* (21 Sept. 1867): 353–6.
78 Letter, 18 July 1893, Add. Mss. 47725 468, in 12:565.
79 Cameron and Jones, "John Snow, the Broad Street Pump and Modern Epidemiology."
80 Cook, *Life of Florence Nightingale*, 2:344.
81 Letter to the chair, Poona Sarvajanik Sabha, Dec. 1891, in 10:363.
82 Letter, 25 Oct. 1892, from E.S. Shakespeare, Add. Mss. 45811 f176.
83 Nightingale, "Remarks of the Barrack and Hospital Improvement Commission on a Report by Dr. Leith," in 9:409–10.
84 Croft, *Notes of Lectures at St. Thomas' Hospital*, chap. XIX.
85 Letter to William R. Robertson, 31 March 1890, BL, Asia, Pacific and Africa Collections, Mss. Eur B263 f28, in 10:710.
86 Letter, 13 June 1893, Add. Mss. 45767 f66.
87 Wellcome Library, Rare Book Collection.
88 Nightingale note, 22 March 1897, Add. Mss. 47764 f64.
89 Franklin letter, 22 April 1897, Add. Mss. 45814 f165.
90 "Miss Florence Nightingale on the Cholera," *Huddersfield Daily Chronicle*, 11 Aug/ 1884, 3.
91 "A Medical Authority's Warning"; "Practical Advice in View"; "Miss Florence Nightingale on the Cholera."
92 "Cholera in Launceston," *Daily Telegraph*, 16 Oct. 1884, 3.
93 "The Cholera," *Times*, 2 Sept. 1892, 9D.
94 "A Medical Authority's Warning," *Dundee Courier & Argus*, 2 Sept. 1892; "More Good Advice," *Sheffield and Rotherham Independent*, 3 Sept. 1892, 6.
95 F.B. Smith, *Florence Nightingale: Reputation and Power*, 200.
96 Shannon, "An Icon and Her Intrigues."
97 Rosenberg, "Introduction."
98 Cantlie, *A History of the Army*, 2:212.
99 Wolstenholme, "Florence Nightingale, New Lamps for Old," 206.
100 Cannadine, *History in Our Time*, 204.
101 Ayliffe and English, *Hospital Infection from Miasmas to MRSA*, 81.

102 Halliday, "Commentary: Dr. John Sutherland."
103 Halliday, *The Great Filth*, 81.
104 Brighton, *Hell Riders*, 306.
105 Examples are Brown, Nolan, and Crawford, "Men in Nursing"; Cordery, "Another Victorian Legacy"; Helmstadter, "Doctors and Nurses," 179; Fealy, McNamara, and Geraghty, "The Health of Hospitals," 3468.

Chapter Eight

1   Census entries 1861–1901, in 12:43.
2   Osler, "Doctor and Nurse," in Osler, *Collected Essays*, 1:37.
3   Cushing, *The Life of Sir William Osler*, 1:133 and 1:703.
4   Machin letter, 16 Oct. 1875, Add. Mss. 47745 f63. On their difficulties, see Helmstadter, "Reforming Hospital Nursing."
5   Nightingale letter, 7 Nov. 1877, Add. Mss. 47745 f173, in 13:541–2.
6   Notes from a meeting, May 1883, Add. Mss. 47747 f241, in 12:373.
7   Osler, *Principles and Practice*, 30–3.
8   Osler, "Medicine in the Nineteenth Century," in Osler, *Collected Essays*, 3:253.
9   Osler, *Principles and Practice*, 33.
10 Ibid., 37.
11 Ibid., 39.
12 Alice Ruddock letter with thanks to Nightingale, 18 March [1897], Add. Mss. 45814 f127.
13 Osler, "Aequanimitas," in Osler, *Collected Essays*, 1:23–40.
14 Osler, "Medicine in the Nineteenth Century," in ibid., 3:238.
15 Ibid., 3:269.
16 Ibid., 3:270.
17 Osler, "Vocation in Medicine and Nursing," 126–7.
18 Osler, in Cushing, *Life of Sir William Osler*, 1:295.
19 See, for instance, Osler Library, Archive Collections, CUS 417.
20 James, "Isabel Hampton and the Professionalization of Nursing," in Baer, *Enduring Issues in American Nursing*, 49–50.
21 James, "Isabel Hampton Robb," in Baer, *Enduring Issues*, 58.
22 Hampton Robb letter, 20 Sept. [1894], Add. Mss. 45812 f189.
23 Hampton Robb letter, 4 Dec. [1896], Add. Mss. 45814 f30.
24 Draft letter [late Dec. 1896], Add. Mss. 45814 f32, in 13:515–16.
25 Letter, 11 Nov. 1916, Osler Library, CUS 417/122.43.
26 Doidge, *The Brain's Way of Healing*, 118; Otter, *The Victorian Eye: A Political History of Light and Vision in Britain*.
27 Cited in Mussey, *Health: Its Friends and Foes*, 46.
28 Brewster, "Researches on Light," 185.

29 R. Rawlinson, "Sanitary Progress," *Builder* 18, no. 900 (5 May 1860): 275–7.
30 Herbert letter, 26 June [1857], Add. Mss. 50134 f171.
31 Nightingale annotation of Quetelet, *Physique sociale*, at 2:184, repeated in her "Essay in Memoriam," in 5:53.
32 Letter, 3 Dec. 1849, Diary, Wellcome, Ms. 9018/8, in 4:169.
33 Nightingale, *Notes on Nursing*, chap. 9, in 12:645.
34 Nightingale, "Nursing the Sick," 1044, in 12:738.
35 Nightingale, "Notes on the Sanitary Construction of Hospitals," in 16:60.
36 Letter, 17 April 1862, Royal Institute of British Architects, in 16:630.
37 Nightingale, in 16:295–307.
38 Letter, 13 May 1874, in 16:13.
39 Letter, 15 Dec. 1885, RSAS, Lea Hurst.
40 Magill et al., "Multistate Point-Prevalence Survey."
41 "Hospital Infection Rates Must Come Down, Says Watchdog," BBC2 online, 17 April 2014 <15 Nov. 2021>.
42 Gindin, "Hospital Acquired Infections in Canada and How to Stop Them."
43 "Hospitals Face Hand-washing Crackdown," *Globe and Mail*, 20 May 2008, A1.
44 Canada, Public Health Agency, "Part B. Hand Hygiene Programs and Continuous Quality Improvement," in *Hand Hygiene Practices in Healthcare Settings*.
45 Nightingale, *Notes on Nursing*, chap. 11, in 12:652.
46 Nightingale, "Nursing the Sick," 1045–7, in 12:742–5.
47 Gawande, "Notes of a Surgeon: On Washing Hands."
48 "Sanitary Ignorance," *New York Times*, 5 Dec. 1898, 6.
49 André Picard, "When Health Care Becomes Unnecessary Care," *Globe and Mail*, 14 July 2015.
50 Denis Campbell, "NHS Wastes over £2.3B a year," *Guardian*, 6 Nov. 2014.
51 World Health Organization, Global Health Risks, Table 1.
52 Pachauri, Foreword, in Griffiths et al., eds, *The Health Practitioner's Guide*, xviii–xix.
53 Ibid.
54 World Health Organization, "Seven Million Premature Deaths."
55 Small, "Florence Nightingale's Public Health Act."
56 Lawrence letter, 5 Jan. 1864, Add. Mss. 45777 f31.

BIBLIOGRAPHY

Collected Works of Florence Nightingale

Nightingale's major works are listed in the bibliography under her name. For unpublished, or difficult-of-access published sources, I refer readers to the sixteen-volume *Collected Works of Florence Nightingale* (Waterloo, ON: Wilfrid Laurier University Press, 2001–12). I edited all the volumes except 4 and 9, which were edited by me (Lynn McDonald) and my wonderful late colleague Dr Gérard Vallée of McMaster University:

Volume 1: *Florence Nightingale: An Introduction to Her Life and Family* (2001)
Volume 2: *Florence Nightingale's Spiritual Journey* (2001)
Volume 3: *Florence Nightingale's Theology: Essays, Letters and Journal Notes* (2002)
Volume 4: *Florence Nightingale on Mysticism and Eastern Religions* (2003)
Volume 5: *Florence Nightingale on Society and Politics, Philosophy, Science, Education and*
Literature (2003)
Volume 6: *Florence Nightingale on Public Health Care* (2004)
Volume 7: *Florence Nightingale's European Travels* (2004)
Volume 8: *Florence Nightingale on Women, Medicine, Midwifery and Prostitution* (2008)
Volume 9: *Florence Nightingale on Health in India* (2006)
Volume 10: *Florence Nightingale on Social Change in India* (2007)
Volume 11: *Florence Nightingale's Suggestions for Thought* (2008)
Volume 12: *Florence Nightingale: The Nightingale School* (2009)
Volume 13: *Florence Nightingale: Extending Nursing* (2009)
Volume 14: *Florence Nightingale: The Crimean War* (2009)
Volume 15: *Florence Nightingale on Wars and the War Office* (2011)
Volume 16: *Florence Nightingale and Hospital Reform* (2012)

Manuscript Sources

Abbreviations, where used in notes, appear at end of entry in parentheses.

Bodleian Library, University of Oxford (Bodleian)
Boston University Archives (Boston)
British Library Additional Manuscripts (Add. Mss.)
British Library Asia, Pacific and Africa Collections, London (BL, Asia)
Cambridge University Archives (Cambridge)
Chiddingstone Castle, Kent
Claydon House, Middle Claydon, Buckinghamshire (Claydon House)
Clendening History of Medicine Library, Kansas University Medical Center, Kansas City (Clendening)
Columbia University Presbyterian Hospital School of Nursing, New York (Columbia)
Dollar, Scotland, Private diary
Edinburgh University Archives
Farr Collection, British Library of Political and Economic Science, London School of Economics and Political Science, London
Florence Nightingale International Foundation, Geneva
Hampshire Record Office, Winchester
Johns Hopkins University Archives, Baltimore
Library of Congress, Washington, DC
London Metropolitan Archives, London (LMA)
Lothian Health Board, Edinburgh (Edinburgh, LHB)
National Library of Scotland, Edinburgh
Osler Library of the History of Medicine, McGill University, Montreal (Osler Library)
Radcliffe College, Schlesinger Library, Boston (Radcliffe)
Royal Archives, Windsor Castle
Royal College of Obstetrics and Gynaecology, London
Royal Free Hospital Archives, London
Royal Surgical Aid Society (RSAS), Lea Hurst, Holloway, Derbyshire
St Bartholomew's Hospital Archives, London
School of Medicine, Mount Sinai, New York
Thomas Fisher Rare Books, University of Toronto (Toronto)
Times Newspaper Limited Archive, London
Waltham Training School for Nurses Collection, Howard Gotlieb Archival Research Center, Boston, Mass.
Wellcome Collection, London (Wellcome)

Wellcome Library, London, Royal Army Medical Corps Archives
   (Wellcome, RAMC)
West Glamorgan Record Office, Swansea
Wiltshire County Record Office, Trowbridge, Pembroke Collection (Wiltshire)
Woodward Library, University of British Columbia (Woodward)

Journals and Newspapers

Adelaide Observer
BBC *Online News*
Berrow's Worcester Journal
British Medical Journal
Builder
Daily News [London]
Daily Telegraph [London]
Derby Mercury
Dundee Courier & Argus
Empire [Sydney, NSW]
Globe and Mail [Toronto]
Guardian
Huddersfield Daily Chronicle
Journal of the American Medical Association
Lancet
Lancet: Infectious Diseases
Leeds Mercury
Medical Times and Gazette
New York Times
St. Thomas's Hospital Gazette
Sheffield and Rotherham Independent
Sydney Mail
Sydney Morning Herald
Times
Toronto Globe

Articles and Books

Abbott, Evelyn, ed. *Letters of Benjamin Jowett, M.A.* London: John Murray,
   1899.
Abel-Smith, Brian. *A History of the Nursing Profession.* London: Heinemann,
   1960.

Acland, Henry. *Memoir on the Cholera at Oxford in the Year 1854, with Considerations Suggested by the Epidemic.* London: John Churchill and J.H. & J. Parker, 1856.

Agnew, R.A.L. "Sir John Forbes (1787–1861) and Miss Florence Nightingale (1820–1910): An Unlikely Association?" *Vesalius* 7 (2001): 36–44.

Allitt, Marie. "What Would Florence Nightingale Prescribe to Fight Covid? Fresh Air." *Guardian*, 11 Feb. 2021.

Anderson, James Wallace. *Lectures on Medical Nursing.* Glasgow: Maclehose & Son, 1883 [1882].

Arikha, Noga. *Passions and Tempers: A History of the Humours.* New York: Harper Perennial, 2008.

Armstrong, Karen. *The Gospel According to Woman: Christianity's Creation of the Sex War in the West.* London: Elm Tree, 1986.

Arneth, F.H. "Evidence of Puerperal Fever Depending upon the Contagious Inoculation of Morbid Matter." *Monthly Journal of Medical Science* 12 (1851): 506–10.

– "Note sur le moyen proposé et employé par M. Semmelweis pour empêcher le développement des épidémies puerpérales dans l'hospice de la maternité de Vienne." *Annales d'hygiène publique et de médicine* 45 (1851): 281–90.

– *Über geburtshilfliche Praxis erläutert durch Ergebnisse der ii. Gebärklinik zu Wien und deren stele Verkleichung mit den statstischen Ausweisen der Anstalten zu Paris, Dublin, u.s.w.* Vienna: Wilhelm Braunhüller, 1851.

Ashley, Evelyn. *Life and Correspondence of Henry John Temple, Viscount Palmerston.* 2 vols. London: R. Bentley, 1879.

Ayers, Gwendoline M. *England's First State Hospitals and the Metropolitan Asylums Board 1867–1930.* London: Wellcome Institute of the History of Medicine, 1971.

Ayliffe, Graham A.J., and Mary P. English. *Hospital Infection from Miasmas to* MRSA. Cambridge: Cambridge University Press, 2003.

Baer, Ellen Davidson, et al., eds. *Enduring Issues in American Nursing.* New York: Springer, 2000.

Balfour, Margaret I., and Ruth Young. *The Work of Medical Women in India.* London: Oxford University Press, 1929.

Baly, Monica E. *Nursing and Social Change.* 2nd ed. London: Heinemann, 1980 [1973].

Baly, Monica E., and H.C.G. Matthew. "Nightingale, Florence (1820–1910)." *Oxford Dictionary of National Biography*, 40: 904–12. Oxford: Oxford University Press, 2004.

Battiscombe, Georgina. *Shaftesbury: A Biography of the Seventh Earl.* London: Constable, 1974.

Baudens, Luciens. *On Military and Camp Hospitals, and the Health of Troops in the Field. Being the results of a commission to inspect the sanitary arrangements of the French Army, and incidentally of other armies in the Crimean War.* Trans. Franklin B. Hough. London: Baillière. Paris: J.B. Baillière et fils, 1862.

Bell, Joseph. *Notes on Surgery for Nurses.* Edinburgh: Oliver & Boyd, 1887.

Bence Jones, Henry. "Report on the Accommodation in St Pancras Workhouse." *Accounts and Papers of the House of Commons* XLIX, 465 (1856).

Bensley, E.H. "The Hospital That Never Was." In *Pages of History.* Reprinted from *Dominion Illustrated,* 12 Jan. 1889.

Blackwell, Elizabeth. *Essays in Medical Sociology.* 2 vols. New York: Arno, 1972; reprint of 1902.

– *The Laws of Life, with Special Reference to the Physical Education of Girls.* New York: Putnam, 1852.

– *Pioneer Work in Opening the Medical Profession to Women: Biographical Sketches.* New York: Schocken Books, 1977 [1895].

Boissier, Pierre. "The Early Years of the Red Cross." *International Review of the Red Cross,* no. 24 (March 1963), 122–39.

Boxall, Robert. *The Uses of Antiseptics in Midwifery: Their Value and Practical Application.* London: H.K. Lewis, 1894.

Boyd, Julia. *The Excellent Doctor Blackwell: The Life of the First Woman Physician.* Stroud, England: Sutton, 2005.

Bradshaw, Ann. *The Nurse Apprentice, 1860–1977.* Aldershot, England: Ashgate, 2001.

Brewster, D. "Researches on Light." *North British Review* 29, no. 57 (Aug. 1858): 177–210.

Brighton, Terry. *Hell Riders: The Truth about the Charge of the Light Brigade.* London: Viking, 2004.

Bristowe, John Syer. "How Far Should Our Hospitals Be Training Schools for Nurses?" *Journal of the Hospitals Association* (1884): 26–35.

– "Letter from Dr. J.S. Bristowe." *Medical Times and Gazette* (20 Feb. 1864): 211.

– *A Treatise on the Theory and Practice of Medicine.* 3rd ed. London: Smith, Elder, 1880 [1867].

British Association for the Advancement of Science. *The Official Guide and Hand-Book to Swansea and its District.* Swansea: Gamwell, 1880.

Brown, R., Peter W. Nolan, and Paul Crawford. "Men in Nursing: Ambivalence in Care, Gender and Masculinity." *Contemporary Nurse: A Journal for the Australian Nursing Profession* 33, no. 2 (Sept. 2009): 120–9.

Burdett, Henry. *Prince, Princess and People: An Account of the Social Progress and Development of our own Times, as Illustrated by the Public Life and Work of*

Their Royal Highnesses the Prince and Princess of Wales, 1863–1889. London: Longmans, 1889.

Burton, Antoinette. "From Child Bride to 'Hindoo Lady': Rukhmabai and the Debate on Sexual Respectability in Imperial Britain." *American Historical Review* 103, no. 4 (1998): 1119–46.

Calkins, Beverly M. "Florence Nightingale: On Feeding an Army." *American Journal of Clinical Nutrition* 50 (1989): 1260–5.

Cameron, Donald, and Ian G. Jones. "John Snow, the Broad Street Pump and Modern Epidemiology." *International Journal of Epidemiology* 12, no. 4 (1983): 393–6.

Canada. Public Health Agency. *Hand Hygiene Practices in Healthcare Settings.* 2012.

Cannadine, David. *History in Our Time.* New Haven, CT: Yale University Press, 1998.

Cantlie, Neil. *A History of the Army Medical Department.* 2 vols. Edinburgh: Churchill Livingstone, 1974.

Centers for Disease Control and Prevention. "Healthcare-associated Infections." 2015.

Chapple, J.A.V., and Arthur Pollard, eds. *The Letters of Mrs. Gaskell.* Manchester: Manchester University Press, 1966.

Chenu, Jean-Charles. *De la mortalité dans l'armée et des moyens d'économiser la vie humaine, extraits des statistiques médico-chirurgicales.* Paris: Hachette, 1870.

– *Rapport au Conseil de Santé des Armées sur les résultats du service médico-chirurgical pendant la campagne d'Orient en 1854–56.* Paris: Victor Masson, 1865.

Cherry, Barbara, and Susan R. Jacob. *Contemporary Nursing: Issues, Trends and Management.* 7th ed. Amsterdam: Elsevier, 2017.

Chung, King-Tom, "Florence Nightingale (1820–1910), Founder of Modern Nursing." *Women Pioneers of Medical Research: Biographies of 25 Outstanding Scientists,* 16–23. Jefferson, NC: McFarland, 2010.

Clark, James, ed. *The Management of Infancy: Physiological and Moral.* [An adaptation of Andrew Combe's *Treatise* (1840).] Edinburgh: Maclachlan & Stewart, 1860.

Cohen, I. Bernard. "Florence Nightingale." *Scientific American* 246 (March 1984): 128–33, 136–7.

– *The Triumph of Numbers: How Counting Shaped Modern Life.* New York: W.W. Norton, 2006.

Combe, Andrew. *The Principles of Physiology Applied to the Preservation of Health and to the Improvement of Physical and Mental Education.* Edinburgh: Adam & Charles Black, 1834.

– *A Treatise on the Physiological and Moral Management of Infancy.* Edinburgh: Maclachlan & Stewart, 1840.

Cook, Edward T. *The Life of Florence Nightingale.* 2 vols. London: Macmillan, 1913.

Cope, Zachary. *Florence Nightingale and the Doctors.* London: Museum, 1958.

– "John Shaw Billings, Florence Nightingale and the Johns Hopkins Hospital." *Medical History: News, Notes and Queries* 1, no. 4 (Oct. 1957): 367–8.

Cordery, Cheryl. "Another Victorian Legacy: Florence Nightingale, Miasmic Theory and Nursing Practice." In Linda Bryder and Derek A. Dow, eds, *New Countries and Old Medicine,* 298–304. Auckland, New Zealand: Auckland Medical History Society, 1995.

Croft, John. *Notes of Lectures at St. Thomas' Hospital.* London: St. Thomas / Blades, East & Blades, 1873.

Cullingworth, Charles James. *The Nurse's Companion: A Manual of General and Monthly Nursing.* London: J. & A. Churchill, 1876.

– *A Short Manual for Monthly Nurses.* London: Churchill, 1884.

Cuningham, J.M. *Cholera: What Can the State Do to Prevent It?* Calcutta: Government Printing, 1884.

Cushing, Harvey. *The Life of Sir William Osler.* 2 vols. Oxford: Clarendon, 1925.

Davico, Rosalba, ed. *The Autobiography of Edward Jarvis (1803–1884).* London: Wellcome Institute, 1992.

Davies, Celia. "Making Sense of the Census in Britain and the U.S.A.: The Changing Occupational Classification and the Position of Nurses." *Sociological Review* 28, no. 3 (1980): 581–609.

De'Ath, G.H. *Cholera: What Can We Do?* Buckingham: Walford & Son, [1892].

De Chaumont, F.S.B. *Lectures on State Medicine.* London: Smith, Elder, 1875.

De Marco, William J. *Performance-Based Medicine: Creating the High-Performance Network to Optimize Managed Care Relationships* Boca Raton, FL: Productivity Press, 2011.

Doidge, Norman. *The Brain's Way of Healing: Remarkable Discoveries and Recoveries from the Frontiers of Neuroplasticity.* Toronto: Penguin Random House, 2015.

Dolan, Josephine A. *History of Nursing.* 12th ed. Philadelphia: W.B. Saunders, 1968 [rev. ed. of Minnie Goodnow, *Outlines of Nursing History* (1916)].

Druitt, Robert. *The Surgeon's Vade Mecum: A Manual of Modern Surgery.* London: Henry Renshaw, 1865.

Duns, John. *Memoir of Sir James Y. Simpson, Bart.* Edinburgh: Edmonston & Douglas, 1873.

Editorial Board, *Zeitschrift der Kaiserliche und Koniglichen Gesellschaft der Arzte zu Wien.* "Continuation of the Findings with regard to the Etiology of Epidemic Puerperal Fever in Maternity Hospitals." Typescript, Vienna, 1848.

Eyler, John M. *Victorian Social Medicine: The Ideas and Methods of William Farr.* Baltimore: Johns Hopkins University Press, 1979.

Fagge, Charles Hilton. *The Principles and Practice of Medicine,* ed. P.H. Pye-Smith. 2nd ed. London: J. & A. Churchill, 1888.

Fancourt, Mary St J. *They Dared to be Doctors: Elizabeth Blackwell, Elizabeth Garrett Anderson.* London: Longmans Green, 1905.

Fealy, Gerard M., Martin S. McNamara, and Ruth Geraghty. "The Health of Hospitals and Lessons from History: Public Health and Sanitary Reform in the Dublin Hospitals, 1858–1898." *Journal of Clinical Nursing* 19 (2010): 3468–76.

Fenwick, Kenneth, ed. *Voice from the Ranks: A Personal Narrative of the Crimean Campaign by a Sergeant of the Royal Fusiliers.* London: Folio Society, 1954.

Forbes, John. *Of Nature and Art in the Cure of Disease.* London: John Churchill, 1857.

Fraser, W.M. *A History of English Public Health, 1834–1939.* London: Baillière, Tindall & Cox, 1950.

Gairdner, T.W. *Public Health in Relation to Air and Water.* Edinburgh: Edmonston & Douglas, 1862 [reprinted as Kevin White, ed. *The Early Sociology of Health and Illness,* vol. 5. London: Routledge, 2001].

Galton, Douglas. *An Address on the General Principles which Should Be Observed in the Construction of Hospitals.* London: Macmillan, 1869.

– *Report to the Right Hon. the Earl de Grey and Ripon, Secretary of State for War, Descriptive of the Herbert Hospital at Woolwich.* London: Eyre & Spottiswoode, 1865.

Garrett, Elizabeth. "Hospital Nursing." *Transactions of the National Association for the Promotion of Social Science* 10 (1866): 472–88.

Garrod, Alfred Baring. *The Essentials of Materia Medica and Therapeutics.* London: Longmans, Green, 1880.

Gawande, Atul. "Notes of a Surgeon: On Washing Hands." *New England Journal of Medicine* 350, no. 3 (2004): 1283–6.

General Orders Issued to the Army of the East from April 30, 1854, to December 31, 1855. London: John W. Parker, 1856.

Gill, Christopher G., and Gillian Gill. "Nightingale in Scutari: Her Legacy Re-examined." *Clinical Infectious Diseases* 40, no. 12 (15 June 2005): 1799–1805.

Godden, Judith. *Lucy Osburn: A Lady Displaced: Florence Nightingale's Envoy to Australia.* Sydney, NSW: Sydney University Press, 2006.

Godden, Judith, and Sue Forsyth. "Defining Relationships and Limiting Power: Two Leaders of Australian Nursing." *Nursing Inquiry* 7, no. 1 (March 2000): 10–19.

Goldie, Sue, ed. *"I Have Done My Duty": Florence Nightingale in the Crimean War, 1854–1856.* Manchester: Manchester University Press, 1987.

Goldman, Lawrence. *Science, Reform and Politics in Victorian Britain: The Social Science Association.* Cambridge: Cambridge University Press, 2002.

Goodnow, Minnie. *Outlines of Nursing History.* Philadelphia: W.B. Saunders, 1916.

Gordon, Alexander. *A Treatise on the Epidemic Puerperal Fever of Aberdeen.* London: G.G. & J. Robinson, 1795.

Graves, Robert James. *A System of Clinical Medicine.* Dublin: Fannin, 1843.

Gray, Henry. *Anatomy, Descriptive and Surgical.* London: John Parker, 1858.

Greenway, Henry. "Improved Hospital Construction." *Medical Times and Gazette* (24 Sept. 1870): 32.

– "On a New Mode of Hospital Construction." *British Medical Journal* (11 May 1872): 495–7.

Griffiths, Jenny, Mala Rao, Fiona Adshead, and Allison Thorpe, eds. *The Health Practitioner's Guide to Climate Change: Diagnosis and Cure.* London: Earthscan, 2009.

Grypma, Sonya. "Florence Nightingale's Changing Image?" *Journal of Christian Nursing* 22, no. 3 (2005): 9–13.

– "Nightingale the Feminist, Statistician and Nurse." *Journal of Christian Nursing* 22, no. 3 (2005): 9–13.

Haffkine, W.M. *Anti-Cholera Inoculation. Report to the Government of India.* Calcutta: Thacker, Spink, 1895.

Hall, John. Letterbook. Wellcome Trust Library, London, Ms. 8520.

– *Observations on the Report of the Sanitary Commissioners in the Crimea, during the Years 1855 and 1856.* London: W. Clowes & Sons, 1857.

Halliday, Stephen, "Commentary: Dr. John Sutherland, *Vibrio cholerae* and 'Predisposing Causes.'" *International Journal of Epidemiology Impact Factor* 31, no. 5 (2002): 912–14.

– *The Great Filth: Disease, Death and the Victorian Life.* Stroud: Sutton, 2007 [2003].

Hamlin, Christopher. *Public Health and Social Justice in the Age of Chadwick: Britain, 1800–1854.* Cambridge: Cambridge University Press, 1998.

Hamlin, Christopher, and Sally Sheard. "Revolutions in Public Health: 1848 and 1998?" *BMJ* 317 (29 Aug. 1988): 587–91.

Hamlin, Cyrus. *My Life and Times.* 2nd ed. Boston: Congregational Sunday School & Publishing Society, 1893.

Hansard. *Parliamentary Debates.* 20 Nov. 1893.

Harford, Tim. "Florence Nightingale: The Pandemic Hero We Need." *Financial Times*, 7 Jan. 2021.

Hart, Ernest. *An Account of the Condition of the Infirmaries of London Workhouses*. London: Chapman & Hall, 1866.

Heath, Christopher, ed. *Dictionary of Practical Surgery, by Various British Hospital Surgeons*. London: Smith, Elder, 1886.

Hegge, Margaret. "Nightingale's Environmental Theory." *Nursing Science Quarterly* 26, no. 3 (July 2013): 211–19.

Helmstadter, Carol. "Doctors and Nurses in the London Teaching Hospitals: Class, Gender, Religion and Professional Expertise, 1850–1890." *Nursing History Review* 5 (1997): 161–97.

– "Florence Nightingale's Opposition to State Registration of Nurses." *Nursing History Review* 15 (2007): 155–66.

– "Reforming Hospital Nursing: The Experience of Maria Machin." *Nursing Inquiry* 13, no. 4 (2007): 249–58.

Hertzler, Ann A. "Florence Nightingale's Influence on Civil War Nutrition." *Nutrition Today* 39, no. 4 (July–Aug. 1997): 157–88.

Hill, Berkeley. *The Essentials of Bandaging*. 2nd ed. London: Smith & Elder, 1869.

Hinton, Mike. "Reporting the Crimean War: Misinformation and Misinterpretation." *Interdisciplinary Studies in the Long Nineteenth Century* 19, no. 20 (2015), doi: https://doi.org/10.16995/ntn.711 <10 Oct. 2021>.

Hoffman, L.E. *Women Who Changed the World: Fifty Inspirational Women Who Shaped History*. London: Quercus, 2006.

Holland, Sydney, Viscount Knutsford. *In Black and White*. London: Edward Arnold, 1926.

Holmes, Oliver Wendell. *Puerperal Fever, as a Private Pestilence*. Boston: Ticknor & Fields, 1855.

Holmes, Timothy, ed. *A System of Surgery, Theoretical and Practical Treatises by Various Authors*. 4 vols. London: J.W. Parker & Son, 1860–64.

Hooper, Robert. *The Anatomist's Vade-Mecum, concerning the Anatomy, Physiology, Morbid Appearances, etc., of the Human Body*. 4th ed. London: John Murray, 1802.

Hoyos, Carola. "How Would Florence Nightingale Have Tackled COVID-19?" *Guardian*, 5 May 2020.

Humphreys, Noel A., ed. *Vital Statistics: A Memorial Volume of Selections from the Reports and Writings of William Farr*. London: Sanitary Institution, 1885.

Humphry, Laurence. *Manual of Nursing: Medical and Surgical*. London and Edinburgh: C. Griffin, 1889.

Hurley, Michael, and Jonah Gindin. "Hospital Acquired Infections in Canada and How to Stop Them." Ontario Council of Hospital Unions, https://slideplayer.com/slide/4350011/ <28 Nov. 2021>.

Husson, Armand. *Étude sur les hôpitaux, considérés sous le rapport de leur construction, de la distribution de leurs bâtiments*. Paris: Paul Dumont, 1862.

Hutchinson, John F. *Champions of Charity: War and the Rise of the Red Cross*. Boulder, CO: Westview, 1996.

Huxley, Thomas Henry. *Elementary Lessons in Physiology*. London: Macmillan, 1866.

Iveson-Iveson, Joan. "A Legend in the Breaking." *Nursing Mirror* (11 May 1983): 26–7.

James, Janet Wilson, "Isabel Hampton and the Professionalization of Nursing." In Ellen Davidson et al., eds, *Enduring Issues in American Nursing*, 42–84. New York: Springer, 2000.

Johnson, Boris. *Johnson's Life of London: The People Who Made the City That Made the World*. London: Harper, 2012 [2011].

Kirby, Percival Robson. *Sir Andrew Smith, M.D., K.C.B.: His Life, Letters and Works*. Cape Town: A.A. Balkema, 1965.

Koch, Robert. "The Etiology of Traumatic Infectious Diseases." In *Investigations into the Etiology of Traumatic Infective Diseases*, trans. W. Watson Cheyne. London: New Sydenham Society, 1880.

Kopf, Edwin W. "Florence Nightingale as Statistician." *Publications of the American Statistical Association* 15 (1916–17): 388–404.

Kuhn, Annette, and Annemarie Wolpe, eds. *Feminism and Materialism: Women and Modes of Production*. London and New York Routledge, 2012 [1978].

Lees, Florence. "The Crown Princess's Lazareth for the Wounded." *Good Words* (1873): 500–5.

– *Handbook for Hospital Sisters*, ed. and preface by Henry Acland. London: Isbister, 1873 and 1874.

– "In a Fever Hospital before Metz." *Good Words* (1873): 322–8.

Le Fort, Léon. *Des hôpitaux: notes sur quelques points de l'hygiène*. Paris: Masson, 1862.

– *Des maternités: étude sur les maternités et les institutions charitables d'accouchement à domicile dans les principaux états de l'Europe*. Paris: Masson, 1866.

– *Oeuvres de Léon Le Fort*, ed. Félix Lejars. 3 vols. Paris: Félix Alcan, 1895.

Leveaux, V.M. "The Correspondence between Dr. Ogle and Florence Nightingale." In *History of the Derbyshire General Infirmary*. Cromford: Scarthin Books, 1999.

Lewis, Percy George. *The Theory and Practice of Nursing: A Textbook for Nurses*. 5th ed. London: Scientific Press, 1893.

Lind, James. *An Essay on the Most Effectual Means of Preserving the Health of Seamen*. 2nd ed. London: D. Wilson, 1762.

Longmore, Thomas. *The Sanitary Contrasts of the British and French Armies during the Crimean War*. London: Griffin, 1883.

Lorentzon, Maria, and Kevin Brown. "Florence Nightingale as 'Mentor of Matrons': Correspondence with Rachel Williams at St. Mary's Hospital." *Journal of Nursing Management* 11, no. 4 (July 2003): 266–74.

Luddy, Maria, ed. *The Crimean Journals of the Sisters of Mercy, 1854–56.* Dublin: Four Courts, 2004.

Lundy, Karen Saucier, and Kaye K. Bender. "And Then There Was Nightingale." In Karen Saucier Lunday and Janes Sharyn, eds, *Community Health Nursing: Caring for the Public's Health,* 79–86. Sudbury, MA: Jones & Bartlett Learning, 2009.

Lyons, Robert D. *A Treatise on Fever, Being Part of a Course of Lectures on the Theory and Practice of Medicine.* Philadelphia: Blanchard & Lea, 1861.

MacCormac, William. *Notes and Recollections of an Ambulance Surgeon, Being an Account of Work done under the Red Cross during the Campaign of 1870.* London: J. & A. Churchill, 1871.

MacDonnell, Freda. *Miss Nightingale's Young Ladies: The Story of Lucy Osburn and Sydney Hospital.* Sydney: Angus & Robertson, 1970.

Mackowiak, Philip A. *Post-Mortem: Solving History's Great Medical Mysteries.* New York: American College of Physicians, 2007.

Magill, Shelley S., et al. "Multistate Point-Prevalence Survey of Health Care–Associated Infections." *New England Journal of Medicine* 370 (March 2014): 1198–1208.

Marshall, Henrietta Elizabeth. *Our Island Story: A History of Britain for Boys and Girls from the Romans to Queen Victoria.* London: Civitas / Galore Park, 1905.

Maurer, Frances A., and Claudia M. Smith. *Community / Public Health Nursing Practice: Health for Families and Populations.* London: Elsevier Health Sciences, 2014.

McCallum, Jack Edward. *Military Medicine: From Ancient Times to the 21st Century.* Santa Barbara, CA: ABC Clio, 2008.

McCrae, Morrice. *Simpson: The Turbulent Life of a Medical Pioneer.* Edinburgh: John Donald, 2010.

McDonald, Lynn, ed. *Florence Nightingale: An Introduction to Her Life and Family.* CWFN, vol. 1. Waterloo, ON: Wilfrid Laurier University Press, 2001.

– ed. *Florence Nightingale and Hospital Reform.* CWFN, vol. 16. Waterloo, ON: Wilfrid Laurier University Press, 2012.

– *Florence Nightingale at First Hand.* London: Continuum Publishing, and Waterloo, ON: Wilfrid Laurier University Press, 2010.

– ed. *Florence Nightingale: The Crimean War.* CWFN, vol. 14. Waterloo, ON: Wilfrid Laurier University Press, 2009.

– ed. *Florence Nightingale: Extending Nursing.* CWFN, vol. 13. Waterloo, ON: Wilfrid Laurier University Press, 2009.

– ed. *Florence Nightingale: The Nightingale School.* CWFN, vol. 12. Waterloo, ON: Wilfrid Laurier University Press, 2009.

– ed. *Florence Nightingale on Public Health Care.* CWFN, vol. 6. Waterloo, ON: Wilfrid Laurier University Press, 2004.

– ed. *Florence Nightingale on Society and Politics, Philosophy, Science, Education and Literature.* CWFN, vol. 5. Waterloo, ON: Wilfrid Laurier University Press, 2003.

– ed. *Florence Nightingale on Wars and the War Office.* CWFN, vol. 15. Waterloo, ON: Wilfrid Laurier University Press, 2011.

– "Florence Nightingale, Statistics and the Crimean War." *Journal of the Royal Statistical Society* Series A 177, part 3 (June 2014): 569–86.

– ed. *Florence Nightingale's Suggestions for Thought.* CWFN, vol. 11. Waterloo, ON: Wilfrid Laurier University Press, 2008.

– "Mythologizing and De-mythologizing." In Sioban Nelson and Anne Marie Rafferty, eds., *Notes on Nightingale: The Influence and Legacy of a Nursing Icon,* 91–114. Ithaca, NY: ILR Press, 2010.

– "Nightingale and the Coronavirus Pandemic: Disease Prevention, Parallels and Principles." *Significance* (30 April 2020), https://www.significancemagazine.com/662 <15 Nov. 2021>.

– "Statistics to Save Lives." *International Journal of Statistics and Probability* 5, no. 1 (2016): 28–35.

McDonald, Lynn, and Gérard Vallée, eds. *Florence Nightingale on Health in India.* CWFN, vol. 9. Waterloo, ON: Wilfrid Laurier University Press, 2006.

– *Florence Nightingale on Mysticism and Eastern Religions.* CWFN, vol. 4. Waterloo, ON: Wilfrid Laurier University Press, 2003.

– *Florence Nightingale on Social Change in India.* CWFN, vol. 10. Waterloo, ON: Wilfrid Laurier University Press, 2007.

Michael, W.H. "The Public Health Act, 1872: Its Defects and Suggested Amendments." *British Medical Journal* (4 April 1874): 443–6.

Mitra, S.M. *The Life and Letters of Sir John Hall, MD, KCB, FRCS.* London: Longmans, Green, 1911.

Morris, Malcolm Alexander. *The Skin and Hair.* London: Cassell, 1886 [1883].

Moten, Matthew. *The Delafield Commission and the American Military Profession.* College Station: Texas A and M University Press, 2000.

Munro, Cindy L. "The 'Lady with the Lamp' Illuminates Critical Care Today." *American Journal of Critical Care* 19, no. 4 (July 2010): 315–17.

Murchison, Charles. "On the Isolation of Infectious Diseases." *Medical Times and Gazette* (20 Feb. 1864): 210–11.

– *Treatise on the Continued Fevers of Great Britain.* London: Parker, 1862.

Mussey, Reuben Dimond. *Health: Its Friends and Foes.* New York: Sheldon, 1862.

New South Wales. *Second Report of the Commission Appointed to Inquire into and Report upon the Working and the Management of the Public Charities of the Colony*, vol. 4. Sydney: New South Wales Legislative Assembly, 1873–74.

Nightingale, Florence. For *Collected Works of Florence Nightingale*, 16 vols (2001–12), please see complete list of volumes at start of bibliography and see volume entries under McDonald, Lynn, editor.

– "Answers to Written Questions Addressed to Miss Nightingale by the Commissioners." In *Report of the Commissioners appointed to Inquire into the Regulations affecting the Sanitary Condition of the Army and the Treatment of the Sick and Wounded*, 361–94. London: HMSO, 1858.

– *Army Sanitary Administration and its Reform under the late Lord Herbert.* London: McCorquodale, 1862.

– "Health and Local Government." Introduction to *Report of the Bucks Sanitary Conference October 1894*, i–ii. Aylesbury: Poulton, 1894.

– "Hospitals." In *Chambers's Encyclopaedia: A Dictionary of Universal Knowledge* 5: 805–7. Edinburgh: W. & R. Chambers, 1890.

– *Introductory Notes on Lying-in Institutions.* London: Longmans, Green, 1871.

– Letter to the Chair, Poona Sarvajanik Sabha. London: Spottiswoode, 1891, reprinted in *Quarterly Journal of the Poona Sarvajanik Sabha* 15, no. 1 (July 1892): 13–17.

– *Letters from Egypt.* London: Spottiswoode, 1854.

– "A Medical Authority's Warning." *Pall Mall Gazette*, 8 Aug. 1884.

– *Method of Improving the Nursing Service of Hospitals.* Printed paper [1868].

– "Miss Florence Nightingale on the Cholera." *The Sanitary Record: A Monthly Journal of Public Health and the Progress of Sanitary Science* 6, no. 73 (15 July 1884): 66.

– *Notes on Hospitals.* 3rd ed. London: Longman, Green, 1863.

– *Notes on Matters Affecting the Health, Efficiency and Hospital Administration of the British Army, Founded Chiefly on the Experience of the Late War.* London: Harrison, 1858.

– *Notes on Nursing: What It Is and What It Is Not.* London: Harrison, 1860.

– *Notes on Nursing: What It Is and What It Is Not.* Rev. ed. London: Harrison, 1860.

– *Notes on Nursing for the Labouring Classes.* London: Harrison, 1861.

– "Notes on the Sanitary Condition of Hospitals, and on Defects in the Construction of Hospital Wards." *Transactions of the National Association for the Promotion of Social Science*, 462–82. London: John W. Parker & Son, 1859.

– "Nurses, Training of." In Robert Quain, ed., *A Dictionary of Medicine.* London: Longmans, Green, 1883, 1038–43; and New York: Appleton, 1890; and London: Longmans, Green, 1894: 1038–43.

– "Nursing the Sick." In Robert Quain, ed., *A Dictionary of Medicine*. London: Longmans, Green, 1883, 1043–9; and New York: Appleton, 1890; and London: Longmans, Green, 1894: 1043–49.

– "Obituary: Dr. Sutherland." *Times*, 24 July 1891, 8D.

– "Practical Advice in View of the Rapid Spread of Cholera: 'Scavenge, Scavenge, Scavenge.'" *Sanitarian* 13 (1884): 114–15.

– "Remarks of the Barrack and Hospital Improvement Commission on a Report by Dr. Leith on the General Sanitary Condition of the Bombay Army," *Parliamentary Papers*, No. 329, 1865.

– "Sanitary Statistics of Native Colonial Schools and Hospitals." *Transactions of the National Association for the Promotion of Social Science* (1863): 475–88.

– "Sick-Nursing and Health-Nursing." In Angela Burdett-Coutts, ed., *Woman's Mission: A Series of Congress Papers on the Philanthropic Work of Women*. 184–205. London: Sampson, Low, Marston, 1893.

– *Subsidiary Notes as to the Introduction of Female Nursing into Military Hospitals in Peace and in War*. London: Harrison & Sons, 1858.

– *Suggestions for Thought to Searchers after Religious Truth*. 3 vols. London: Eyre & Spottiswoode, 1860.

– "Suggestions on the Subject of Providing Training and Organizing Nurses for the Sick Poor in Workhouse Infirmaries." Report of the Committee appointed to consider Cubic Space of Metropolitan Workhouses. Paper No. 16. HMSO. 19 Jan. 1867: 64–76.

– "Trained Nurses for the Sick Poor." *Times*, 14 April 1876, 6CD.

– "An Unpublished Letter of Florence Nightingale," *St. Thomas' Hospital Gazette* 27, no. 8 (Feb. 1920): 247–8.

Norris, Rachel. *Norris's Nursing Notes: Being a Manual of Medical and Surgical Information for the Use of Hospital Nurses*. London: Sampson Low, Marston, 1891.

Nuland, Sherwin B. *The Doctors' Plague: Germs, Childbed Fever, and the Strange Story of Ignác Semmelweis*. New York: Norton, 2003.

Nutting, M. Adelaide, and Lavinia L. Dock. *A History of Nursing: The Evolution of Nursing Systems from the Earliest Times to the Foundation of the First English and American Training Schools for Nurses*. 4 vols. New York: G.P. Putman's Sons, 1907–12.

Olmsted, Frederick Law. *The Sanitary Commission, Report of the Resident Secretary*. 1861.

Osler, William. *The Collected Essays of Sir William Osler*, ed. John P. McGovern and Charles G. Roland. 3 vols. Birmingham: Classics of Medicine Library, 1985.

– *The Principles and Practice of Medicine*. New York: D. Appleton & Co., 1892.

– "Vocation in Medicine and Nursing." In *Essays on Vocation*, ed. Basil Mathews. London: Oxford University Press, 1919.

Otter, Chris. *The Victorian Eye: A Political History of Light and Vision in Britain, 1800–1910*. Chicago: University of Chicago, 2008.

Paget, James. *St. Bartholomew's Hospital and School Fifty Years Ago: An Address Given at a Meeting of the Abernethian Society*. London: Adlard, 1885.

Paget, Stephen, ed. *Memoirs and Letters of Sir James Paget*. London: Longmans Green, 1901.

[Parkes, Edmumd A.] *On Personal Care of Health*. London: Society for Promoting Christian Knowledge, 1876.

Parkes, Edmund Alexander. *A Manual of Practical Hygiene, Prepared especially for Use in the Medical Services of the Army*. London: John Churchill, 1864.

Parsons, Malcolm. *The General Infirmary at Leeds: A Pictorial History*. York: Wm. Sessions, 2003.

Pincoffs, Peter. *Experiences of a Civilian in Eastern Military Hospitals with Observations on the English, French and Other Medical Departments*. London: Williams & Norgate, 1857.

Pollock, C.E. "Florence Nightingale, O.M., R.R.C.," *Journal of the Royal Army Medical Corps* 15, no. 4 (Oct. 1910): 383–93.

Ponting, Clive. *The Crimean War: The Truth behind the Myth*. London: Chatto & Windus, 2004.

Porter, Whitworth. *Life in the Trenches*. London: Longman, Brown, 1856.

Pringle, John. *Observations on the Diseases of the Army in Camp and Garrison*. 3rd ed. London: Millar, 1761 [1752].

Purvis, June, ed. *Women's History: Britain, 1850–1945*. New York: St Martin's Press, 1995.

Quetelet, L.A.J. *Physique sociale ou Essai sur le développement des facultés de l'homme*. 2 vols. Brussels: Muquardt, 1869.

Quinn, Vincent, and John Prest, eds. *"Dear Miss Nightingale": A Selection of Benjamin Jowett's Letters to Florence Nightingale 1860–1893*. Oxford: Clarendon, 1987.

Rafferty, Anne Marie. *The Politics of Nursing Knowledge*. London: Routledge, 1996.

Raju, W.E. Dhanakoti. *The Elements of Hygiene, or, Easy Lessons on the Laws of Health*. Madras: Foster Press, 1875.

"The Rational Construction of Hospitals." *Scientific American* new series 21 (20 Nov. 1869): 329.

Reid, Douglas Arthur. *Memories of the Crimean War: January 1855 to June 1856*. London: St Catherines Press, 1911.

Reverby, Susan M. *Ordered to Care: The Dilemma of American Nursing, 1850–1945*. Cambridge: Cambridge University Press, 1987.

Richards, Laura E. *Florence Nightingale: The Angel of the Crimea, a Story for Young People*. New York: Floating Press, 2014 [1945].

– "Letters of Florence Nightingale." *Yale Review* 24 (Dec. 1934): 327–30.
– *Samuel Gridley Howe.* New York: D. Appleton-Century, 1935.
Richards, Laura E., Maud Howe Elliott, and Florence Howe Hall. *Julia Ward Howe 1819–1910.* 2 vols. Boston: Houghton Mifflin, 1916.
Richardson, B.W. [B.W.R.] "Commentary on Hospital Mortality." *Medical Times and Gazette* (5 March 1864): 262–3.
Richardson, Robert G., ed. *Nurse Sarah Anne: With Florence Nightingale at Scutari.* London: John Murray, 1977.
Richardson, Ruth. "Middlesex Hospital Outpatients Wing / Strand Union Workhouse." *History Today* 43, no. 9 (Sept. 1993): 61–3.
Rigby, Edward. *A System of Midwifery.* London: Lea & Blanchard, 1841.
Robb, Isabel Hampton. *Nursing: Its Principles and Practice for Hospital and Private Use.* Philadelphia: W.B. Saunders, 1893.
Roberton, John. "On the Defects, with Reference to the Plan of Construction and Ventilation, of Most of our Hospitals for the Reception of the Sick and Wounded." *Transactions of the Manchester Statistical Society* (1855–6): 133–48.
– "On the Need of Additional as Well as Improved Hospital Accommodation." *Transactions of the Manchester Statistical Society* (1857–8): 23–48.
Robinson, Frederick. *Diary of the Crimean War.* London: Richard Bentley, 1856.
Robinson, Robert. Narrative typescript, British Library, Add. Mss. 45797 ff82–101.
Rogers, Joseph. *Joseph Rogers, M.D.: Reminiscences of a Workhouse Medical Officer*, ed. and preface by Thorold Rogers. London: T. Fisher Unwin, 1889.
Rosenberg, Charles. "Introduction, Florence Nightingale." In *Florence Nightingale on Hospital Reform*, ed. Charles Rosenberg. New York: Garland, 1989.
Rothstein, William G. *American Medical Schools and the Practice of Medicine: A History.* New York: Oxford University Press, 1987.
Routh, C.H.F. "On the Causes of the Endemic Puerperal Fever of Vienna." *Medico-Chirurgical Transactions* 2nd series, 14 (1849): 27–40.
Royle, Trevor. *Crimea: The Great Crimean War, 1854–1856.* New York: St Martin's Press, 2000.
Rumsey, Henry Wyldbore. *Essays on State Medicine in Great Britain and Ireland.* New York: Arno, 1977; reprint of London: J. Churchill, 1856.
Scharlieb, Mary. *Reminiscences.* London: Williams & Norgate, 1924.
Scotland, Thomas, and Steven Heys. *Wars, Pestilence and the Surgeon's Blade: The Evolution of British Military Medicine and Surgery during the Nineteenth Century.* Solihull, England: Helion, 2013.
Scrive, Gaspard. *Relation médico-chirurgicale de la Campagne d'Orient du 31 mars 1854, occupation de Gallipoli au 6 juillet 1856, évacuation de la Crimée.* Paris: Victor Masson, 1857.

Semmelweis, Ignaz P. *Die Aetiologie, der Begriff und die Prophylaxis des Kindbettfebers*. Pest and Wien, 1861.
– *The Etiology, Concept and Prophylaxis of Childbed Fever*, trans. K. Codell Carter. Madison: University of Wisconsin Press, 1983.
– "Höchst wichtige Erfahrungen über der in Gebäranstalten epidemischen Puerperalfieber" (Very Important Findings on the Etiology of Epidemic Puerperal Fevers in Maternity Hospitals). *Zeitschrift der Kaiserliche und Koniglichen Gesellschaft der Arzte zu Wien* 4, no. 2 (1847–48): 242–4.
Shannon, Richard. "An Icon and Ker Intrigues." *Times Literary Supplement* (28 May 1982): 571–3.
Shelly, Judith Allen, and Arlene B. Miller. *Values in Conflict: Christian Nursing in a Changing Profession*. Downers' Grove, IL: Intervarsity Press, 1991.
Shepherd, John. *The Crimean Doctors: A History of the British Medical Services in the Crimean War*. 2 vols. Liverpool: Liverpool University Press, 1991.
Sieveking, E.H. *The Training Institutions for Nurses and the Workhouses: An Attempt to Solve One of the Social Problems of the Present Day*. London: Williams & Norgate, 1849.
Simon, John. *English Sanitary Institutions, Reviewed in their Course of Development, and in some of their Political and Social Relations*. London: Cassell, 1890.
– "An Introductory Report on the Preventability of Certain Kinds of Premature Death." *Papers Relating to the Sanitary State of the People of England*, i–xlviii. London: General Board of Health, 1858.
– *Public Health Reports,* ed. Edward Seaton. Vol. 2. London: J. & A. Churchill, 1887.
Simpson, James Y. "Effects of Hospitalism upon the Mortality of Limb-Amputations." *British Medical Journal* 1, no. 422 (30 Jan. 1869): 93–4.
– "On the Relative Danger to Life from Limb-Amputations, in St. Bartholomew's Hospital, London, and in Country Practice." *British Medical Journal* 1, no. 435 (1 May 1869): 393–6.
Simpson, Myrtle Lillias. *Simpson the Obstetrician: A Biography*. London: Gollancz, 1972.
Singh, Simon, and Edzard Ernst. *Trick or Treatment: Alternative Medicine on Trial*. London: Bantam, 2008.
Skretkowicz, Victor, ed. *Florence Nightingale's Notes on Nursing*. London: Baillière Tindall, 1996.
Small, Hugh. *Florence Nightingale: Avenging Angel*. London: Constable, 1998.
– "Florence Nightingale's Public Health Act, COVID-19 and the Empowerment of Local Government." *History and Policy* (12 Oct. 2020).
Smith, Andrew, ed. *Medical and Surgical History of the British Army which Served in Turkey and the Crimea*. 2 vols. London: Harrison, 1858.

Smith, F.B. *Florence Nightingale: Reputation and Power*. London: Croom Helm, 1982.

Smith, Fred. *A Short History of the Royal Army Medical Corps*. Aldershot: Gale & Polden, 1929.

Smith, Thomas Southwood. *Philosophy of Health, or, an Exposition of the Physical and Mental Constitution of Man*. 2 vols. London: 1836–37.

South, John Flint. *Facts Relating to Hospital Nurses, Also Observations on Training Establishments for Hospitals*. London: Richardson Bros., 1857.

– *Household Surgery, or Hints on Emergencies*. London, 1850.

– *A Short Description of the Bones*. London W. Jackson, 1825.

Soyer, Alexis. *Soyer's Culinary Campaign: Being Historical Reminiscences of the Late War*. London: G. Routledge, 1857.

Speck, Reinhard S. "Cholera." In Kenneth J. Kiple, ed., *Cambridge World History of Human Disease*, 642–9. Cambridge: Cambridge University Press, 1993.

Spriggs, Edmund Antony. "Hector Gavin, MD, FRCSE (1815–1855): His Life, His Work for the Sanitary Movement and His Accidental Death in the Crimea." *Medical History* 28 (1984): 283–92.

Steven, John Lindsay. "A Lecture on the Duties and Training of the Medical Nurse." *Glasgow Medical Journal* 31, no. 5 (1889): 330–7.

Stillé, Charles Janeway. *History of the United States Sanitary Commission, Being the General Report of its Work during the War of the Rebellion*. Philadelphia: J.B. Lippincott, 1866.

Swayne, Joseph Griffiths. *Obstetric Aphorisms: for the Use of Students Commencing Midwifery Practice*. London: J. & A. Churchill, 1856.

Tanner, Thomas Hawkes. *An Index of Diseases and Their Treatment*. London: Henry Renshaw, 1866.

Taylor, Jeremy. *The Rebirth of the Norfolk and Norwich Hospital, 1874–1883: An Architectural Exploration*. London: Wellcome Unit for the History of Medicine, 2000.

Tenon, Jacques-René. *Memoirs on Paris Hospitals*, ed. Dora B. Weiner. Canton, MA: Science History, 1996 [1788].

Thomas, D.P. "The Demise of Bloodletting." *Journal of the Royal College of Physicians of Edinburgh* 44 (2014): 72–7.

Topinard, Paul. *Quelques aperçus sur la chirurgie anglaise*. Paris, 1860.

Treves, Frederick. *The Influence of Clothing on Health*. London: Cassell & Co., 1886.

Tulloch, Alexander. *The Crimean Commission and the Chelsea Board, Being a Review of the Proceedings and Report of the Board*. London: Harrison, 1857.

Turner, A. Logan. *Story of a Great Hospital: The Royal Infirmary of Edinburgh, 1729–1929*. Edinburgh: Mercat, 1979.

Twining, Louisa. *Recollections of Workhouse Visiting and Management during Twenty-five Years.* London: C. Kegan Paul, 1880.

Tyson, Edith, ed. *Letters from the Crimea: Captain Jasper Hall of the 4th (or King's Own) Regiment of Foot, to his Sister and Father.* Lancaster Museum Monograph, 2000.

United Kingdom. *Report of the Commission of Inquiry* [Supply Commission] *into the Supplies of the British Army in the Crimea. 1856.* XX, 1, 497.

– *Report of the Commissioners Appointed to Inquire into the Regulations Affecting the Sanitary Condition of the Army, the Organisation of Military Hospitals and the Treatment of the Sick and Wounded* [Royal Commission on the Crimean War]. 2 vols. London: HMSO, 1858.

– *Report of the Pathology of the Diseases of the Army in the East. Parliamentary Papers* 1857 2229.

– *Report of the Proceedings of the Sanitary Commissioners* [Sanitary Commission] *dispatched to the Seat of War in the East. Parliamentary Papers.* March 1857 [2196] IX.

– *Report of the Royal Commission on the Sanitary State of the Army in India.* 2 vols. 1863.

– *Report upon the State of the Hospitals of the British Army in the Crimea and Scutari.* London: Eyre & Spottiswoode, 1855.

– *Second Report from the Select Committee on the Army before Sebastopol, With Minutes of Evidence and Appendix. Parliamentary Papers.* Ordered 30 March 1855.

Vicinus, Martha. *Independent Women: Work and Community for Single Women, 1850–1920.* Chicago: University of Chicago Press, 1985.

Wagenaar, Cor, ed. *The Architecture of Hospitals.* Amsterdam: NAI, 2006.

Watson, James Kenneth. *A Handbook for Nurses.* London: Scientific Press, 1899.

Watson, Thomas. *Lectures on the Principles and Practice of Physic.* 2 vols. London, 1843.

Watson, William N. Boog. "An Edinburgh Surgeon of the Crimean War – Patrick Heron Watson (1832–1907)." *Medical History* 10, no. 2 (April 1966): 166–75.

Wells, T. Spencer. *On Ovarian and Uterine Tumours: Their Diagnosis and Treatment.* London: J. & A. Churchill, 1882.

White, Rosemary. "Some Political Influences Surrounding the Nurses Registration Act 1919 in the United Kingdom." *Journal of Advanced Nursing* 1 (1976): 209–17.

Widmer, Carolyn Ladd. "Grandfather and Florence Nightingale." *American Journal of Nursing* 55, no. 5 (May 1955): 569–71.

Williams, Rachel, and Alice Fisher. *Hints for Hospital Nurses*. Edinburgh: Maclachlan & Stewart, 1877.

Winkelstein, Warren. "Florence Nightingale: Founder of Modern Nursing and Hospital Epidemiology." *Epidemiology* 20, no. 2 (2009): 311.

Winslow, Charles-Edward A. "Florence Nightingale and Public Health Nursing." *Public Health Nursing* 46 (1946): 330–2.

Wolstenholme, G.E.W. "Florence Nightingale, New Lamps for Old." In R.M. Shaw et al., eds, *All Heal: A Medical and Social Miscellany*, 201–15. London: Wm. Heinemann, 1971.

Woodham-Smith, Cecil. *Florence Nightingale, 1820–1910*. London: Constable, 1986 [1950].

Worcester, Alfred. *A New Way of Training Nurses*. Boston: Cupples & Hurd, 1888.

– *Nurses and Nursing*. Cambridge, MA: Harvard University Press, 1927.

World Health Organization. "Global Health Risks, Mortality and Burden of Disease Attributable to Selected Major Risks." World Health Organization, 2009, https://apps.who.int/iris/handle/10665/44203 <28 Nov. 2021>.

– "Seven Million Premature Deaths Annually Linked to Air Pollution." *Public Health, Environmental and Social Determinants of Health* (PHE), issue 63 (March 2014).

Wylie, Walker Gill. *Hospitals: Their History, Organization and Development*. New York: Appleton, 1876.

INDEX